2010
YEAR BOOK OF
GASTROENTEROLOGY™

The 2010 Year Book Series

Year Book of Anesthesiology and Pain Management™: Drs Chestnut, Abram, Black, Gravlee, Lien, Mathru, and Roizen

Year Book of Cardiology®: Drs Gersh, Cheitlin, Elliott, Gold, Graham, and Suri

Year Book of Critical Care Medicine®: Drs Dellinger, Parrillo, Balk, Dorman, Dries, and Zanotti-Cavazzoni

Year Book of Dermatology and Dermatologic Surgery™: Dr Del Rosso

Year Book of Diagnostic Radiology®: Drs Osborn, Abbara, Birdwell, Elster, Manaster, Oestreich, Offiah, Rosado de Christenson, and Walker

Year Book of Emergency Medicine®: Drs Hamilton, Bruno, Handly, Mullin, Quintana, and Ramoska

Year Book of Endocrinology®: Drs Schott, Apovian, Clarke, Eugster, Ludlam, Meikle, Ovalle, Schinner, Schteingart, and Toth

Year Book of Gastroenterology™: Drs Talley, Ambikaipaker, Bollipo, DeVault, Harnois, Pearson, Picco, Rombeau, Scolapio, and Smith

Year Book of Hand and Upper Limb Surgery®: Drs Yao, and Steinmann

Year Book of Medicine®: Drs Barker, Garrick, Gersh, Khardori, LeRoith, Seo, Talley, and Thigpen

Year Book of Neonatal and Perinatal Medicine®: Drs Fanaroff, Benitz, Donn, Neu, Papile, Polin, and van Marter

Year Book of Neurology and Neurosurgery®: Drs Klimo, and Rabinstein

Year Book of Obstetrics, Gynecology, and Women's Health®: Drs Dungan, and Shulman

Year Book of Oncology®: Drs Arceci, Bauer, Gordon, Lawton, and Thigpen

Year Book of Ophthalmology®: Drs Rapuano, Cohen, Flanders, Hammersmith, Milman, Myers, Nelson, Penne, Pyfer, Sergott, Shields, and Vander

Year Book of Orthopedics®: Drs Morrey, Beauchamp, Huddleston, Swiontkowski, and Trigg

Year Book of Otolaryngology-Head and Neck Surgery®: Drs Sindwani, Balough, Franco, Gapany, and Mitchell

Year Book of Pathology and Laboratory Medicine®: Drs Raab, Parwani, Bejarano, and Bissell

Year Book of Pediatrics®: Dr Stockman

Year Book of Plastic and Aesthetic Surgery™: Drs Miller, Gosain, Gurtner, Gutowski, Ruberg, Salisbury, and Smith

Year Book of Psychiatry and Applied Mental Health®: Drs Talbott, Ballenger, Buckley, Frances, Krupnick, and Mack

Year Book of Pulmonary Disease®: Drs Barker, Jones, Maurer, Raza, Tanoue, and Willsie

Year Book of Sports Medicine®: Drs Shephard, Cantu, Feldman, Jankowski, Khan, Lebrun, Nieman, Pierrynowski, and Rowland

Year Book of Surgery®: Drs Copeland, Behrns, Daly, Eberlein, Fahey, Huber, Jones, Mozingo, and Pruett

Year Book of Urology®: Drs Andriole, and Coplen

Year Book of Vascular Surgery®: Drs Moneta, Gillespie, Starnes, and Watkins

2010
The Year Book of GASTROENTEROLOGY™

Editor-in-Chief
Nicholas J. Talley, MD, PhD
Pro Vice-Chancellor, Faculty of Health, University of Newcastle, Callaghan, New South Wales, Australia; Adjunct Professor of Medicine, Mayo Clinic, Jacksonville, Florida; Adjunct Professor of Medicine, Mayo Clinic, Rochester, Minnesota; and Adjunct Professor, University of North Carolina, Chapel Hill, North Carolina

ELSEVIER
MOSBY

ELSEVIER
MOSBY

Vice President, Continuity: Kimberly Murphy
Senior Editor: Kerry Holland
Production Supervisor, Electronic Year Books: Donna M. Skelton
Electronic Article Manager: Emily Ogle
Illustrations and Permissions Coordinator: Dawn Vohsen

2010 EDITION

Composition by TNQ Books and Journals Pvt Ltd, India

Editorial Office:
Elsevier
1600 John F. Kennedy Blvd.
Suite 1800
Philadelphia, PA 19103-2899

International Standard Serial Number: 0739-5930
International Standard Book Number: 978-0-323-06831-4

Associate Editors

Vimalan Ambikaipaker, MB, ChB
Advanced Trainee, Department of Gastroenterology and General Medicine, John Hunter Hospital, Newcastle, New South Wales, Australia

Steven Bollipo, FRACP
Director of Gastroenterology and Endoscopy, John Hunter Hospital, Newcastle, New South Wales, Australia

Kenneth R. DeVault, MD
Professor and Chair, Department of Medicine, Mayo Clinic, Jacksonville, Florida

Denise M. Harnois, DO
Assistant Professor, Department of Medicine, Mayo Clinic, Jacksonville, Florida

Randall K. Pearson, MD
Associate Professor of Medicine, Department of Gastroenterology and Hepatology, Mayo Clinic, Rochester, Minnesota

Michael F. Picco, MD, PhD
Assistant Professor of Medicine, Department of Gastroenterology and Hepatology, Mayo Clinic, Jacksonville, Florida

John L. Rombeau, MD
Professor of Surgery, Department of Surgery, Temple University Hospital, Philadelphia, Pennsylvania

James S. Scolapio, MD
Professor of Medicine, Division of Gastroenterology and Hepatology, Mayo Clinic, Jacksonville, Florida

C. Daniel Smith, MD
Professor and Chair, Department of Surgery, Mayo Clinic, Jacksonville, Florida

Table of Contents

Journals Represented

Journals represented in this YEAR BOOK are listed below.

American Journal of Clinical Nutrition
American Journal of Gastroenterology
American Journal of Surgery
American Journal of Surgical Pathology
American Surgeon
Annals of Internal Medicine
Annals of Surgery
Annals of Surgical Oncology
Archives of Internal Medicine
Archives of Surgery
British Journal of Cancer
British Journal of Surgery
British Medical Journal
Clinical Cancer Research
Clinical Gastroenterology and Hepatology
Clinical Infectious Diseases
Critical Care Medicine
Digestive Diseases and Sciences
Diseases of the Colon and Rectum
European Journal of Cancer
Gastroenterology
Gastrointestinal Endoscopy
Gut
Hepatology
Journal of Clinical Psychiatry
Journal of Pediatric Gastroenterology and Nutrition
Journal of Rheumatology
Journal of the American College of Surgeons
Journal of the American Medical Association
Journal of Thoracic and Cardiovascular Surgery
Journal of Vascular and Interventional Radiology
Lancet
Liver Transplantation
Nature
Neurology
New England Journal of Medicine
Pediatric Emergency Care
Pediatrics
Radiology
Surgery
Transplantation Proceedings
World Journal of Surgery

STANDARD ABBREVIATIONS

The following terms are abbreviated in this edition: acquired immunodeficiency syndrome (AIDS), cardiopulmonary resuscitation (CPR), central nervous system

(CNS), cerebrospinal fluid (CSF), computed tomography (CT), deoxyribonucleic acid (DNA), electrocardiography (ECG), health maintenance organization (HMO), human immunodeficiency virus (HIV), intensive care unit (ICU), intramuscular (IM), intravenous (IV), magnetic resonance (MR) imaging (MRI), ribonucleic acid (RNA), and ultrasound (US).

Note

The Year Book of Gastroenterology is a literature survey service providing abstracts of articles published in the professional literature. Every effort is made to assure the accuracy of the information presented in these pages. Neither the editors nor the publisher of the Year Book of Gastroenterology can be responsible for errors in the original materials. The editors' comments are their own opinions. Mention of specific products within this publication does not constitute endorsement.

To facilitate the use of the Year Book of Gastroenterology as a reference tool, all illustrations and tables included in this publication are now identified as they appear in the original article. This change is meant to help the reader recognize that any illustration or table appearing in the Year Book of Gastroenterology may be only one of many in the original article. For this reason, figure and table numbers will often appear to be out of sequence within the Year Book of Gastroenterology.

Introduction

Welcome to a new edition of YEAR BOOK OF GASTROENTEROLOGY, now in its 27th year. With experts from around the world, we have surveyed the American and international literature across the fields of gastroenterology, hepatology, and endoscopy. From those publications, we have chosen the most important and intriguing articles for abstracting and commentary. Here you will find the best summary of our subspecialty available, from landmark articles to practical diagnostics and therapeutics.

A top-level survey of some of the key literature included is illuminating. For example, while surgery has become ascendant in the management of achalasia, new data support pneumatic dilatation, especially in older patients. Esophageal dilatation has had a bad name in eosinophilic esophagitis, but if carried out appropriately can produce long-term benefit. More evidence supporting endoscopic resection followed by thermal ablation of early neoplasia complicating Barrett's esophagus is presented.

The frightening figures signalling a dramatic rise in obesity appear to finally be flattening out in the United States, but now nearly one third of Americans are obese, and the health care implications remain enormous. Thiopurines are dramatically associated with lymphoproliferative disorders, a finding with implications for their use in inflammatory bowel disease. Extending colon cancer surveillance intervals is debated, based on new data. Clopidogrel may not need to be stopped before routine polypectomy. Constipation may be the earliest presenting feature of Parkinson's disease. Early colonoscopy seems useful in the management of lower gastrointestinal bleeding.

Perhaps half of patients with an intraductal mucinous neoplasm (IPMN) of the pancreas have an extrapancreatic neoplasm, especially colon cancer or Barrett's cancer, suggesting the need for more aggressive screening in these patients. Potential novel roles for rifaximin, a nonabsorbable antibiotic, are described. Other new data support administration of cisplatin and gemcitabine for the rare but deadly cancer of the biliary tract, as this improves survival. These and many other relevant contributions await you in this book.

The commentators have worked tirelessly with the editor to sift through the ever-increasing literature in order to bring you the medical literature that has mattered the most in the last year. We very much hope you will enjoy the new edition, and we would also greatly welcome your feedback as we begin to prepare for next year.

Nicholas J. Talley, MD, PhD

1 Esophagus

Achalasia

Long-term Outcome of Pneumatic Dilation in the Treatment of Achalasia

Hulselmans M, Vanuytsel T, Degreef T, et al (Ctr for Gastroenterological Res, Leuven, Belgium; et al)

Clin Gastroenterol Hepatol 8:30-35, 2010

Background & Aims.—Achalasia is treated with pneumatic dilation or Heller myotomy, but studies suggest poor long-term outcomes. We analyzed long-term outcomes after initial pneumatic dilation and studied factors associated with failure.

Methods.—A total of 209 patients (111 men; mean age, 51.2 ± 1.4 years) with achalasia who were treated with pneumatic dilation between 1992 and 2002 were followed. Outcomes were correlated with demographics, presenting symptoms, manometric features, and treatment variables by using χ^2 and Student *t* tests.

Results.—All patients were initially treated with consecutive esophageal dilations up to balloon diameters of 3.0 (26%), 3.5 (41%), or 4.0 cm (33%). After dilations, mean lower esophageal sphincter (LES) pressure had decreased from 31.3 ± 1.3 to 14.0 ± 0.7 mm Hg ($P < .0001$); dysphagia decreased from 96% to 26%; and 49% had gained an average of 4.6 ± 0.5 kg (weight loss at presentation was 10.6 ± 0.7 kg in 39%). During follow-up, 66% required no additional treatment, whereas 23% underwent repeat dilations after 79 ± 8 months. Patients without recurrence were older (41.2 ± 2.1 vs 56.6 ± 1.6 years; $P < .0001$) and had lower post-treatment LES pressure (17.8 ± 1.2 vs 12.9 ± 0.6 mm Hg; $P < .005$). After 70-month follow-up, balloon dilation yielded good or excellent outcomes in 72% of patients. In nonresponders, rescue surgery yielded higher success rates than botulinum toxin therapy (84% vs 44%). Patient satisfaction ranged from good to excellent in 81% of patients.

Conclusions.—Treating achalasia with initial dilation and then surgery for short-term failures yielded good long-term results in more than 70%

and treatment satisfaction in more than 80% of patients. Management of dilation failures is more problematic.

▶ This is an impressive study reporting long-term follow-up in 209 patients with achalasia treated with pneumatic dilation. The authors found good results and satisfaction in 70% to 80% of the patients. Their perforation rate was 2.9%, and all 6 were managed without surgery. Patients with recurrences were retreated, and only 13 ended up with a myotomy. The authors suggest that initial dilation should be considered a preferred strategy in achalasia.

How did these authors achieve such good results and are they generalizable? They are a high-volume expert center that follows a set algorithm. They always begin with a 30-mm dilator and then progress to a larger dilator (35 or 40 mm) only in the case of failure. They also have determined that resting higher lower esophageal sphincter pressure after dilation was predictive of the need for future additional therapy. There were a few areas where their treatment differed from the typical US treatment. Dilations were performed as inpatient and contrast imaging was not routine but only done in the case of symptoms, which potentially could have missed some asymptomatic leaks that likely would be of minimal consequence. They also confirmed previous studies suggesting better outcomes with pneumatic dilation in older patients.

This article confirms pneumatic dilation as a viable treatment for achalasia. It would seem that this illness is ideally treated in a center with expertise in both endoscopic and surgical treatment. Perforation is rare but can occur, and appropriate surgical backup when performing pneumatic dilation is still recommended despite the safety reported in this study.

K. R. DeVault, MD

Esophageal Motility Disorders

Efficacy of Venlafaxine for Symptomatic Relief in Young Adult Patients With Functional Chest Pain: A Randomized, Double-Blind, Placebo-Controlled, Crossover Trial

Lee H, Kim JH, Min B-H, et al (Sungkyunkwan Univ School of Medicine, Seoul, Korea; Konkuk Univ School of Medicine, Seoul, Korea; et al)
Am J Gastroenterol 105:1504-1512, 2010

Objectives.—Esophageal hypersensitivity is currently believed to have a crucial role in the pathogenesis of functional chest pain (FCP). The aim of this study was to evaluate the clinical efficacy of venlafaxine, a serotonin–norepinephrine reuptake inhibitor (SNRI), for FCP in young adult patients.

Methods.—Patients diagnosed with FCP were randomized to either an extended-release formulation of venlafaxine (75 mg hora somni) or a placebo for 4 weeks. After a washout period of 2 weeks, patients crossed over to the other arm of the study. The primary efficacy variable was the number of patients with > 50% improvement in symptom scores. The secondary efficacy variables were (i) the symptom intensity score during each week, (ii) quality of life (QOL), (iii) the Beck Depression Inventory (BDI) score, and (iv) side effects.

Results.—A total of 43 patients (37 men, mean age 23.5 ± 1.9 years) completed the study. A positive response was observed in 52.0% of patients during venlafaxine treatment; 4.0% had a positive response with placebo treatment as assessed by the intention-to-treat analysis (venlafaxine vs. placebo: odds ratio 26.0; 95% confidence interval 5.7–118.8; $P < 0.001$). Results of Short-Form 36 (SF-36) indicated that patients who received venlafaxine treatment had a significantly greater improvement in body pain and emotional role compared with those who received placebo treatment ($P = 0.002$ and $P = 0.002$, respectively). No significant change was noted in the depression score after venalafaxine or placebo treatment. One patient withdrew from the study because of sleep disturbance and loss of appetite while receiving venlafaxine.

Conclusions.—Venlafaxine, an SNRI antidepressant, significantly improved symptoms in young adult patients with FCP.

▶ This trial compared a serotonin-norepinephrine reuptake inhibitor antidepressant with placebo in young patients with functional chest pain. The authors found a positive response in 52% of treated patients compared with only 4% of placebo, although complete response was less than 20% on therapy and did not occur at all on placebo. The response in this study did not seem to be related to baseline or any improvement in questionnaire-monitored depression. Many health care providers currently treat functional gastrointestinal (GI) disorders such as functional chest pain with antidepressants, despite relatively limited data from well-designed trials. This crossover trial provides additional support for that practice. There are several limitations to wide application of these results. This was a very young population (20-29 years), and it is unclear whether similar results could be expected in older patients. The authors also carefully selected the patients by replacing reflux and esophageal dysmotility with endoscopy, pH testing, and manometry, which is reasonable but perhaps different from empirically treating patients who may or may not have been through a similar evaluation. The placebo response rate in this study was also lower than in most studies of functional GI disorders, with the reason for this difference being unclear.

Despite those differences, it is becoming increasingly clear that antidepressants are beneficial in functional GI disorders. In chest pain, for example, trazodone, imipramine, and other antidepressants have demonstrated efficacy. Venlafaxine is now another agent that can be tried to help in these often frustrated patients. Gastroenterologists should take time to learn about the indications, dosage, and potential side effects of this class of agents in order to use them safely and effectively in their practices.

K. R. DeVault, MD

Barrett's Esophagus

The Risk of Esophageal Adenocarcinoma After Antireflux Surgery

Lagergren J, Ye W, Lagergren P, et al (Karolinska Institutet, Stockholm, Sweden)

Gastroenterology 138:1297-1301, 2010

Background & Aims.—The question of a possible preventive effect of antireflux surgery on the development of esophageal or cardia adenocarcinoma remains unsettled. We aimed to clarify whether antireflux surgery prevents later development of esophageal adenocarcinoma.

Methods.—We performed a Swedish population-based cohort study of antireflux surgery from 1965 to 2006. Follow-up evaluation for cancer and censoring for death and emigration were achieved up to December 31, 2006, through linkages to nationwide registers of cancer, population, and emigration. The cancer incidence in the antireflux surgery cohort was compared with that in the corresponding Swedish population. Relative risks were presented as standardized incidence ratios (SIRs), that is, the observed number of cancer cases in the antireflux surgery cohort divided by the expected number.

Results.—The antireflux surgery cohort comprised 14,102 persons, contributing 120,514 person-years at risk. Overall risk of esophageal adenocarcinoma (n = 39) was increased 12-fold (SIR, 12.3; 95% confidence interval [CI], 8.7–16.8). No risk decrease with time after antireflux surgery was found ($P = .86$). After a postsurgical follow-up evaluation of 15 years or more, the SIR was 14.6 (95% CI, 7.0–26.8). For the corresponding overall risk of cardia adenocarcinoma (n = 21) the SIR was 4.4 (95% CI, 2.7–6.7), without any major decrease in risk with time ($P = .20$); the SIR was 3.1 (95% CI, 0.6–9.1) after at least 15 years of follow-up evaluation. No association between antireflux surgery and gastric adenocarcinoma or esophageal squamous cell carcinoma was identified.

Conclusions.—Antireflux surgery cannot be considered to prevent the development of esophageal or cardia adenocarcinoma among persons with reflux.

▶ This is a very important study looking for a potential protective effect of antireflux surgery toward esophageal adenocarcinoma (EAC). The authors used the powerful Swedish population database to evaluate over 14 000 patients undergoing reflux surgery from 1965 to 2006 and compared them with the entire population. They found a 12-fold increased risk of EAC in the surgery group and also found that the risk persisted for up to 15 years after surgery.

Many groups have advocated aggressive acid control in patients with gastroesophageal reflux disease as a potential method for decreasing the incidence of EAC. Because Barrett's esophagus is the primary risk factor for EAC and reflux is the major risk factor for Barrett's esophagus, the hypothesis that acid control decreases cancer is attractive. Unfortunately, data to support this are almost entirely lacking. This population-based study provides additional data that contradict the idea that reflux control is preventive for cancer. Because EAC is a fairly rare cancer (even among those with reflux and/or Barrett's esophagus), randomized controlled trials are almost impossible, and population studies like this are the best data currently available. This study could not control for baseline severity of reflux nor were there data with regard to the presence or absence of Barrett's esophagus prior to surgery. In fact, even if there were such data, they likely would not be helpful because advances in both equipment and understanding have changed our approach so much since the 1960s that endoscopic data from then would be uninterruptible. Despite these 2 weaknesses, this study provides the best look at this question to date.

This and other studies indicate that surgical and medical control of reflux in patients with Barrett's esophagus should be considered as a method to control symptoms and not as a cancer-prevention strategy. An exception to this indication is patients who have undergone ablation since they experience a rapid return of Barrett's esophagus if their acid is not controlled. In addition, there are emerging data suggesting that a combination of acid control and aspirin may be beneficial (at least with intermediate markers). Based on this study and others, we can now confidently counsel patients that they should not undergo reflux surgery when their only concern is the risk of subsequent EAC.

K. R. DeVault, MD

Medications (NSAIDs, Statins, Proton Pump Inhibitors) and the Risk of Esophageal Adenocarcinoma in Patients With Barrett's Esophagus

Nguyen DM, Richardson P, El-Serag HB (Veterans Affairs Med Ctr, Houston, TX)

Gastroenterology 138:2260-2266, 2010

Background & Aims.—Limited evidence suggests that proton pump inhibitors (PPI), nonsteroidal anti-inflammatory drugs (NSAID)/aspirin, and statins may be associated with a low risk of esophageal neoplasia. However, the possible effect these medications may have on the risk of esophageal adenocarcinoma (EAC) in patients with existing Barrett's esophagus (BE) is unclear.

Methods.—We conducted a nested case-control study in a cohort of patients with BE identified in the national Department of Veterans' Affairs computerized databases. Cases with incident EAC were matched by incidence density sampling to controls with BE who remained without EAC at the date of the EAC diagnosis for the corresponding case. We identified prescriptions for PPI, NSAIDs/aspirin, and statins that were filled between BE diagnosis and EAC diagnosis. Incidence density ratios were calculated using conditional logistic regression models that adjusted for race, outpatient encounters, a disease comorbidity index, and socioeconomic status.

Results.—In a cohort of 11,823 patients with first-time BE diagnosis, we examined 116 EAC cases and 696 matched controls. Most cases and controls had at least one filled PPI prescription (95% vs 94%; $P=.5$).

In this setting of almost universal PPI use, filled NSAID/aspirin prescriptions were associated with a reduced risk of EAC (adjusted incidence density ratio, 0.64; 95% confidence interval, 0.42–0.97). Filled statin prescriptions also were associated with a reduction in EAC risk (0.55; 95% confidence interval, 0.36–0.86), with a significant trend toward greater risk reduction with longer duration of statin use. However, the strong inverse associations with even short periods of use raise concerns of uncontrolled confounding.

Conclusions.—This observational study indicates that in patients with BE using PPI, NSAID/aspirin, or statin therapy might reduce the risk of developing EAC.

▶ These authors have performed a nested case-control study to evaluate the role of several medications in the outcome of patients with Barrett's esophagus. From a database of 11 000 patients, they identified 116 cancer cases and 696 matched controls. Almost all patients were on acid suppression, and the use of nonsteroidal anti-inflammatory drugs, such as aspirin or long-term statins, was associated with a reduction in the risk of developing esophageal adenocarcinoma.

Most patients identified with Barrett's esophagus did not develop cancer, but a subset of patients developed dysplasia, which will develop into cancer. Short-term placebo-controlled trials have suggested a decrease in malignant markers when patients with Barrett's esophagus are treated with aspirin or nonsteroidal agents. To my knowledge, similar data from humans have not been reported with statins. There are several ongoing clinical trials looking at aspirin in Barrett's esophagus. It will be several years before convincing data from these trials are available. For now, the use of aspirin in a patient with Barrett's esophagus who is already on a proton pump inhibitor presents a very low risk of an adverse event and should be considered. The correct dose of aspirin is not clear, but pulmonary data suggest that a full dose (325 mg) may be needed.

K. R. DeVault, MD

Gastroesophageal Reflux

Arbaclofen Placarbil Decreases Postprandial Reflux in Patients With Gastroesophageal Reflux Disease

Gerson LB, Huff FJ, Hila A, et al (Stanford Univ School of Medicine, CA; XenoPort Inc, Santa Clara, CA; Med Univ of South Carolina, Charleston; et al)
Am J Gastroenterol 105:1266-1275, 2010

Objectives.—Arbaclofen placarbil (AP), previously designated as XP19986, is an investigational prodrug of the active R-isomer of baclofen, a γ-aminobutyric acid agonist reflux inhibitor. The aim of this study was to assess the efficacy and safety of AP for decreasing meal-induced reflux episodes in patients with gastroesophageal reflux disease (GERD).

Methods.—We conducted a multicenter, randomized, double-blind, crossover study comparing single doses of AP with placebo. Different patients were enrolled at each of four escalating AP doses: 10, 20, 40, and 60 mg. Enrolled patients had GERD symptoms at least three times a week and 20 reflux episodes on impedance/pH monitoring over a period of 2 h. During study visits separated by periods of 3–7 days, patients received single doses of AP or placebo, followed by high-fat meals 2 and 6 h after treatment. The primary end point was the number of reflux episodes over 12 h after treatment.

Results.—A total of 50 patients were treated; efficacy analysis included 44 patients who received both AP and placebo and had technically satisfactory impedance/pH data. For the combined data from all dose cohorts, there was a statistically significant ($P = 0.01$) decrease in reflux episodes over 12 h after treatment with AP compared with placebo. The mean (s.d.) number of reflux episodes over 12 h after AP treatment was 50.5 (27.2), with a mean reduction of 10.4 (23.9) episodes (17%) compared with placebo, for which a mean (s.d.) number of 60.9 (35.3) episodes was observed. Heartburn events associated with reflux were reduced during treatment with AP compared with placebo. AP seemed to be the most efficacious in the 60-mg dose group, and was well tolerated at all dose levels.

Conclusions.—AP decreased reflux and associated symptoms with good tolerability in patients with GERD.

▶ In most cases gastroesophageal reflux disease (GERD) is a motility illness and is usually not characterized by excess acid secretion but by a functional deficit at the esophagogastric junction. In some patients this is an anatomical defect (hiatal hernia), but in most cases reflux events are initiated by what has been described as transient lower esophageal sphincter relaxation (TLESR). Recently, some downsides of chronic acid suppression have been identified, and there is much active research ongoing into the agents that prevent rather than simply neutralize acid reflux.

Arbaclofen placarbil (AP) is a prodrug of baclofen that appears to have activity against TLESR with a better safety profile than baclofen itself. This study evaluated 4 doses of AP (10, 20, 40, and 60 mg) or placebo given to patients with symptomatic GERD. The dose was given 2 hours prior to the ingestion of a high-fat meal, and reflux was monitored with a combined pH impedance catheter. To be included in the study, patients were required to have greater than 20 reflux events in the 2 hours after the meal during the placebo portion of the study. AP was able to decrease reflux events across all dose ranges, but for individual doses, a significant reduction was only seen at 60 mg. This held for heartburn-producing and asymptomatic reflux episodes. There were no significant adverse events.

This study confirmed a modest decrease in postprandial reflux events with AP. Whether or not this or other similar agents will find efficacy as the therapy for GERD remains to be determined. Thus far, physiological studies have shown modest changes with baclofen-like or other similar agents, but appropriately powered symptom-based efficacy studies have not yet been reported for most agents. It appears that some manufacturers are seeking an indication as an add-on to the proton pump inhibitor (PPI) therapy in partially responsive patients. These patients often have significant functional overlay and may be particularly difficult to treat. It is likely that some of these agents will be approved in the not-too-distant future and will provide an important addition to our therapeutic armamentarium, but it is unlikely that they will replace PPI in most patients.

K. R. DeVault, MD

Characteristics of Reflux Episodes and Symptom Association in Patients With Erosive Esophagitis and Nonerosive Reflux Disease: Study Using Combined Impedance–pH Off Therapy

Savarino E, Tutuian R, Zentilin P, et al (Univ of Genoa, Italy; Univ Hosp Bern, Switzerland; et al)

Am J Gastroenterol 105:1053-1061, 2010

Objectives.—We sought to compare reflux and symptom association patterns in patients with nonerosive reflux disease (NERD), erosive esophagitis (EE), and in healthy volunteers (HVs).

Methods.—Patients with EE and NERD underwent combined impedance–pH monitoring. Normal values were defined on the basis of previously collected data from 48 HVs. We evaluated distal esophageal acid exposure time (AET), number and type of reflux episodes (acid, nonacid), acid and bolus clearance times, proximal extension of reflux episodes, and symptom association probability (SAP).

Results.—Distal AET (percentage time, pH < 4) was higher ($P < 0.01$) in 58 EE patients (median 7.4%, 25–75th percentile 4.2–9.9%) compared with 168 NERD patients (4.2% (1.2–6.4%)) and 48 HVs (0.7% (0.2–1.4%)). Patients with EE and NERD had a higher ($P < 0.01$) number of acid reflux episodes compared with HVs (51 (37–66) vs. 34 (22–51) vs. 17 (8–31); $P < 0.05$), but a similar number of nonacid reflux episodes (22 (15–39) vs. 23 (15–38) vs. 18 (14–26); $P =$ NS). The percentage of reflux episodes reaching the proximal esophagus was higher ($P < 0.01$) in EE patients (57% (45–73%)) than in NERD patients (45% (36–60%)) and HVs (33% (19–46%)). A positive SAP for heartburn or regurgitation was found in 161 of 168 (96%) NERD and 54 of 58 (93%) EE patients ($P =$ NS).

Conclusions.—Acid reflux episodes, volume, and acid clearance are important factors in the pathogenesis of reflux-induced lesions. Nonacid reflux contributes less to esophageal mucosa damage, but is involved in the development of reflux symptoms in both NERD and EE patients.

▶ The authors studied combined impedance-pH monitoring in 58 patients with erosive esophagitis (EE), 168 patients with nonerosive reflux disease (NERD), and 48 healthy volunteers. The patients had more acid reflux events than the healthy volunteers, but there were similar numbers of nonacid events in all 3 groups. Positive symptom associations were noted in both the NERD and EE groups.

Until recently, an ambulatory reflux monitoring was limited to recording acid exposure in the esophagus. The advent of combined impedance-pH monitoring has for the first time allowed us to monitor the reflux of material of neutral or near neutral pH. Many studies have concentrated on performing this monitoring while patients were on acid suppressants to evaluate for residual, ongoing, neutralized reflux. This study took a different approach measuring both acid and impedance events in patients who were not on acid suppressants. It is interesting that with worsening mucosal disease, the number of acid reflux events increased, but the number of nonacid events were relatively stable between controls and the patients with reflux disease. The symptom association data were even more interesting. Predictably, in both EE and NERD, those with increased acid exposure tended to have more symptoms produced by acid than nonacid events. On the other hand, in those with normal acid exposure (19% of EE and 47% of nonerosive, all of which required a positive symptom association probability), the chances of an acid or nonacid event producing symptoms were roughly equal.

The authors conclude that monitoring of both acid and nonacid reflux is important in the evaluation of patients with reflux symptoms and that a portion of positive tests would be missed if only acid is monitored. I agree with the majority of the findings of this study but remain concerned with the concept of diagnosing a patient with gastroesophageal reflux disease who has normal acid exposure and a negative symptom association using acid only while tested off medications. These nonacid-only refluxers may represent a portion of patients suggested to have a hypersensitive esophagus, and it is not clear whether medical therapy using prokinetic agents or surgical therapy will control symptoms of this group; therefore, care should be taken in making therapeutic decisions based on the finding of a positive symptom association of nonacid reflux in a patient who is not on acid suppressants.

K. R. DeVault, MD

Iatrogenic Gastric Acid Suppression and the Risk of Nosocomial *Clostridium difficile* Infection

Howell MD, Novack V, Grgurich P, et al (Beth Israel Deaconess Med Ctr, Boston, MA; Harvard Clinical Res Inst, Boston, MA; Froedtert Hosp, Milwaukee, WI)

Arch Intern Med 170:784-790, 2010

Background.—The incidence and severity of *Clostridium difficile* infections are increasing. Acidsuppressive therapy has been suggested as a risk factor for *C difficile*, but this remains controversial.

Methods.—We conducted a pharmacoepidemiologic cohort study, performing a secondary analysis of data collected prospectively on 101 796 discharges from a tertiary care medical center during a 5-year period. The primary exposure of interest was acid suppression therapy, classified by the most intense acid suppression therapy received (no acid suppression, histamine$_2$-receptor antagonist [H_2RA] therapy, daily proton pump inhibitor [PPI], and PPI more frequently than daily).

Results.—As the level of acid suppression increased, the risk of nosocomial *C difficile* infection increased, from 0.3% (95% confidence interval [CI], 0.21%-0.31%) in patients not receiving acid suppressive therapy to 0.6% (95% CI, 0.49%-0.79%) in those receiving H_2RA therapy, to 0.9% (95% CI, 0.80%-0.98%) in those receiving daily PPI treatment, and to 1.4% (1.15%-1.71%) in those receiving more frequent PPI therapy. After adjustment for comorbid conditions, age, antibiotics, and propensity score–based likelihood of receipt of acid-suppression therapy, the association persisted, increasing from an odds ratio of 1 (no acid suppression [reference]) to 1.53 (95% CI, 1.12-2.10) (H_2RA), to 1.74 (95% CI, 1.39-2.18) (daily PPI), and to 2.36 (95% CI, 1.79-3.11) (more frequent PPI). Similar estimates were found with a matched cohort analysis and with nested case-control techniques.

Conclusions.—Increasing levels of pharmacologic acid suppression are associated with increased risks of nosocomial *C difficile* infection. This evidence of a dose-response effect provides further support for the potentially causal nature of iatrogenic acid suppression in the development of nosocomial *C difficile* infection.

▶ There have been several metabolic and infectious complications recently associated with long-term proton pump inhibitor (PPI) therapy. One of these is *Clostridium difficile* infection. This article is a large retrospective analysis of over 100 000 hospital discharges at a single institution. These data once again support the association between PPI therapy and *C difficile*. There was a clear dose response with a rate of 0.3% in patients not on acid suppression up to 1.4% in patients treated with greater than once daily PPI. After adjusting for comorbidities, a statistical increase in odds ratio was noted to be present, and the odds ratio increased as treatment moved from histamine$_2$-receptor antagonist (1.53) to daily PPI (1.74) to high-dose PPI (2.36).

How should providers react to studies like this, which suggest a small but statistically significant risk with PPI therapy? First, this study and others confirm that *C difficile* is not only associated with antibiotic therapy, older age, and multiple comorbidities but also associated with PPI use. Interestingly, high-dose PPI had an odds ratio (2.36) intermediate between low-risk antibiotics (1.82) and high-risk antibiotics (3.37). Secondly, up to 60% of the population is exposed to acid suppression medication, and over 15% of PPI prescriptions are for greater than once daily dosing, despite minimal evidence of improved efficacy at higher doses. Finally, *C difficile* infection is increasing and becoming a greater public health issue.

The authors made several valid conclusions. Each patient should have their acid suppression tailored to control symptoms or mucosal disease at the minimally effective dose. Also, not all hospitalized patients need stress ulcer prophylaxis. Finally, this issue needs continued study to develop better cost-benefit ratios in both the outpatient and inpatient environments.

K. R. DeVault, MD

Miscellaneous

Anti-interleukin-5 antibody treatment (mepolizumab) in active eosinophilic oesophagitis: a randomised, placebo-controlled, double-blind trial

Straumann A, Conus S, Grzonka P, et al (Kantonsspital, Olten, Switzerland; Univ of Bern, Switzerland; et al)

Gut 59:21-30, 2010

Objective.—Eosinophilic oesophagitis (EoO) is a clinicopathological condition defined by proton pump inhibitor-refractory oesophageal symptoms combined with oesophageal eosinophilia. The pharmacodynamic effect of mepolizumab (a humanised anti-interleukin-5 monoclonal antibody) in EoO was evaluated.

Methods.—Eleven adults with active EoO (>20 peak eosinophil number/high power field (hpf) and dysphagia) were randomised to 750 mg of mepolizumab ($n = 5$) or placebo ($n = 6$) and received two intravenous infusions, 1 week apart. Those not in complete remission (<5 peak eosinophil number/hpf) after 8 weeks received two further doses 4 weeks apart, 1500 mg of mepolizumab or placebo. The effect of mepolizumab was assessed clinically, endoscopically, histologically, and via blood and tissue biomarkers.

Results.—As assessed by immunofluorescence, a marked reduction of mean oesophageal eosinophilia ($p = 0.03$) was seen in the mepolizumab group (−54%) compared with the placebo group (−5%) 4 weeks after initiation of treatment. No further reduction of eosinophil numbers was observed in response to the two additional infusions in either group. Mepolizumab reduced tenascin C ($p = 0.033$) and transforming growth factor β1 ($p = 0.05$) expression in the oesophageal epithelial layer 13 weeks after initiation of treatment. Clinically, limited improvement of symptoms was seen, although a trend was seen between 4 and 13 weeks after initiation of mepolizumab treatment. Mepolizumab was well tolerated.

Conclusions.—Mepolizumab significantly reduced eosinophil numbers in oesophageal tissues in adult patients with active EoO, and changes in the expression of molecules associated with oesophageal remodelling were reversed. Minimal clinical improvement was achieved in a subgroup of patients with EoO. Mepolizumab had an acceptable safety profile, even at the high 1500 mg dose level.

Trial Registration Number.—NCT00274703.

▶ This study examined the use of an anti-interleukin-5 (anti-IL-5) antibody (mepolizumab) in a small number of patients ($n = 11$) with eosinophilic esophagitis (EOE). The authors were able to demonstrate significant improvement in eosinophil infiltration (54% reduction vs 5% with placebo) and other changes associated with inflammatory markers. The treatment appeared to be safe and well tolerated, but the study was not powered to effectively evaluate clinical response.

EOE is an inflammatory condition of the esophagus that appears to be rapidly increasing in incidence. The classic presentation is dysphagia to solids, but some patients present with chest pain, heartburn, and other nonspecific symptoms. Initial treatment of EOE may include a trial of acid suppression or a trial of topical or systemic steroids. Mepolizumab is a fully humanized anti-IL-5 myocardial antibody that has been effective in several disorders characterized by eosinophilic infiltration.

When should agents of this type be considered in EOE? Most of these patients have symptoms that are transient or that can be managed with agents that have a good safety profile such as proton pump inhibitors, topical steroids, or both. In addition, recent studies have confirmed efficacy and reasonable safety for esophageal dilation. The authors suggest that controlling inflammation may decrease esophageal remodeling, although this concept certainly remains theoretical. Mepolizumab and other immunomodulators are usually well tolerated but have a clear side effect profile, including, in rare cases, lymphoma. It would seem prudent to reserve systemic agents like this one and even systemic steroids for severe or refractory cases and continue to use proton pump inhibitors, topical steroids, and careful dilation in the majority.

K. R. DeVault, MD

Esophageal Dilation in Eosinophilic Esophagitis: Effectiveness, Safety and Impact on the Underlying Inflammation

Schoepfer AM, Gonsalves N, Bussmann C, et al (McMaster Univ, Hamilton, Ontario, Canada; Northwestern Univ School of Medicine, Chicago, IL; Kantonsspital Lucerne, Switzerland; et al)

Am J Gastroenterol 105:1062-1070, 2010

Objectives.—Esophageal dilation often leads to long-lasting relief of dysphagia in eosinophilic esophagitis (EoE). The aim of this study was to define the effectiveness, safety, and patient acceptance of esophageal dilation in EoE. In addition, we examined the influence of dilation on the underlying esophageal inflammation.

Methods.—Two databases including 681 EoE patients were reviewed. Cohort 1 consisted of patients treated with dilation alone, whereas cohort 2 included patients treated with a combination of dilation and antieosinophilic medication. Patients from cohort 1 underwent a prospective histological reexamination and an evaluation using a questionnaire.

Results.—In total, 207 EoE patients were treated with esophageal dilation, 63 in cohort 1 and 144 in cohort 2. Dilation led to a significant increase in esophageal diameter and to an improvement in dysphagia in both the cohorts ($P < 0.001$). After dilation, dysphagia recurred after 23 ± 22 months in cohort 1 and 20 ± 14 months in cohort 2. No esophageal perforation or major bleeding occurred. Among the patients surveyed, 74 % reported retrosternal pain after dilation; however, all were agreeable to repeated dilation if required. Eosinophil peak infiltration, eosinophil load, and EoE-associated histological signs were not significantly affected by esophageal dilation.

Conclusions.—Esophageal dilation is highly effective in providing long-lasting symptom relief and can be performed safely with a high degree of patient acceptance. However, dilation is associated with postprocedural pain in most patients and does not influence the underlying inflammatory process. Symptom improvement despite persistence of inflammation suggests that tissue remodeling contributes substantially to symptom generation in EoE.

▶ This study examined the safety and efficacy of esophageal dilation in patients with eosinophilic esophagitis (EOE). A total of 207 patients underwent dilation and were divided into those dilated in combination with medical therapy for EOE (n = 122) and those dilated alone (n = 63). Both groups experienced long-term improvement (mean of 20-23 months), but there was a large intra-subject variation in duration (14-22 months). Postprocedural pain was common (74%), but there were no perforations or major bleeding. The duration of response did not differ between the groups that underwent dilation alone or had dilation with medical therapy.

This study is somewhat limited by its retrospective design but still adds to our understanding of this common disorder. One of the important shortcomings of this article is lack of standard treatment in the medically treated cohort, which could have included topical or systemic steroids, leukotriene receptor antagonists, mast cell stabilizers, other immunomodulators, or various combinations. The method of dilation was also only partially standardized, with some undergoing balloon dilation and others undergoing Savary-type dilation. The goal was to achieve a 16- to 17-mm lumen with an increase of 3 mm per dilation session. Dilation did not change the histological evidence of inflammation except in the group where there was combined therapy with other topical and systemic agents.

This study provides support for esophageal dilation if carried out in a systematic and conservative fashion. Dilation may actually be the treatment most likely to produce long-term benefit and remains a first-line option for EOE patients presenting with dysphagia.

K. R. DeVault, MD

Depth of Submucosal Invasion Does Not Predict Lymph Node Metastasis and Survival of Patients With Esophageal Carcinoma

Badreddine RJ, Prasad GA, Lewis JT, et al (Mayo Clinic College of Medicine, Rochester, MN)

Clin Gastroenterol Hepatol 8:248-253, 2010

Background & Aims.—There is controversy over the outcomes of esophageal adenocarcinoma with superficial submucosal invasion. We evaluated the impact of depth of submucosal invasion on the presence of metastatic lymphadenopathy and survival in patients with esophageal adenocarcinoma.

Methods.—Pathology reports of esophagectomy samples collected from 1997 to 2007 were reviewed. Specimens from patients with esophageal adenocarcinoma and submucosal invasion were reviewed and classified as superficial (upper 1 third, sm1) or deep (middle third, sm2 or deepest third, sm3) invasion. Outcomes studied were presence of metastatic lymphadenopathy and overall survival. Variables of interest were analyzed as factors that affect overall and cancer-free survival using Cox proportional hazards modeling. A multivariate model was constructed to establish independent associations with survival.

Results.—The study included 80 patients; 31 (39%) had sm1 carcinoma, 23 (29%) had sm2 carcinoma, and 26 (33%) had sm3 carcinoma. Superficial and deep submucosal invasion were associated with substantial rates of metastatic lymphadenopathy (12.9% and 20.4%, respectively). The mean follow-up time was 40.5 ± 4 months and the mean overall unadjusted survival time was 53.8 ± 4.1 months. Factors significantly associated with reduced survival time included the presence of metastatic lymph nodes (hazard ratio [HR], 2.89; confidence interval [CI], 1.13–6.88) and esophageal cancer recurrence (HR 6.39, CI 2.40–16.14), but not depth of submucosal invasion.

Conclusions.—Patients with sm1 esophageal carcinoma have substantial rates of metastatic lymphadenopathy. Endoscopic treatment of superficial submucosal adenocarcinoma is not advised for patients that are candidates for surgery.

▶ The treatment of esophageal carcinoma is in a state of flux. Several years ago, the only options were surgery, radiation, and chemotherapy or some combination. Now, we have made advances in screening, imaging, and endoscopic therapy, allowing the identification of more superficial lesions. Many lesions can now be resected endoscopically to provide both better staging and potential endoscopic cures. It is clear that if a lesion is invasive, then endoscopic therapy is not curative, and it is becoming clear that if a lesion is confined to the mucosa (essentially high-grade dysplasia), then endoscopic cure is possible. What is less clear is the situation with tumors invading into the submucosa but not deeper (sm1, 2, or 3). In this study, lymph node (LN) involvement was assessed in patients with tumors invading into the superficial submucosa (sm1) or deeper submucosa (sm1 or 2). LNs were positive for malignant cells in 12.9% of the sm1 tumors and 20.4% of the sm2-3 tumors.

Although this is a fairly small study (80 patients), the results and conclusions must be respected. Patients discovered to have submucosal invasion at surgery or by endoscopic mucosal resection should understand their risk of metastatic disease and should be offered additional therapy, if clinically appropriate. Some high-risk surgical patients may elect to not have more definitive surgery or even undergo radiation and chemotherapy, but they must understand their 12% to 20% risk of developing recurrent disease and that it is possible chemotherapy and radiation followed by surgery may (although certainly not proven) decrease that risk at the expense of increased early risk of morbidity and mortality.

K. R. DeVault, MD

Diagnostic Criteria for Eosinophilic Esophagitis: A 5-year Retrospective Review in a Pediatric Population

Lai AL, Girgis S, Liang Y, et al (Univ of Alberta, Edmonton, Canada; Alberta Res Centre for Child Health Evidence, Edmonton, Canada; et al)

J Pediatr Gastroenterol Nutr 49:63-70, 2009

Background.—The diagnostic criterion based on the number of eosinophils (Eos) per high-power field (HPF) does not appear to capture all patients with eosinophilic esophagitis (EE).

Objectives.—To determine whether EE has been underrecognized at our institution, clinical variables predicting EE, and whether the Luna eosinophil granule (LEG) stain detects eosinophils better than hematoxylin and eosin (HE).

Materials and Methods.—Esophageal biopsies of 202 children younger than 18 years old from 2000 to 2004 were reviewed and Eos/HPF was recorded. Clinical variables from charts were reviewed and a marginal logit model was used to determine significance. LEG stains for 60 randomly selected patients were prepared and compared to HE originals.

Results.—EE diagnoses have risen from none in 2000 to 23 in 2004. The clinically significant variables that predicted EE were improvement from EE treatment (160 times more likely to have EE; $P < 0.0005$), final endoscopic diagnosis of EE (31 times; $P = 0.004$), absence of vascular pattern on endoscopy (20 times; $P = 0.008$), and vertical furrows on endoscopy (29 times; $P = 0.039$). LEG stain appeared to be superior to HE in detecting low Eos/HPF (mean 24.82 and 38.53, respectively). Peak counts of eosinophils in the most involved HPF significantly correlated with highest average count of eosinophils per HPF in the most involved specimen (Pearson correlation 0.958).

Conclusions.—Misdiagnosed EE cases decreased but prevalence appeared to increase. LEG potentially can be a more sensitive stain. The key variables that predict EE were typical endoscopic findings and improvement from specific EE treatment.

▶ This is a great article to review as patients with eosinophilic esophagitis (EE) may present with dysphagia and heartburn, which are common patient symptoms that we see in our gastrointestinal (GI) practice. The results of this study agree with previous studies that both clinical and histological features as well as response to treatment help establish a correct diagnosis of EE. I would encourage all gastroenterologists and all GI pathologists to read this article as it has important clinical application.

J. S. Scolapio, MD

Esophageal Disorders

Kahrilas PJ, Smout AJPM (Northwestern Univ, Chicago, IL; Academic Med Ctr, Amsterdam, The Netherlands)

Am J Gastroenterol 105:747-756, 2010

Background.—Patients who have upper gastrointestinal (GI) symptoms require a careful clinical history. Many have a relatively mild, non-life-threatening illness, and a careful history can reveal the proper management. Patients likely to have a more serious underlying disease require further steps to determine the right treatment. Physicians should include questions about dietary history, smoking, and alcohol consumption when collecting the history. The major symptoms of esophageal disorders related to functional esophageal disorders are heartburn, chest pain, dysphagia, and globus.

Disorders.—Heartburn or pyrosis is the most common symptom reported by patients with esophageal complaints. Characteristics include discomfort or burning sensation behind the sternum that comes from the epigastrium and can radiate neckward. This intermittent symptom generally occurs within 60 minutes of eating, while exercising, or when recumbent. Drinking water or taking antacids relieves the discomfort, but frequent recurrences can interfere with daily living. When heartburn is the predominant or only symptom, gastroesophageal reflux disease (GERD) is the most likely diagnosis.

Chest pain is another common symptom and resembles pain of cardiac origin, a possibility that should be explored first. The similarity of cardiac pain to esophageal chest pain is probably because these organs share a nerve plexus and the esophageal wall nerve endings discriminate poorly among stimuli. Esophageal pain is usually described as a sense of pressure in the mid chest that radiates to the mid back, arms, or jaws. The specific mechanism causing esophageal chest pain is not yet known, but esophageal spasm and contractile abnormalities are not likely explanations. Chest pain is more likely to indicate GERD than esophageal dysmotility.

Dysphagia is found in over 30% of persons with GERD and results from peptic stricture, a Schatzki ring, peristaltic dysfunction, or mucosal inflammation related to esophagitis. It can also occur with no apparent abnormality, which is usually the result of abnormal sensitivity to bolus movement during peristalsis. Patients describe the sensation of having food "stick" on the way down the esophagus or remain in the chest. Different types of dysphagia are possible, with purely solid food versus liquid and solid, episodic versus constant, and progressive versus static. Liquid-solid food dysphagia suggests a motor aberration of the esophagus; solid-only dysphagia is likely the result of a structural abnormality and requires further investigation. Episodic dysphagia represents a slightly compromised esophageal lumen and is manifest as complete obstruction or no compromise at all. Progressive solid-food dysphagia plus weight loss is the classic finding in esophageal cancer. About 30% of distal esophageal obstructions are perceived as cervical dysphagia and suggest oropharyngeal swallowing disorder, but these patient-reported sensations are highly unreliable.

In globus sensation or globus hystericus the patient perceives a lump or fullness in the throat that is unrelated to swallowing. Often swallowing relieves the symptom. It often is found in individuals with anxiety or obsessive-compulsive disorders but can also be caused by GERD.

Diagnosis and Management.—History and physical examination are the first steps to take in reaching a diagnosis. A proton pump inhibitor (PPI) trial at a standard dose once or twice a day for 2 to 4 weeks can be instituted. Once a satisfactory response has been established, the dose can be reduced to the least amount that maintains that treatment response. In the absence of a satisfactory response, other tests can be conducted, depending on the symptoms. These can include endoscopy with appropriate biopsy, high-resolution manometry, pH or impedance-pH monitoring while withholding PPI therapy, videofluoroscopic swallowing study, or a trial of antireflux therapy, as indicated.

▶ This is an excellent review article on esophageal disorders that all clinical gastroenterologists should read. It covers the topics of heartburn, noncardiac chest pain, dysphagia, and globus. This article is written in a way that is very easy to follow. Each topic is presented in a case-based format followed by a legend algorithm that is very easy to follow. The legend describes each disease state in a clear and concise manner that is easy for the reader to follow. I find this style of presentation a great way to review the subject of esophageal disorders.

J. S. Scolapio, MD

2 Gastrointestinal Motility Disorders/ Neurogastroenterology

Gastric Motility

Delayed Radionucleotide Gastric Emptying Studies Predict Morbidity in Diabetics With Symptoms of Gastroparesis

Hyett B, Martinez FJ, Gill BM, et al (Brigham and Women's Hosp, Boston, MA; Beth Israel Deaconess Med Ctr, Boston, MA)

Gastroenterology 137:445-452, 2009

Background & Aims.—The aim of this study was to evaluate the prognostic value of gastric emptying studies on the morbidity associated with diabetic gastroparesis.

Methods.—This was a parallel cohort study of 3 groups. Group A (n = 94) contained diabetic patients (type 1 and type 2) with classic symptoms of gastroparesis (including early satiety, postprandial fullness, bloating, abdominal swelling, nausea, vomiting, and retching) and delay in radionucleotide gastric emptying study. Group B (n = 94) contained diabetic subjects with classic symptoms of gastroparesis but negative scintigraphy. Group C (n = 94) contained diabetic subjects without symptoms of gastroparesis. Data were gathered on the number of days hospitalized and hospitalizations, office visits, emergency department visits, death rate, glycosylated hemoglobin levels, medications, and past medical history.

Results.—Group A had significantly more hospital days per 1000 patient days (25.5) than both group B (5.1; $P < .01$) and group C (2.3; $P < .01$). Group A also had significantly more hospitalizations, office visits, and emergency department visits than both group B and group C. Deaths and mean glycosylated hemoglobin levels did not differ between the groups. Patients in group A were more likely to have cardiovascular disease (19.2% vs 6.4%, A vs C; $P < .05$), hypertension (63% vs 43%, A vs C; $P = .005$), and retinopathy (33% vs 11.7%, A vs C; $P < .001$).

Conclusions.—A delayed radionucleotide gastric emptying study predicts negative health outcomes in diabetic patients with symptoms of gastroparesis. We identified a correlation between diabetic gastroparesis and cardiovascular disease, hypertension, and retinopathy that may indicate an underlying vascular etiology.

▶ In this retrospective parallel cohort study, a group of patients with diabetes and upper gastrointestinal (GI) symptoms with and without delayed gastric emptying were compared in terms of their outcomes. Despite similar clinical presentations, there was a striking correlation between definite gastroparesis and bad outcomes, including coronary artery disease, hypertension, and retinopathy. Even after normalizing for hemoglobin A_{1C} levels, gastroparesis appeared to be an independent marker for increased morbidity. There was also a trend for increased mortality in those with gastroparesis, although the study wasn't powered for this difference and it didn't reach statistical significance. These observations, if true, are very concerning; they suggest diabetic patients deserve to have their gastric emptying assessed and be more aggressively managed if gastric emptying is delayed. However, it is possible that these findings are all due to confounding factors. For example, there was a longer duration of diabetes in the gastroparesis group, and thus the finding of gastroparesis may simply represent a marker of longer diabetes exposure and hence worse outcomes, rather than gastroparesis itself being directly causally related to worse outcomes.

N. J. Talley, MD, PhD

Full-thickness biopsy findings in chronic intestinal pseudo-obstruction and enteric dysmotility

Lindberg G, Törnblom H, Iwarzon M, et al (Karolinska Univ Hosp, Huddinge, Stockholm, Sweden; et al)

Gut 58:1084-1090, 2009

Background and Aims.—Small bowel manometry is increasingly used in the clinical investigation of patients with symptoms of intestinal motor dysfunction. Enteric dysmotility (ED) has been suggested as a new diagnostic term for patients with abnormal intestinal motor activity but no radiological signs of chronic intestinal pseudo-obstruction (CIP). Histopathological features of adult patients with ED and CIP have been compared in a large case series to study differences and similarities between the two diagnostic groups.

Methods.—Routine staining and an extensive panel of immunohistochemical stains on transversal and tangential cuts from full-thickness biopsies of the small bowel were used.

Results.—39 females and 11 males with CIP and 58 females and 7 males with ED were investigated. The underlying lesion was more often a visceral myopathy (22% vs 5%) or neuromyopathy (30% vs 12%) in patients with CIP than in those with ED, whereas the predominant lesion in ED was neuropathy with inflammation.

Conclusion.—CIP in adults is associated with very different underlying pathology, whereas ED is more homogeneously associated with neuropathy in the enteric nervous system. Neuropathy of enteric ganglia with inflammation seems to be the most common cause for measurable disturbances of intestinal motor function.

▶ This is a very important and novel study from Sweden because the management of patients with severe intestinal motility disorders remains incredibly problematic. Different terms have been used to describe patients who have severe unexplained gastrointestinal (GI) symptoms; these are usually classified as functional, although patients who continue to vomit and lose weight on medical therapy are at the extreme end of the functional bowel disease spectrum. In this article, Lindberg and colleagues studied a group of patients with severe unexplained GI symptoms by small bowel manometry study, which found no evidence of mechanical obstruction but was still abnormal; they refer to these patients as having enteric dysmotility. The patients did not have chronic idiopathic intestinal pseudo-obstruction (CIIP); by definition, patients with CIIP have chronic signs mimicking mechanical obstruction but no evidence of mechanical obstruction on appropriate investigations. It is important to note that these patients are clinically different from those presenting with irritable bowel syndrome. The investigators performed full thickness biopsies and noted an inflammatory neuropathy with infiltration of lymphocytes in the ganglia of the myenteric plexus in most of the patients with enteric dysmotility, defining the pathology for the first time. Similar findings were seen in CIIP. The data suggest that the enteric dysmotility group is pathologically part of the spectrum of pseudo-obstruction, is relatively rare, and is usually caused by a visceral neuropathy.

Another very interesting observation was that small bowel manometry poorly differentiated between neuropathic and myopathic conditions in this cohort, that suggesting current algorithms using small bowel manometry may be of little help. Manometry can assist in identifying a severe disease subset but doesn't define the pathology.

In terms of therapeutic options, there is no clear-cut therapy proven to reverse the visceral neuropathy and inflammatory changes identified in this study. Whether patients with severe disease and an enteric ganglionitis would benefit from aggressive immunosuppressive therapy now needs testing.

N. J. Talley, MD, PhD

***Helicobacter pylori*–positive Versus *Helicobacter pylori*–negative Idiopathic Peptic Ulcers in Children With Their Long-Term Outcomes**

Tam YH, Lee KH, To KF, et al (The Chinese Univ of Hong Kong, China)
J Pediatr Gastroenterol Nutr 48:299-305, 2009

Objectives.—The aim of this study is to investigate the differences in the characteristics between *Helicobacter pylori*–positive and *H pylori*–negative primary ulcers in Chinese children.

Patients and Methods.—We conducted a retrospective review of children with primary peptic ulcers. Demographic data, clinical presentations, endoscopic features, histological findings, *H pylori* prevalence, and ulcer recurrences were studied.

Results.—Forty-three Chinese children with primary peptic ulcers were diagnosed over 8 years and were reviewed. There were 31 boys and 12 girls (median age 12 years, range 3–16 years). Thirty children (70%) presented with acute gastrointestinal bleeding, whereas only 19 had a history of epigastric pain. Twenty-three patients (53.5%) were *H pylori* positive. *H pylori*–positive ulcers developed in older children (median age 12 vs 10 years, $P < 0.05$) and affected more males (91.3% vs 50%, $P < 0.01$) than the *H pylori*–negative group. The annual ulcer recurrence rates were estimated to be 5.2% (95% CI 4.2–6.3) and 11.4% (95% CI 9.1–13.6) for positive and negative groups, respectively ($P < 0.05$). Multivariate logistic regression suggested *H pylori*–negative status and ulcer size > 1 cm were independent risk factors for recurrence.

Conclusions.—Our report suggests that *H pylori*–negative primary ulcers exist in children with their own distinct features. In contrast to *H pylori*–positive ulcers, *H pylori*–negative ulcers develop in younger children, affect both sexes equally, and carry a higher recurrence risk.

▶ Peptic ulcer disease is uncommon in childhood, and *Helicobacter pylori*-negative causes unexplained peptic ulcer disease even more rarely. This retrospective study from Hong Kong identified 20 cases of *H pylori*-negative ulcers in children and compared these with 23 *H pylori*-positive cases. A number of differences were identified between the *H pylori*-negative and *H pylori*-positive ulcer cases. In particular, the gender distribution was equal in the *H pylori*-negative group, although the symptom presentation was very similar. Notably, recurrence was higher in the *H pylori*-negative group than in the treated *H pylori*-positive group, adding further evidence that long-term acid-suppression therapy may be required in children to control idiopathic ulcer disease. Notably, 3 quarters of the children in the *H pylori*-negative group still had chronic inflammation on antral biopsy and whether this was due to a missed *H pylori* infection or other infectious processes is unknown. More effort is needed to understand idiopathic peptic ulcer disease in children and adults.

N. J. Talley, MD, PhD

Gastric Electrical Stimulation in Intractable Nausea and Vomiting: Assessment of Predictive Factors of Favorable Outcomes

Gourcerol G, Chaput U, LeBlanc I, et al (Univ of Rouen, France)

J Am Coll Surg 209:215-221, 2009

Background.—Gastric electrical stimulation (GES) represents a new therapy in patients with intractable vomiting and nausea. We aimed to determine preoperative factors associated with positive response during GES. Thirty-three consecutive patients received implants for medically refractory nausea or vomiting or both.

Study Design.—Symptoms, Quality of Life (QOL), and gastric emptying (GE) were monitored before and 6 months after implantation. Compared with baseline, dyspeptic symptoms including nausea and vomiting, and QOL all improved at 6 months, yielding a significant weight gain while the GE rate remained unchanged. Twenty-four patients reported improvement; nine remained unimproved at 6 months.

Results.—In multivariate analysis, baseline QOL and appetite alterations were predictive of improvement; previous history of gastric surgery was associated with failure. Surprisingly, patients with initial delayed GE (21 of 33) displayed similar improvement compared with patients with normal GE. Likewise, basal GE was not found to be predictive of positive outcomes, QOL, or symptoms improvement.

Conclusions.—Patients with severe symptoms and altered QOL at inclusion particularly benefit from GES; delay in GE is not predictive of positive outcomes. This suggests that indication for GES should be based on clinical settings rather than initial GE, and then possibly extended to patients with normal GE.

▶ In patients with severe gastroparesis who have vomiting and weight loss, gastric electrical stimulation (GES) is a potential rescue therapy once medical approaches have been exhausted. In this uncontrolled surgical series, GES appeared to improve symptoms although body mass index did not significantly increase, and gastric emptying also did not improve as expected. One difference in this study is that patients with normal gastric emptying were included, which might suggest a possible benefit for GES in severe functional dyspepsia characterized by nausea and vomiting, which has failed to respond to all other treatments. However, the uncontrolled nature of these observations severely limits their interpretation.

N. J. Talley, MD, PhD

H. pylori Eradication Prevents the Progression of Gastric Intestinal Metaplasia in Reflux Esophagitis Patients Using Long-Term Esomeprazole

Yang H-B, Sheu B-S, Wang S-T, et al (Natl Cheng Kung Univ Med Ctr, Tainan, Taiwan, Republic of China)

Am J Gastroenterol 104:1642-1649, 2009

Objectives.—This study aimed to determine whether *Helicobacter pylori* eradication limits the progression of precancerous changes, manifested as intestinal metaplasia (IM), in patients with reflux esophagitis using long-term esomeprazole.

Methods.—Three hundred twenty-five reflux esophagitis patients were enrolled and randomly assigned to (i) the *H. pylori*–positive eradication group receiving 1-week triple therapy ($n = 105$); (ii) *H. pylori*–positive non-eradication controls (n = 105); and (iii) *H. pylori*–negative controls (n = 115). All the patients received continuous esomeprazole until sustained symptomatic response, and when possible, shifted to on-demand therapy (ODT) thereafter. Serial gastroscopy was scheduled on enrollment and at the end of the first and second years to assess the prevalence and progression or regression of gastric atrophy (AT) and IM.

Results.—There were 93 patients in the *H. pylori*–eradication group, 83 in the non-eradication controls, and 100 in the negative controls to complete the study. The negative controls had no progression of AT and IM during follow-up. For the *H. pylori*–positive eradication group, there was significant regression of AT and IM during follow-up ($P < 0.05$). In the *H. pylori*–positive non-treated controls, the prevalence rates of AT and IM were significantly greater on the second year than on enrollment ($P < 0.05$). During the second-year follow-up, the patients in the eradication group achieved more regression and less development of AT and IM than did the non-eradication controls ($P < 0.001$).

Conclusions.—In patients using long-term esomeprazole for reflux esophagitis, screening for and eradicating *H. pylori* infection are necessary in order to limit the progression or cause the regression of gastric precancerous changes.

▶ It remains controversial whether patients who require long-term acid suppression therapy (eg, those with gastroesophageal reflux disease) should be tested for *Helicobacter pylori* and treated if infected to prevent the risk of progression of gastric precancerous lesions, most notably intestinal metaplasia. Current US guidelines do not recommend testing for *H pylori* in this setting,[1] although the Maastricht III consensus conference advised eradication of *H pylori* in patients with reflux esophagitis who need long-term proton pump inhibitor (PPI) therapy.[2]

In this elegant randomized controlled trial, there was no evidence of progression of intestinal metaplasia atrophic gastritis in those who were *H pylori*–negative treated with acid suppression, but in *H pylori*–infected persons, there was a significantly greater prevalence of these findings even in the second year of follow-up. The data strongly suggest that long-term PPI therapy increases the risk of progression of significant precancerous changes in the setting of continued *H pylori* infection. The findings in this study do not seem likely to be explained by sampling error, although this is possibly a confounder.

Notably, this study came from Taiwan where *H pylori* is known to be more virulent than in the west (based on the cag pathogenicity island). Previous work from the west suggests that intestinal metaplasia was not a significant risk in *H pylori*–infected individuals prescribed PPI, but this may reflect the fact that patients in western countries tend to be infected with less virulent strains.[3] Thus, the guidelines may need to be reconsidered. The current data do suggest that in regions with a high prevalence of *H pylori*–related gastric cancer (and there are pockets of these in the United States), *H pylori* should be tested and treated before long-term treatment with acid suppression therapy is considered.

N. J. Talley, MD, PhD

References

1. Chey WD, Wong BC. Practice Parameters Committee of the American College of Gastroenterology. American College of Gastroenterology guideline on the management of *Helicobacter pylori* infection. *Am J Gastroenterol.* 2007;102: 1808-1825.
2. Malfertheiner P, Megraud F, O'Morain C, et al. Current concepts in the management of *Helicobacter pylori* infection: the Maastricht III Consensus Report. *Gut.* 2007;56:772-781.
3. Kuipers EJ, Nelis GF, Klinkenberg-Knol EC, et al. Cure of *Helicobacter pylori* infection in patients with reflux oesophagitis treated with long term omeprazole reverses gastritis without exacerbation of reflux disease: results of a randomised controlled trial. *Gut.* 2004;53:12-20.

High Incidence of Mortality and Recurrent Bleeding in Patients With *Helicobacter pylori*–Negative Idiopathic Bleeding Ulcers

Wong GL-H, Wong VW-S, Chan Y, et al (The Chinese Univ of Hong Kong, China; Hong Kong SAR, China)

Gastroenterology 137:525-531, 2009

Background & Aims.—The long-term prognosis of peptic ulcers associated with neither *Helicobacter pylori* nor nonsteroidal anti-inflammatory drugs (NSAIDs) is unknown.

Methods.—This 7-year prospective cohort study recruited patients with bleeding ulcers from January to December 2000. *H pylori*–negative idiopathic bleeding ulcers were defined as having tested negative for *H pylori*, having no exposure to aspirin or analgesics within 4 weeks before endoscopy, and having no other identifiable causative factors. After ulcers healed, patients were divided into 2 groups: patients with prior *H pylori*–negative idiopathic bleeding ulcers (*H pylori*–negative idiopathic ulcer cohort; n = 120) and those with *H pylori*–positive, NSAID-negative bleeding ulcers who received eradication therapy (*H pylori* ulcer cohort;

n = 213). Both groups were followed for ≤7 years without gastroprotective therapy. The primary endpoints were recurrent ulcer bleeding and mortality.

Results.—The 7-year cumulative incidence of recurrent ulcer bleeding was 42.3% (95% CI, 36.5%–48.1%) in the *H pylori*–negative idiopathic ulcer cohort and 11.2% (95% CI, 8.8%–13.6%) in the *H pylori* ulcer cohort (a difference of 31.1%; 95% CI, 27.7%–34.5%; $P < .0001$). Significantly more patients died in the *H pylori*–negative idiopathic ulcer cohort (87.6%; 95% CI, 83.0%–92.2%) than in the *H pylori* ulcer cohort (37.3%; 95% CI, 34.0%–40.6%) with a difference of 50.3% (95% CI, 49.0%–51.6%; $P < .0001$).

Conclusions.—Patients with history of *H pylori*–negative idiopathic bleeding ulcers have a high risk of recurrent ulcer bleeding and mortality.

▶ Since the recognition that *Helicobacter pylori* is causally linked to peptic ulcer disease (PUD), it has become standard practice to ensure *H pylori* is eradicated in all patients with a current or past history of peptic ulcer whether or not they have had upper gastrointestinal bleeding. However, there is a well-recognized group of patients with PUD who have no obvious evidence of *H pylori* infection and have no known exposure to nonsteroidal anti-inflammatory drugs (NSAIDs). In these patients with an idiopathic ulcer who have experienced an upper gastrointestinal bleed, the natural history is unknown and currently long-term acid-suppression therapy is not routinely recommended.

In this large well-conducted cohort study from Hong Kong, 120 patients with *H pylori*-negative idiopathic ulcer bleeding were followed for up to 7 years as was a control cohort with *H pylori*-related ulcer bleeding who underwent *H pylori* eradication therapy. The investigators observed that those with *H pylori*-negative idiopathic bleeding ulcers were about 4 times more likely to have a recurrent ulcer bleed; these data are consistent with observations from Denmark in albeit a much smaller cohort.[1]

The causes of ulcer disease in this *H pylori*-negative cohort are unknown. It may be that there is occult infection that has been missed, although this seems unlikely in most cases. Surreptitious use of NSAIDs is also possible, although the authors meticulously tried to exclude this possibility short of measuring serum salicylate levels. Overall, these data strongly suggest that *H pylori*-negative bleeding ulcer patients need life-long acid-suppression therapy to prevent ulcer recurrence, and this should become the standard of care.

N. J. Talley, MD, PhD

Reference

1. Bytzer P, Teglbjaerg PS. Danish Ulcer Study Group. *Helicobacter pylori*-negative duodenal ulcers: prevalence, clinical characteristics, and prognosis–results from a randomized trial with 2-year follow-up. *Am J Gastroenterol.* 2001;96:1409-1416.

Incidence of Gastrointestinal Symptoms in Children With Autism: A Population-Based Study

Ibrahim SH, Voigt RG, Katusic SK, et al (Mayo Clinic, Rochester, MN)
Pediatrics 124:680-686, 2009

Objective.—To determine whether children with autism have an increased incidence of gastrointestinal symptoms compared with matched control subjects in a population-based sample.

Design/Methods.—In a previous study including all of the residents of Olmsted County, Minnesota, aged <21 years between 1976 and 1997, we identified 124 children who fulfilled criteria on the basis of *Diagnostic and Statistical Manual of Mental Disorders, Fourth Edition*, for a research diagnosis of autism. Two matched control subjects were identified for each case subject. Through the Rochester Epidemiology Project, all medical diagnoses, are indexed for computerized retrieval. Gastrointestinal diagnoses before 21 years of age were grouped into 5 categories: (1) constipation; (2) diarrhea; (3) abdominal bloating, discomfort, or irritability; (4) gastroesophageal reflux or vomiting; and (5) feeding issues or food selectivity. The cumulative incidence of each category was calculated by using the Kaplan-Meier method. Cox proportional hazards models were fit to estimate the risk ratios (case subjects versus control subjects) and corresponding 95% confidence intervals.

Results.—Subjects were followed to median ages of 18.2 (case subjects) and 18.7 (control subjects) years. Significant differences between autism case and control subjects were identified in the cumulative incidence of constipation (33.9% vs 17.6%) and feeding issues/food selectivity (24.5% vs 16.1). No significant associations were found between autism case status and overall incidence of gastrointestinal symptoms or any other gastrointestinal symptom category.

Conclusions.—As constipation and feeding issues/food selectivity often have a behavioral etiology, data suggest that a neurobehavioral rather than a primary organic gastrointestinal etiology may account for the higher incidence of these gastrointestinal symptoms in children with autism.

▶ Autism represents a chronic neurodevelopment disorder that is not curable using current methods. A link between autism and gastrointestinal (GI) disease has been suggested, but this is highly controversial.[1] Some have suggested that there may be a chronic intestinal inflammatory process that leads to intestinal permeability changes that in turn contribute both to common GI problems and the primary features of autism. One theory even has suggested that measles, mumps, and rubella vaccine causes an enterocolitis that produces a leaky gut that is of primary importance in the development of autism, although most authorities now dispute the idea (and this theory has even been challenged through the legal system).[2]

This is a novel population-based work from Olmstead County, Minnesota, documenting for the first time the incidence of GI symptoms in children with autism. Notably, there was not an increased rate of celiac disease or other GI disorders, contradicting previous nonpopulation studies, which have suggested that GI problems may be very common in autism. The only 2 symptoms linked to autism were constipation and feeding issues, which may be explained by behavioral factors in autism rather than by primary GI disease. These data do not support the contention that treatment of GI problems in children with autism is likely to change the natural history of the condition.

N. J. Talley, MD, PhD

References

1. Levy SE, Souders MC, Ittenbach RF, Giarelli E, Mulberg AE, Pinto-Martin JA. Relationship of dietary intake to gastrointestinal symptoms in children with autistic spectrum disorders. *Biol Psychiatry.* 2007;61:492-497.
2. Dyer C. US parents take government to court over MMR vaccine. *BMJ.* 2007;334: 1241.

Proton pump inhibitors and risk of gastric cancer: a population-based cohort study

Poulsen AH, Christensen S, McLaughlin JK, et al (Inst of Cancer Epidemiology, Copenhagen, Denmark; Aarhus Univ Hosp, Denmark; International Epidemiology Inst, Rockville MD)

Br J Cancer 100:1503-1507, 2009

Proton pump inhibitor (PPI) use leads to hypergastrinaemia, which has been associated with gastrointestinal neoplasia. We evaluated the association between PPI use and risk of gastric cancer using population-based health-care registers in North Jutland, Denmark, during 1990–2003. We compared incidence rates among new users of PPI ($n = 18\,790$) or histamine-2-antagonists (H2RAs) ($n = 17\,478$) and non-users of either drug. Poisson regression analysis was used to estimate incidence rate ratios (IRRs) adjusted for multiple confounders. We incorporated a 1-year lag time to address potential reverse causation. We identified 109 gastric cancer cases among PPI users and 52 cases among H2RA users. After incorporating the 1-year lag time, we observed IRRs for gastric cancer of 1.2 (95% CI: 0.8–2.0) among PPI users and 1.2 (95% CI: 0.8–1.8) among H2RA users compared with non-users. These estimates are in contrast to significant overall IRRs of 9.0 and 2.8, respectively, without the lag time. In lag time analyses, increased IRRs were observed among PPI users with the largest number of prescriptions or the longest follow-up compared with H2RA users or non-users. Although our results point to a major influence of reverse causation and confounding by indication on the association between PPI use and gastric cancer incidence, the finding of increased incidence among PPI users with most prescriptions and longest follow-up warrants further investigation.

▶ Gastrin is a well-known trophic hormone, and hypergastrinaemia is associated with an increased risk of gastric carcinoids and adenocarcinoma. While proton pump inhibitors (PPIs) elevate gastrin levels moderately, the association between PPIs and gastric cancer is controversial. In this Danish population-based cohort study, new uses of PPIs and new uses of H2-receptor antagonists were identified to determine whether gastric cancer rates were increased. A 1-year lag time was incorporated to adjust for confounding by indication; there was no significant association between any of the acid-suppressing drug classes and gastric cancer. The finding of gastric cancer was largely confined to those who had no history of *Helicobacter pylori* eradication supporting an effect of confounding by indication. The data support other epidemiological studies that have failed to find an association of PPI use with gastric cancer once confounding was taken into account.[1] Although these data are not definitive, it appears reasonable for clinicians to reassure their patients that there is no risk of gastric cancer from long-term PPI use based on the best available evidence.

N. J. Talley, MD, PhD

Reference

1. García Rodríguez LA, Lagergren J, Lindblad M. Gastric acid suppression and risk of oesophageal and gastric adenocarcinoma: a nested case control study in the UK. *Gut*. 2006;55:1538-1544.

Efficacy of Linaclotide for Patients With Chronic Constipation

Lembo AJ, Kurtz CB, MacDougall JE, et al (Beth Israel Deaconess Med Ctr, Boston, MA; Ironwood Pharmaceuticals Inc., Cambridge, MA)

Gastroenterology 138:886-895, 2010

Background & Aims.—Linaclotide is a minimally absorbed peptide agonist of the guanylate cyclase-C receptor that stimulates intestinal fluid secretion and transit and reduces pain in animal models. We assessed the safety and efficacy of a range of linaclotide doses in patients with chronic constipation.

Methods.—We performed a multicenter, double-blind, placebo-controlled, parallel-group study of 310 patients with chronic constipation. Patients were randomly assigned to groups given 75, 150, 300, or 600 μg oral linaclotide or placebo once daily for 4 weeks. Symptom assessments included spontaneous bowel movements (SBMs), complete SBMs, stool consistency, straining, abdominal discomfort, and bloating. Severity of constipation, adequate relief of constipation, global relief of constipation, treatment satisfaction, quality of life, adverse events, clinical laboratory data, and electrocardiogram results were assessed.

Results.—All doses of linaclotide improved the weekly rate of SBM (primary end point) compared with placebo; the increases in overall weekly number of SBMs from baseline were 2.6, 3.3, 3.6, and 4.3 for linaclotide doses of 75, 150, 300, and 600 μg, respectively, compared with 1.5 for placebo ($P \leq .05$ for each pair-wise comparison of a linaclotide dose to placebo). Likewise, linaclotide significantly improved the weekly rate of complete SBM, stool consistency, straining, abdominal discomfort, bloating, global assessments, and quality of life. The most common and only dose-related adverse event was diarrhea (only 6 patients discontinued treatment because of diarrhea).

Conclusions.—Linaclotide therapy was associated with few adverse events and produced rapid and sustained improvement of bowel habits, abdominal symptoms, global relief, and quality of life in patients with chronic constipation.

▶ Linaclotide is a novel drug that appears to be largely locally acting, which suggests that the side-effect profile will be very favorable. The drug binds to the guanylate cyclase-C receptor on the intestinal enterocytes and by activating the receptor triggers the release of chloride and bicarbonate as well as water into the intestinal lumen (through activation of the cystic fibrosis transmembrane conductance regulator). In this well-conducted randomized controlled trial, linaclotide substantially increased stool frequency as well as reduced abdominal discomfort and bloating versus placebo. There were no serious adverse events, although the higher dose (600 μg per day) was more likely to induce diarrhea. Based on the data, a dose of 150 or 300 μg of linaclotide daily appears optimal for chronic constipation. The impact on abdominal pain and bloating also suggests that this drug may have a benefit in irritable bowel syndrome (IBS). If the results hold up in constipation and IBS, linaclotide appears highly likely to represent an excellent addition to the gastroenterologists' armamentarium for constipation.

N. J. Talley, MD, PhD

Food Intolerance, Diet Composition, and Eating Patterns in Functional Dyspepsia Patients

Carvalho RVB, Lorena SLS, de Souza Almeida JR, et al (Universidade Estadual de Campinas-UNICAMP, São Paulo, Brazil)
Dig Dis Sci 55:60-65, 2010

The aims of this study are to investigate dietary factors, food intolerance, and the body mass index data, as an indicator of nutritional status, in functional dyspepsia patients. Forty-one functional dyspepsia patients and 30 healthy volunteers answered a standardized questionnaire to identify eating habits and food intolerance, and then completed a 7-day alimentary diary. There was no significant difference in daily total caloric intake between patients and controls. Patients associated their symptoms with the ingestion of several foods, but in general maintained their regular intake, with the exception of a small reduction in the proportion of fat in comparison with controls (median 28 vs. 34%; $P = 0.001$). No patient was underweight. In conclusion, our results suggest that food intolerance has no remarkable influence on food pattern and nutritional status in most functional dyspepsia patients. Further studies are necessary to clarify the role of fat in the generation of dyspeptic symptoms.

▶ There is accumulating evidence that patients with functional dyspepsia (FD) have meal-induced symptoms, yet relatively little is known about the importance of different dietary constituents in terms of symptom generation.[1] This Brazilian study evaluated both nutritional status and dietary constituents in patients with FD compared with healthy volunteers recruited from hospital staff. A variety of items were associated with dyspeptic symptoms, including high-fat foods, coffee, and wheat-containing foods. Wheat intolerance has also been linked to irritable bowel syndrome in the absence of celiac disease and deserves further investigation in both upper and lower functional gastrointestinal disorders.[2] The data here confirm other studies suggesting that coffee-induced symptoms may be a common explanation for dyspeptic symptoms,[3] although interestingly, in this study most patients still consumed coffee regularly despite their symptoms. Some physicians mistakenly believe that fatty food intolerance occurs from gallstones (which can lead to unnecessary cholecystectomy), but a high fat intake was linked to postprandial fullness in FD in this study. Their results are consistent with work from other groups suggesting that fatty food intolerance (which can slow gastric emptying) is an important precipitating factor in FD.[4] Potentially, food allergy might also be important in the genesis of FD; a link between this syndrome and duodenal eosinophilia has been reported.[5]

In patients referred to tertiary referral centers, being underweight has been linked to FD, perhaps secondary to failure of gastric fundus relaxation after a meal. However, this was not observed in this study of patients with FD attending a general gastroenterology clinic. One of the limitations of this work is that the patients in the control group were significantly younger than the cases, which may indicate that dietary patterns could be different because of age rather than disease.

The results overall suggest that food elimination diets are worth trialing in FD. Further work in this area is critical, and most importantly, research into the efficacy of food restriction diets is urgently needed.

N. J. Talley, MD, PhD

References

1. Pilichiewicz AN, Horowitz M, Holtmann GJ, et al. Relationship between symptoms and dietary patterns in patients with functional dyspepsia. *Clin Gastroenterol Hepatol.* 2009;7:317-322.
2. Carroccio A, Brusca I, Mansueto P, et al. A cytologic assay for diagnosis of food hypersensitivity in patients with irritable bowel syndrome. *Clin Gastroenterol Hepatol.* 2010;8:254-260.
3. Boekema PJ, Samsom M, van Berge Henegouwen GP, et al. Coffee and gastrointestinal function: facts and fiction. A review. *Scand J Gastroenterol Suppl.* 1999; 230:35-39.
4. Pilichiewicz AN, Horowitz M, Holtmann GJ, et al. Relationship between symptoms and dietary patterns in patients with functional dyspepsia. *Clin Gastroenterol Hepatol.* 2009;7:317-322.

5. Walker MM, Salehian SS, Murray CE, et al. Implications of eosinophilia in the normal duodenal biopsy - an association with allergy and functional dyspepsia. *Aliment Pharmacol Ther.* 2010;31:1229-1236.

Onset and Risk Factors for Fecal Incontinence in a US Community

Rey E, Choung RS, Schleck CD, et al (Mayo Clinic College of Medicine, Rochester, MN)

Am J Gastroenterol 105:412-419, 2010

Objectives.—The natural history of fecal incontinence (FI) in community subjects is uncertain and the onset rate is unknown. The aim of the study is to estimate the prevalence, new-onset rate, and risk factors for FI in community subjects.

Methods.—A random sample of 2,400 community subjects aged ≥50 years was surveyed in 1993, using a validated questionnaire. Responders were recontacted in 2003. FI was defined as self-reported problems with leakage of stool. Onset rate was calculated as the proportion of subjects without FI who became new cases. Logistic regression models were constructed to identify predictive factors for developing FI and changes in bowel habit associated with the onset of FI.

Results.—Overall, 1,540 (64%) subjects responded to the initial survey, and 674 (44%) of them responded to the second survey a median of 9 (8.8–9.5) years later. The prevalence of FI in the first survey was 15.3% (13.4–17.3%). In the second survey, 37 reported incident FI; thus, the onset rate of FI was 7.0% (5.0–9.6) per 10 years. Predictive factors at baseline for the onset of FI were self-reported diarrhea (odds ratio (OR) = 3.8 (1.5, 9.4)), incomplete evacuation (OR = 3.4 (1.2, 9.8)), and pelvic radiation (OR = 5.1 (1.01, 25.9)). Development of urgency was the primary predictor among the set of predictors reflecting changes in bowel symptoms that were associated with the onset of FI (OR = 24.9 (10.6, 58.4)).

Conclusions.—The onset rate of FI is approximately 7% per 10 years in community subjects aged ≥50 years. Prevention may be possible if bowel habit is appropriately managed in high-risk individuals.

▶ While there is a considerable body of literature defining the prevalence (or frequency) of fecal incontinence at a particular time point in the United States population, information on the incidence (or new onset) of fecal incontinence in the community has been unavailable. Because fecal incontinence is a potentially devastating problem for both patients and their families, knowledge of the incidence and risk factors remains particularly important.

In this population-based study from Olmsted County, MN, 15% of people living in the community reported a problem with leakage of stool, and this was more common in women. Interestingly, only 8% had consulted a physician for leakage of stools, indicating this is very much a hidden problem uncovered only by specific questioning.

The incidence of fecal incontinence was calculated to be 7% over a 10-year period or just under 1% per year. Importantly, a change in bowel pattern to urgency was identified to be associated with the new onset of fecal incontinence. Based on these data, attention to identification of symptoms of fecal urgency at gastrointestinal consultation appears to be important, as treatment of this symptom (eg, with loperamide) may prevent the development of fecal incontinence in those otherwise predisposed because of previous pelvic irradiation, presence of a rectocele, or other risk factors.

N. J. Talley, MD, PhD

Chronic Intestinal Pseudo-Obstruction Related to Viral Infections

De Giorgio R, Ricciardiello L, Naponelli V, et al (Univ of Bologna, Italy; et al)

Transplant Proc 42:9-14, 2010

Chronic intestinal pseudo-obstruction (CIPO), one of the most severe gastrointestinal motility disorders, is a condition characterized by a clinical picture mimicking small bowel occlusion with related symptoms and signs in the absence of demonstrable mechanical obstruction. Analysis of full-thickness biopsy samples may unravel structural changes of the neuromuscular layer involving the whole gut, although the midgut is usually worst affected. Intestinal pseudo-obstruction can occur in association with systemic neurological, endocrine, and connective tissue diseases or malignancy but, when no recognizable etiology is found, CIPO is referred to as idiopathic (CIIPO). The latter form can be diagnosed early in life due to a genetic etiology or in adulthood when a viral origin may be considered. This review addresses the hypothesis that some systemic neurotrophic viral infections can affect the enteric nervous system thereby altering normal peristaltic activity. Available data are reviewed, focusing specifically on herpesviruses or polyomaviruses (JC virus). These suggest that in comparison to a proportion of CIIPO patients, healthy controls rarely harbor viral DNA in the myenteric plexus, leaving open the possibility that a viral infection might have an etiologic role in the development of CIIPO. The review thus provides some new perspectives in the pathophysiology and perhaps targeted treatment of CIIPO.

► This is an excellent and very interesting article that I believe most gastroenterologists would enjoy reading. Chronic intestinal pseudo-obstruction (CIPO) is characterized by small bowel obstructive symptoms in the absence of a mechanical obstruction. I would like to point out that it is very important to exclude a mechanical obstruction with radiographic testing and sometimes surgical exploration before labeling a patient with CIPO. As stated in this article, most cases of CIPO are the result of a systemic neurological condition and systemic connective tissue disease, such as scleroderma or malignancy. This article, however, discusses the various neurotropic viruses that are capable of infecting the enteric nervous system. The most plausible viruses include the herpes virus and the JC virus. To date, a direct causative link between a particular infection and CIPO has not been established. Nevertheless, this review gives an update on the current evidence for possible involvement of various viruses that may cause CIPO.

J. S. Scolapio, MD

Impact of Capsule Endoscopy Findings on Patient Outcomes

Kim S, Kedia PS, Jaffe DL, et al (Univ of Pennsylvania School of Medicine, Philadelphia)

Dig Dis Sci 54:2441-2448, 2009

Background and Aims.—There is limited data on the impact of capsule endoscopy (CE) findings on patient outcomes. The aim of our study is to evaluate the impact of CE findings on further diagnostic work-up, treatment, and symptom resolution.

Methods.—A retrospective chart review of patients who underwent CE at a single tertiary care center over a 3-year period was performed. CE findings were classified as positive, suspicious, or negative. Therapeutic interventions were medical, endoscopic, surgical, other, or none. Symptoms were considered resolved when the patient had cessation of symptoms for at least 6 months post-CE.

Results.—A total of 193 patients were studied. The overall diagnostic yield of CE was 37%. There were 97 (50%) patients who had further diagnostic testing following CE; (40 with positive, 22 with suspicious, 35 with negative CE findings). There were 76% patients who received treatment post-CE (59% with positive, 43% with suspicious, 49% with negative CE findings). Overall symptom resolution was seen in 71% of patients (59% with positive, 68% with suspicious, 70% with negative CE findings). There was no statistically significant difference in diagnostic work-up, treatment, and symptom resolution between patients with positive, suspicious, and negative findings. Patients with obscure overt GI bleeding were less likely to have further diagnostic work-up ($P = 0.001$), and had the highest rate of symptom resolution as compared to other indications ($P < 0.001$).

Conclusions.—There is no significant difference in outcomes amongst patients with positive, suspicious, and negative CE findings. Patients with obscure overt GI bleeding had more favorable outcomes as compared to other indications.

▶ In this article the authors evaluate the impact of capsule endoscopy (CE) findings on need for further diagnostic work up and treatment. Although this is an important study, its major weakness is that it is a single-center, retrospective study of only 193 patients. It is not clear from this study the experience of the gastrointestinal physicians reading the CE and the length of time they spent interpreting the CE video. Perhaps the most important message to learn from this study is that patients with a negative CE can still have missed small bowel pathology that requires further testing to make a diagnosis. In this study, further testing following a negative CE found clinically significant lesions in 14% of patients. If the pretest probability of a lesion and the etiology of a patient's symptoms are high, further testing, including a double-balloon enteroscopy, should be done.

J. S. Scolapio, MD

Gastroparesis

Gastric Neuromuscular Pathology in Gastroparesis: Analysis of Full-Thickness Antral Biopsies

Harberson J, Thomas RM, Harbison SP, et al (Temple Univ School of Medicine, Philadelphia, PA)

Dig Dis Sci 55:359-370, 2010

Background.—Pathologic assessment of gastric tissue in patients with gastroparesis is limited.

Aims.—To evaluate gastric histopathology in patients with gastroparesis.

Methods.—Full-thickness antral biopsies were obtained in 28 patients with gastroparesis. Control specimens were obtained from patients undergoing gastric resection. H&E and immunohistochemical stained slides were reviewed for the presence of inflammation, ganglion cells, and interstitial cells of Cajal (ICCs).

Results.—A mild lymphocytic infiltrate in the myenteric plexus was present in 6 out of 14 patients with diabetic gastroparesis (DG), one of 14 idiopathic gastroparesis (IG) and 0 of eight controls. Significant reductions in total nerve cell bodies were seen in gastroparesis patients (2.2 ± 0.3 per hpf; $p = 0.0002$) compared to controls (3.2 ± 0.12). This was seen in both DG (2.4 ± 0.32) and IG (2.0 ± 0.2). Sixteen patients (ten IG and six DG) had a reduction of ganglion cells (<2.3 cells/hpf). C-kit staining showed a reduction of ICCs in six patients (five IG and one DG). Four patients (three IG and one DG) had abnormal ICC morphology on C-kit staining with more rounded morphology and less dendritic processes.

Conclusions.—This study shows several pathologic abnormalities in the gastric tissue in some patients with refractory gastroparesis. An inflammatory infiltrate was present in nearly half of the patients with diabetic gastroparesis. There was a reduction in nerve cell bodies in both idiopathic and diabetic gastroparesis. A reduced number of ICCs were found in the myenteric plexus. Thus, histologic abnormalities in gastroparesis are heterogeneous and include myenteric inflammation, decreased innervation, and reduction of ICCs.

► In this elegant descriptive study, 28 patients with gastroparesis undergoing gastric electrical stimulation therapy had full-thickness antral biopsies obtained; both idiopathic and diabetic gastroparesis were evaluated. Perhaps not surprisingly, the pathology indicated a very heterogeneous group of conditions occuring in patients with gastroparesis with abnormalities in interstitial cells of Cajal and ganglion cells, evidence of inflammation of nerve cells. Most notably, half of the specimens did not have pathological changes identified in the antrum whether from cases of idiopathic or diabetic gastroparesis; these findings suggest that there are functional explanations for gastroparesis in a subset of cases that remain to be identified (eg, hormonal or central abnormalities). The finding of an inflammatory lymphocytic infiltrate in the myenteric plexus in a subset of gastroparesis patients is of particular interest. It is possible that use of corticosteroids in patients with gastroparesis who have myenteric plexitis could be beneficial, and small uncontrolled case series have supported this potential approach.[1] However, it remains to be established that steroids are efficacious in gastroparesis; presumably only a subset could respond (perhaps those early in the disease course), and these may only be the cases with inflammatory change (plexitis). Directly characterizing the histology of patients with gastroparesis to tailor therapy is likely to be beneficial in the future; the lack of uniform histology probably explains the heterogeneity of response to current standard medical and electrical therapies.

N. J. Talley, MD, PhD

Reference

1. De Giorgio R, Guerrini S, Barbara G, et al. Inflammatory neuropathies of the enteric nervous system. *Gastroenterology.* 2004;126:1872-1883.

Irritable Bowel Syndrome

A Treatment Trial of Acupuncture in IBS Patients

Lembo AJ, Conboy L, Kelley JM, et al (The Beth Israel Deaconess Med Ctr, Boston, MA; Harvard Med School, Boston, MA; Massachusetts General Hosp, Boston; et al)
Am J Gastroenterol 104:1489-1497, 2009

Objectives.—This study aimed to compare the effects of true and sham acupuncture in relieving symptoms of irritable bowel syndrome (IBS).

Methods.—A total of 230 adult IBS patients (75% females, average age: 38.4years) were randomly assigned to 3 weeks of true or sham acupuncture (6 treatments) after a 3-week "run-in" with sham acupuncture in an "augmented" or "limited" patient–practitioner interaction. A third arm of the study included a waitlist control group. The primary outcome was the IBS Global Improvement Scale (IBS-GIS) (range: 1–7); secondary outcomes included the IBS Symptom Severity Scale (IBS-SSS), the IBS Adequate Relief (IBS-AR), and the IBS Quality of Life (IBS-QOL).

Results.—Although there was no statistically significant difference between acupuncture and sham acupuncture on the IBS-GIS (41 vs. 32%, $P = 0.25$), both groups improved significantly compared with the waitlist control group (37 vs. 4%, $P = 0.001$). Similarly, small differences that were not statistically significant favored acupuncture over the other three outcomes: IBS-AR (59 vs. 57%, $P = 0.83$), IBS-SSS (31 vs. 21%,

$P = 0.18$), and IBS-QOL (17 vs. 13%, $P = 0.56$). Eliminating responders during the run-in period did not substantively change the results. Side effects were generally mild and only slightly greater in the acupuncture group.

Conclusions.—This study did not find evidence to support the superiority of acupuncture compared with sham acupuncture in the treatment of IBS.

▶ Alternative therapies are commonly sought by patients with irritable bowel syndrome (IBS) as conventional therapy is considered unsatisfactory by many sufferers. In this high quality National Institutes of Health (NIH) funded trial, acupuncture was compared with sham acupuncture. There were 2 types of sham acupuncture: one with a limited patient practitioner encounter and one where there was an augmented patient-practitioner encounter, which included a warm, friendly, and supportive patient practitioner interaction. In the present report, those who received sham acupuncture were rerandomized to either acupuncture or sham acupuncture, and these results were reported to be completely negative. The addition of a supportive patient-physician relationship did not improve the responder rate with acupuncture. These results strongly suggest that acupuncture is not an option that should be considered for patients with IBS.

The trial design included the removal of patients who had responded to sham acupuncture before the rerandomization process. The authors had hoped that removing these sham responders would increase the gap between active treatment and control but found the exact opposite. These data support the view that the removal of placebo responders in a clinical trial (eg, by doing a run-in study) may actually impair finding real differences if they exist (supporting the current Rome III clinical trial design recommendations).

N. J. Talley, MD, PhD

Bloating and Distension in Irritable Bowel Syndrome: The Role of Gastrointestinal Transit

Agrawal A, Houghton LA, Reilly B, et al (Univ of Manchester, UK; et al)
Am J Gastroenterol 104:1998-2004, 2009

Objectives.—Patients with irritable bowel syndrome and constipation (IBS-C) show more abdominal distension than do those with diarrhea. Because constipation is often associated with delayed gastrointestinal transit, this study aimed at establishing whether patients with delayed transit show more distension and bloating than do those with normal transit.

Methods.—Abdominal girth was recorded for 24 h using abdominal inductance plethysmography (AIP) in 30 IBS-C (Rome II criteria) patients (aged 18–68 years; 27 women) and in 30 healthy volunteers (21–58 years of age; 26 women). Within 2 weeks of this recording, orocecal and colonic transits were assessed. Orocecal transit was determined from the increase in breath hydrogen after a standard meal, and colonic transit from the number of radio-opaque markers identified on a plain abdominal X-ray. Bloating severity was assessed hourly during AIP recording using a 0–5 scale.

Results.—IBS-C patients showed more bloating and distension than did healthy volunteers ($P < 0.001$). They also had prolonged colonic ($P < 0.001$) and orocecal ($P = 0.05$) transits than did healthy volunteers, such that 47 and 17%, respectively, had colonic and orocecal transit times greater than the normal reference range. Those with delayed colonic ($P = 0.025$) and orocecal ($P = 0.13$) transits had greater distension but not bloating ($P = 0.63$ and $P = 0.48$, respectively) compared with those with normal transit. Moreover, distension directly correlated with orocecal ($\mathrm{r} = 0.40$; $\mathrm{P} = 0.03$) and colonic ($r = 0.51$; $P = 0.004$) transit times and inversely with stool consistency ($r = -0.43$; $P = 0.07$).

Conclusions.—IBS-C patients with delayed transit show greater abdominal distension than do those with normal transit. Therefore, drugs that accelerate transit may be expected to alleviate this troublesome problem.

▶ One of the most difficult symptom complexes to manage in adult gastroenterology is bloating and visible distention. Some of these patients have irritable bowel syndrome (IBS) and others have functional abdominal bloating, but whatever the underlying diagnosis, the symptom complex is often resistant to treatment, in part reflecting our inadequate understanding of the pathophysiology. This study suggests that patients with IBS and constipation (IBS-C) are at particular risk of bloating and distention and are more likely to have slow colonic transit (the slow orocecal transit time also largely reflects colonic transit). Slow colonic transit could lead to bacterial flora change in the small intestine and colon that in turn could lead to greater fermentation of food products, producing excess gas and leading to the sensation of bloating.

The findings further emphasize that in IBS-C the sensation of bloating and reported distention is real; the measurement device applied (abdominal inductance plethysmography) showed that the girth in IBS-C was significantly and objectively increased over the girth in healthy volunteers at the end of first day of measurement.

The data suggest that in patients with bloating and distention, reasonably aggressive treatment of constipation may potentially provide some help although this is not established yet by trial data. Some probiotic compounds may be able to change the flora and may also promote increased transit, effects which could be beneficial for bloating. The role of nonabsorbable antibiotics (eg, rifaximin) is as yet unclear.

N. J. Talley, MD, PhD

Comprehensive Self-Management for Irritable Bowel Syndrome: Randomized Trial of In-Person vs. Combined In-Person and Telephone Sessions

Jarrett ME, Cain KC, Burr RL, et al (Univ of Washington, Seattle; et al)

Am J Gastroenterol 104:3004-3014, 2009

Objectives.—Psychological and behavioral therapies are being increasingly used for symptom management in patients with irritable bowel syndrome (IBS). The aims of this study were to compare two delivery modes for a comprehensive self-management (CSM) intervention, primarily by telephone vs. entirely in person, and to compare each with usual care (UC).

Methods.—Adults with IBS were recruited through community advertisement. Subjects ($N = 188$) were randomly assigned to three groups: one in which all nine weekly CSM sessions were delivered in person, one in which six of the nine sessions were conducted over telephone, and one in which subjects received UC. Primary outcome measures were a gastrointestinal (GI) symptom score based on six symptoms from a daily diary and disease-specific quality of life (QOL). These and other outcomes were assessed at baseline and at 3, 6, and 12 months after randomization. Mixed model analyses tested for differences between the three groups in each outcome variable at the three follow-up occasions, controlling for the baseline level of each outcome.

Results.—Both GI symptom score and QOL showed significantly greater improvement in the two CSM groups than in the UC group ($P < 0.001$), with the magnitude of this difference being quite similar for the three follow-up time points. The two CSM groups experienced a very similar degree of improvement, and there were no statistically significant differences between the two.

Conclusions.—A CSM program is efficacious whether delivered primarily by telephone or totally in person, and there is no evidence that replacing six of the in-person sessions by telephone sessions reduces the efficacy of the intervention.

▶ More data have been accumulating that psychological therapies provide significant benefit for patients with the irritable bowel syndrome (IBS).[1] However, one of the major barriers to their widespread utilization is the time, complexity, and cost of the intervention. In this well-performed randomized trial, research nurses were trained to provide cognitive behavioral therapy with education, relaxation, and diet advice as part of a self-management program. Building on previous work from the same investigators who had shown that such an intensive management program was superior to usual care, this study assessed whether utilization of most of the program over the telephone was comparable to an in-person program. Importantly, they still included a usual care control group. Overall, both methods of delivering the program appeared to be efficacious compared with usual care. There are, however, limitations of the work that readers need to be aware of. First, blinding was impossible, and this may have impacted the apparent success. However, it is notable that 9 months after the end of treatment, long-term benefits were still seen in the active intervention groups. Furthermore, this is still a costly approach as the first 2 sessions were still in person for the telephone group. Finally, this study was performed by experts, and whether their results would translate elsewhere is unknown. The search for a cost-effective mode of delivering psychological therapy continues, but these results look promising.

N. J. Talley, MD, PhD

Reference

1. Ford AC, Talley NJ, Schoenfeld PS, Quigley EM, Moayyedi P. Efficacy of antidepressants and psychological therapies in irritable bowel syndrome: systematic review and meta-analysis. *Gut.* 2009;58:367-378.

Efficacy of Sacral Nerve Stimulation for Fecal Incontinence in Patients with Anal Sphincter Defects

Boyle DJ, Knowles CH, Lunniss PJ, et al (Centre for Academic Surgery [Gastrointestinal Physiology Unit], Barts and The London School of Medicine and Dentistry, UK)

Dis Colon Rectum 52:1234-1238, 2009

Purpose.—Sacral nerve stimulation has traditionally been used to treat patients with fecal incontinence with intact anal sphincters. This rationale has been challenged, but it remains unknown if its efficacy is related to the extent of the sphincter injury.

Methods.—This was a prospective study of 15 patients with sphincter defects (9 combined, 2 external only, and 4 internal only) undergoing sacral nerve stimulation for fecal incontinence. Endoanal ultrasound scans were reviewed and defects scored (0–16) with use of a system published by two independent observers. These were correlated with the following outcomes: 1) reduction in fecal incontinence episodes, 2) reduction in soiling, 3) improvement in Cleveland Clinic scores, and 4) improvement in ability to defer defecation. All patients were studied after temporary stimulation and again at three to six months after permanent implantation.

Results.—Thirteen patients (87%) progressed to permanent stimulation. Median fecal incontinence episodes per two weeks decreased from 15 (range, 1–53) to 3 (range, 0–16; $P = 0.01$). Median soiling episodes were reduced from 10 (range, 1–14) to 6 (range, 0–14; $P = 0.009$). Median Cleveland Clinic scores decreased from 12 (range, 9–18) to 9 (range, 4–14; $P = 0.0005$). The ability to defer defecation was improved significantly ($P = 0.05$). There were no relationships between sphincter defect scores and outcome measures after sacral nerve stimulation ($r^2 = 0.001–0.10$; $P = 0.28–0.94$).

Conclusion.—Sacral nerve stimulation is an effective treatment in patients with fecal incontinence who have anal sphincter defects, and outcome is not associated with severity of sphincter disruption.

► In patients with fecal incontinence but no anal sphincter defect, where medical treatment fails, the alternatives are surgery or sacral nerve stimulation. Sacral nerve stimulation has now been shown to be safe and effective in the short term. Long-term data in 52 patients showed that the efficacy of sacral nerve stimulation can be maintained for at least 5 years, which is very encouraging. Furthermore, sacral nerve stimulation can lead to improvement of urinary incontinence and retention, which often coexists with fecal incontinence in severe cases. However, there are treatment failures and continence is not perfect; about 75% of patients maintain at least a 50% improvement, whereas only 18% had 100% improvement with complete continence of stool.

Work from London further suggests that even those with definitive anal sphincter defects can respond to sacral nerve stimulation, and this is a viable alternative to surgery that appears to have a low success rate. Previous work has focused on patients with intact sphincters, although they may have had weak pressures. The encouraging results in patients with actual sphincter defects suggest that sacral stimulation is a viable alternative, although how it works in this situation remains uncertain. There is a need for a randomized controlled trial of sphincter repair versus sacral nerve stimulation, although whether this will ever be done is unclear.

N. J. Talley, MD, PhD

Exposure to Severe Wartime Conditions in Early Life Is Associated With an Increased Risk of Irritable Bowel Syndrome: A Population-Based Cohort Study

Klooker TK, Braak B, Painter RC, et al (Academic Med Ctr, Amsterdam, The Netherlands; et al)

Am J Gastroenterol 104:2250-2256, 2009

Objectives.—Stressful events during early life have been suggested to play an important role in the development of the irritable bowel syndrome (IBS). In this study, we evaluate whether an exposure to severe wartime conditions during gestation and in early life are associated with an increased prevalence of IBS.

Methods.—We assessed the prevalence of IBS using the Rome II questionnaire among 816 men and women (aged 58 ± 1 years) who were born as term singletons in Wilhelmina Gasthuis, Amsterdam, The Netherlands around the time of World War II.

Results.—Of a total of 816 participants, 9.6% ($n = 78$, 52F) met the criteria for IBS. Exposure to severe wartime conditions *in utero* was not associated with the prevalence of IBS in adulthood (8.3%). Early-life exposure to severe wartime conditions was associated with an increased prevalence of IBS. The prevalence of IBS among individuals exposed up to 0.5 years of age, 1 year of age, and 1.5 years of age was 8.1%, 12.5%, and 15.3%, respectively. The increased IBS prevalence was not associated with an increased stress response.

Conclusions.—Our data indicate that exposure to severe wartime conditions in early life is associated with an increased risk of developing IBS. To what extent this is attributable to the stressful environment of war, to severe undernutrition, or to the increased prevalence of infectious diseases is, however, unclear.

▶ The etiopathogenesis of the irritable bowel syndrome (IBS) is uncertain, although both environmental factors and genetic factors appear to be relevant. This fascinating birth cohort study assessed Dutch children born during World War II, when there was a short period of severe famine. These cases were compared with individuals who were conceived just after the war ended. Although exposure to wartime conditions between the ages of 1 to 18 months doubled the risk of IBS, this was not explained by changes in stress response (hypothalamic-pituitary-adrenal [HPA] axis) or weight. This contrasts a twin study from Norway, which suggested that a very low birth weight (less than 1500 g) in combination with genetic factors was important in terms of later risk of IBS.[1] However, in the Dutch study, most cases were not of very low birth weight. Notably, there was no change in the HPA axis found in this study; this particular pathway is being investigated for therapeutic intervention in IBS (with rather disappointing results to date). A period of undernutrition in early childhood may perhaps increase the risk of exposure to infectious diseases, but there is no evidence that IBS has increased in developing nations.[2] It is possible that the increased risk of IBS with exposure to wartime conditions in the first months after birth might be related to an increased risk in visceral hypersensitivity; animal data suggest that paternal separation in early childhood can lead to visceral hypersensitivity.[2] What the environment does to our children (including our actions as parents) may influence their outcomes much later in life.

N. J. Talley, MD, PhD

References

1. Bengtson MB, Rønning T, Vatn MH, Harris JR. Irritable bowel syndrome in twins: genes and environment. *Gut.* 2006;55:1754-1759.
2. Rey E, Talley NJ. Irritable bowel syndrome: novel views on the epidemiology and potential risk factors. *Dig Liver Dis.* 2009;41:772-780.

Fecal Incontinence in US Adults: Epidemiology and Risk Factors

Whitehead WE, Borrud L, Goode PS, et al (Univ of North Carolina at Chapel Hill; Ctrs for Disease Control and Prevention, Hyattsville, MD; Veterans Affairs Med Ctr, Birmingham, AL; et al)

Gastroenterology 137:512-517, 2009

Background & Aims.—The study aims were to estimate the prevalence of different types and frequencies of fecal incontinence (FI), describe demographic factors, and identify risk factors.

Methods.—The National Health and Nutrition Examination Survey (NHANES) assesses health status in the civilian noninstitutionalized US population. The validated Fecal Incontinence Severity Index was added to NHANES in 2005–2006. Participants were 2229 women and 2079 men aged 20 years or older. FI was defined as accidental leakage of solid, liquid, or mucus at least once in the preceding month. Sampling weights were used to obtain prevalence estimates for the national population. Multivariate logistic regression identified independent risk factors.

Results.—The estimated prevalence of FI in noninstitutionalized US adults is 8.3% (95% confidence interval, 7.1–9.5) and consists of liquid stool in 6.2%, solid stool in 1.6%, and mucus in 3.1%. It occurs at least weekly in 2.7%. Prevalence is similar in women (8.9%) and men (7.7%) and increases with age from 2.6% in 20 to 29 year olds up to 15.3% in participants aged 70 years and older. FI is not significantly associated with race/ethnicity, education, income, or marital status after adjusting for age. Independent risk factors in women are advancing age, loose or watery stools, more than 21 stools per week, multiple chronic illnesses, and urinary incontinence. Independent risk factors in men are age, loose or watery stools, poor self-rated health, and urinary incontinence.

Conclusions.—FI is a prevalent age-related disorder. Chronic diarrhea is a strong modifiable risk factor that may form the basis for prevention and treatment.

▶ More data on the illness burden of fecal incontinence are welcome, as this malady is often hidden by those afflicted because of embarrassment. At least in noninstitutionalized adults, around about 8% of the population report at least one episode of fecal incontinence monthly, 3% report an episode at least weekly, and nearly 1% having daily fecal incontinence.

A few of the other observations are worthy of emphasis. First, urinary incontinence often coexists with fecal incontinence as confirmed by these data; it is important to take the history for both disorders as this may alter management. Second, fecal incontinence is often associated with coexistent diarrhea, and based on clinical experience, effectively treating the diarrhea appears to be critically important for the management of the fecal incontinence in many cases. The identification of diarrhea and effectively managing it is likely to reduce the illness burden of fecal incontinence in the population, which is remarkably high.

N. J. Talley, MD, PhD

Increased Frequency of Gastrointestinal Symptoms in Patients with Fibromyalgia and Associated Factors: A Comparative Study

Pamuk ÖN, Ümit H, Harmandar O (Trakya Univ Med Faculty, Edirne, Turkey)

J Rheumatol 36:1720-1724, 2009

Objective.—To determine the frequency and severity of gastrointestinal (GI) symptoms in patients with fibromyalgia (FM).

Methods.—We included 152 women with FM (mean age 45.4 ± 12.2 yrs), 98 women with rheumatoid arthritis (RA; mean age 45.5 ± 12.3 yrs), and 60 healthy female controls (mean age 44 ± 11.3 yrs). All patients were questioned about the severity of their chronic widespread pain, symptoms of FM, symptoms of dyspepsia, using a visual analog scale (VAS), and anxiety-depression scale. Patients were asked self-reported (yes/no), symptom-based (≥ 2 criteria) constipation and severity of constipation questions, and about the severity of quality of life (QOL) disturbance secondary to dyspepsia and constipation.

Results.—Patients with FM had higher symptom severities for belching, reflux, bloating, sour taste, and vomiting than patients with RA and controls (all p values < 0.01). Patients with FM had significantly more dyspepsia-related QOL disturbances than the other 2 groups (p < 0.01). FM and RA patients had more frequent self-reported constipation than controls (respectively, 42.1%, 48%, 21.7%; p < 0.01). The frequency of symptom-based constipation was significantly higher in the RA group (49%) than in FM (29.6%) and control groups (23.3%) (p < 0.01). Constipation-related QOL disturbance was significantly higher in patients with FM than in controls (p < 0.01).

Conclusion.—In patients with FM, the severity scores of dyspepsia symptoms, constipation, and dyspepsia-related QOL disturbance were higher than in patients with RA and controls. The higher GI symptom severity in patients with FM might have negative effects on their QOL.

▶ It is well known that the irritable bowel syndrome is associated with fibromyalgia. This interesting piece of work now documents an association of fibromyalgia with dyspepsia for the first time, and this knowledge is potentially relevant in terms of planning management. However, it is unknown if pregabalin, used for fibromyalgia and neuropathy, has any efficacy in functional dyspepsia. Whether the disease association is explained by comorbid psychiatric or psychological disorders or whether there is a common pathogenic factor in dyspepsia and fibromyalgia (such as an infectious process or genetic predisposition) is unknown.

N. J. Talley, MD, PhD

Psychosocial Distress and Somatic Symptoms in Community Subjects With Irritable Bowel Syndrome: A Psychological Component Is the Rule

Choung RS, Locke GR III, Zinsmeister AR, et al (Mayo Clinic College of Medicine, Rochester)

Am J Gastroenterol 104:1772-1779, 2009

Objectives.—Psychosocial factors may drive people with irritable bowel syndrome (IBS) to seek health care, but whether psychological factors are causally linked to IBS is controversial. One hypothesis is that IBS is a heterogeneous syndrome comprising two distinct conditions, one psychological and the other biological. However, it is unclear how many people with IBS in the community have little somatization and minimal psychosocial distress. The aim of our study was to estimate the proportion of people with IBS in a representative US community, who have low levels of somatic and psychological symptoms.

Methods.—The cohort comprised subjects from three randomly selected population studies from Olmsted County, Minnesota. All of them filled out a validated gastrointestinal (GI) symptom questionnaire, the Symptom Checklist-90-R (SCL-90-R), and the Somatic Symptom Checklist (SSC) comprising 11 somatic complaint items. Logistic regression models were used to evaluate the associations between somatic symptoms/psychosocial factors and IBS, adjusting for age and gender.

Results.—Of the 501 eligible subjects, 461 (92%) provided complete data (mean age = 56 years, 49% female). IBS (Rome II criteria) was associated with both higher SSC and Global Severity Index (GSI of SCL-90-R) scores. Among subjects with high (>75th percentile) SSC scores, 43% reported IBS vs. 10% of those with low (<25th percentile) SSC scores. Among those with high (>60) GSI scores, 23% reported IBS vs. 6% with low (<40) GSI scores. Specifically, none of the IBS subjects had both low SSC and low GSI scores.

Conclusions.—Psychological factors and somatization are strongly associated with IBS in the community. However, IBS may not be related to low psychological distress and/or somatization.

▶ The role of psychological factors in the pathogenesis of irritable bowel syndrome (IBS) remains highly controversial. Originally, IBS was considered to be primarily a psychological (or psychosomatic) disorder. However, landmark studies in the 1980s suggested that psychosocial factors and IBS were not related to the condition itself but rather induced increased illness behavior (and hence greater consulting with doctors) leading to the clinical impression (bias) that IBS patients are more psychosocially disturbed than controls.[1] This study from the Mayo Clinic, however, strongly suggests that those with IBS living in the community indeed are much more likely to suffer with a psychological disorder. Most notably, the investigators did not find a single community subject with IBS who had low psychological distress and low somatic complaint scores! Among the somatic complaints by this population sample were headache, backache, insomnia, fatigue, general stiffness, heart palpitations, and eye pain. These symptoms were all more likely to occur in those with classical IBS; however, IBS sufferers were not more likely to report having asthma, hypertension, or weakness. Overall, these data strongly suggest that psychological factors, in particular somatization, is of major importance in IBS; moreover, any psychological association with IBS is not likely to be explained only by health care-seeking behavior. Central (brain) dysfunction is likely to be important in the pathogenesis of IBS, and this needs attention in terms of management approaches in clinical practice.

N. J. Talley, MD, PhD

Reference

1. Drossman DA, McKee DC, Sandler RS, et al. Psychosocial factors in the irritable bowel syndrome. A multivariate study of patients and nonpatients with irritable bowel syndrome. *Gastroenterology.* 1988;95:701-708.

Soluble or insoluble fibre in irritable bowel syndrome in primary care? Randomised placebo controlled trial

Bijkerk CJ, de Wit NJ, Muris JWM, et al (Univ Med Ctr Utrecht, Netherlands; Maastricht Univ, Netherlands; et al)

BMJ 339:b3154, 2009

Objective.—To determine the effectiveness of increasing the dietary content of soluble fibre (psyllium) or insoluble fibre (bran) in patients with irritable bowel syndrome.

Design.—Randomised controlled trial.

Setting.—General practice.

Participants.—275 patients aged 18-65 years with irritable bowel syndrome.

Interventions.—12 weeks of treatment with 10 g psyllium (n = 85), 10 g bran (n = 97), or 10 g placebo (rice flour) (n = 93).

Main Outcome Measures.—The primary end point was adequate symptom relief during at least two weeks in the previous month, analysed after one, two, and three months of treatment to assess both short term and sustained effectiveness. Secondary end points included irritable bowel syndrome symptom severity score, severity of abdominal pain, and irritable bowel syndrome quality of life scale.

Results.—The proportion of responders was significantly greater in the psyllium group than in the placebo group during the first month (57% *v* 35%; relative risk 1.60, 95% confidence interval 1.13 to 2.26) and the second month of treatment (59% *v* 41%; 1.44, 1.02 to 2.06). Bran was more effective than placebo during the third month of treatment only (57% *v* 32%; 1.70, 1.12 to 2.57), but this was not statistically significant in the worst case analysis (1.45, 0.97 to 2.16). After three months of treatment, symptom severity in the psyllium group was reduced by 90 points, compared with 49 points in the placebo group (P = 0.03) and 58 points in the bran group ($P = 0.61$ versus placebo). No differences were found with respect to quality of life. Fifty four (64%) of the patients allocated to psyllium, 54 (56%) in the bran group, and 56 (60%) in the placebo group completed the three month treatment period. Early dropout was most common in the bran group; the main reason was that the symptoms of irritable bowel syndrome worsened.

Conclusions.—Psyllium offers benefits in patients with irritable bowel syndrome in primary care.

Trial Registration.—Clinical trials NCT00189033.

▶ This is a high-quality randomized trial that further explores the potential benefits of fiber in the irritable bowel syndrome (IBS), an approach that has become controversial.[1] Although it is common practice to prescribe fiber for patients with IBS, the recommendation has been called into question by work showing that many patients started on fiber actually can have worse symptoms, especially bloating. This excellent research conducted in primary care clearly demonstrates that psyllium (a soluble fiber product) improves global IBS symptoms and reduces the severity of IBS symptoms. A subtype analysis of the constipation-dominant group showed that psyllium was still better than placebo; while the clinical trial included patients with constipation, diarrhea, or mixed bowel habit, the results are not presented for the diarrhea and alternating groups separately to determine whether psyllium was beneficial here (and the study was not powered to look at such differences). Psyllium was compared with insoluble fiber (bran) that failed to show any efficacy in the first 2 months of treatment, although in the third month bran then appeared to be more efficacious than placebo. It was notable that the bran was more likely to worsen symptoms, especially at the beginning of treatment. The trial did not test whether starting with a very small amount of fiber and slowly building it up would be a better approach than just adding in the supplementation at full dose. However, in clinical practice prescribing fiber with a "start low, go slow" approach appears to be optimal. Overall, these data support the view that psyllium rather than bran represents reasonable first-line therapy for IBS, particularly in the constipation subtype and may be worth trying regardless of subtype.

N. J. Talley, MD, PhD

Reference

1. Ford AC, Talley NJ, Spiegel BM, et al. Effect of fibre, antispasmodics, and peppermint oil in the treatment of irritable bowel syndrome: systematic review and meta-analysis. *BMJ*. 2008;337:a2313.

Constipation

Long-Term Outcome of Sacral Nerve Stimulation for Fecal Incontinence
Altomare DF, Ratto C, Ganio E, et al (Univ of Bari, Italy; Catholic Univ, Rome, Italy; S. Rita Hosp, Vercelli, Italy; et al)
Dis Colon Rectum 52:11-17, 2009

Purpose.—Sacral nerve stimulation is a safe and effective procedure for fecal incontinence. We investigated whether its efficacy is maintained long term.

Patients and Methods.—Sixty patients with fecal incontinence underwent permanent sacral nerve stimulation. Patients' data were prospectively recorded in the national registry of the Italian Group of sacral nerve stimulation. The severity of fecal incontinence was evaluated by the Wexner score, and data were collected in a bowel function diary. Quality of life was evaluated by the Italian version of the Medical Outcomes Survey Short Form (SF-36) questionnaire.

Results.—Fifty-two patients were available for long-term follow-up lasting at least 5 years. Compared with baseline, the Wexner score decreased significantly after definitive implantation (from 15 ± 4 to 5 ± 5, $P < 0.001$). At least 50 percent improvement in continence was achieved in 74 percent of the patients, and at least 70 percent improvement (median value) was achieved in 50 percent. The mean number of solid/liquid incontinence episodes decreased significantly from 0.5 (±0.5) to 0.1 (±0.3) per day ($P = 0.004$). Quality of life improved in all domains. The overall mean improvement in SF-36 scores was 39.8 percent. Both mean resting and squeeze anal pressures increased significantly, and maximum volume tolerated decreased significantly.

Conclusions.—Sacral nerve stimulation maintains its efficacy long term, not only in regard to control of symptoms but also regarding quality of life.

▶ In patients with fecal incontinence but no anal sphincter defect where medical treatment fails, the alternatives are surgery or sacral nerve stimulation. Sacral nerve stimulation has now been shown to be safe and effective in the short term. Long-term data in 52 patients showed that the efficacy of sacral nerve stimulation can be maintained for at least 5 years, which is very encouraging. Furthermore, sacral nerve stimulation can lead to improvement of urinary incontinence and retention, which often coexists with fecal incontinence in severe cases. However, there are treatment failures and continence is not perfect; about 75% of patients maintain at least a 50% improvement, whereas only 18% had 100% improvement with complete continence of stool.

Work from London further suggests that even those with definitive anal sphincter defects can respond to sacral nerve stimulation, and this is a viable alternative to surgery that appears to have a low success rate. Previous work has focused on patients with intact sphincters, although they may have had weak pressures. The encouraging results in patients with actual sphincter defects suggest that sacral stimulation is a viable alternative, although how it works in this situation remains uncertain. There is a need for a randomized controlled trial of sphincter repair versus sacral nerve stimulation, although whether this will ever be done is unclear.

N. J. Talley, MD, PhD

Medical records documentation of constipation preceding Parkinson disease: A case-control study

Savica R, Carlin JM, Grossardt BR, et al (Mayo Clinic, Rochester, MN)
Neurology 73:1752-1758, 2009

Objective.—Parkinson disease (PD) may affect the autonomic nervous system and may cause constipation; however, few studies have explored constipation preceding the motor onset of PD. We investigated constipation preceding PD using a case-control study design in a population-based sample.

Methods.—Using the medical records-linkage system of the Rochester Epidemiology Project, we identified 196 subjects who developed PD in Olmsted County, MN, from 1976 through 1995. Each incident case was matched by age (± 1 year) and sex to a general population control. We reviewed the complete medical records of cases and controls in the medical records-linkage system to ascertain the occurrence of constipation preceding the onset of PD (or index year).

Results.—Constipation preceding PD or the index year was more common in cases than in controls (odds ratio [OR] 2.48; 95% confidence interval [CI] 1.49 to 4.11; $p = 0.0005$). This association remained significant after adjusting for smoking and coffee consumption (ever vs never), and after excluding constipation possibly induced by drugs. In addition, the association remained significant in analyses restricted to constipation documented 20 or more years before the onset of motor symptoms of PD. Although the association was stronger in women than in men and in patients with PD with rest tremor compared with patients with PD without rest tremor, these differences were not significant.

Conclusions.—Our findings suggest that constipation occurring as early as 20 or more years before the onset of motor symptoms is associated with an increased risk of Parkinson disease.

► The concept that Parkinson disease, a neurodegenerative disorder, may first manifest with symptoms of constipation before the classical diagnostic neurological symptoms and signs is supported by this well-done medical records linkage case-control study. Surprisingly, constipation could be experienced 20 or more years before the first onset of the symptoms of Parkinson disease. The results are biologically plausible because the neuropathology of Parkinson disease include changes in the autonomic nervous system, which clearly can alter gastrointestinal tract function. Of course, there are other potential explanations for the association, including the fact that there may be a third unknown causal factor that manifests with both constipation and later Parkinson disease. Such a causal factor might represent for example a genetic susceptibility to both conditions. Gastroenterologists should be aware of this association and be on the lookout in their patients with long-standing constipation for early signs of Parkinson disease.

N. J. Talley, MD, PhD

Phenotypic Variation of Colonic Motor Functions in Chronic Constipation

Ravi K, Bharucha AE, Camilleri M, et al (Mayo Clinic and Mayo Foundation, Rochester, MN)

Gastroenterology 138:89-97, 2010

Background & Aims.—Colonic motor disturbances in chronic constipation (CC) are heterogeneous and incompletely understood; the relationship between colonic transit and motor activity is unclear. We sought to characterize the phenotypic variability in chronic constipation.

Methods.—Fasting and postprandial colonic tone and phasic activity and pressure-volume relationships were assessed by a barostat manometric assembly in 35 healthy women and 111 women with CC who had normal colon transit (NTC; n = 25), slow transit (STC; n = 19), and defecatory disorders with normal (DD-normal; n = 34) or slow transit (DD-slow; n = 33). Logistic regression models assessed whether motor parameters could discriminate among these groups. Among CC, phenotypes were characterized by principal components analysis of these measurements.

Results.—Compared with 10th percentile values in healthy subjects, fasting and/or postprandial colonic tone and/or compliance were reduced in 40% with NTC, 47% with STC, 53% with DD-normal, and 42% with DD-slow transit. Compared with healthy subjects, compliance was reduced ($P \leq .05$) in isolated STC and DD but not in NTC. Four principal components accounted for 85% of the total variation among patients: factors 1 and 2 were predominantly weighted by fasting and postprandial colonic phasic activity and tone, respectively; factor 3 by postprandial high-amplitude propagated contractions; and factor 4 by postprandial tonic response.

Conclusions.—Fasting and/or postprandial colonic tone are reduced, reflecting motor dysfunctions, even in NTC. Colonic motor assessments allow chronic constipation to be characterized into phenotypes. Further studies are needed to evaluate the relationship among these phenotypes, enteric neuropathology, and response to treatment in CC.

▶ Patients who have no structural or metabolic cause for constipation traditionally have been subdivided into 3 subgroups: slow transit constipation, pelvic floor dysfunction, and those who have normal transit plus no evidence of a defecatory disorder. This work suggests that such a classification is simplistic; clear-cut fasting and postprandial motor disturbances were identified in most of the patients studied with chronic constipation, regardless of subtype.

Notably, those with normal colonic transit often had reduced fasting and postprandial colonic tone. This work suggests that therapeutic targeting of the subgroups may need to be reconsidered, although until there are better noninvasive techniques for subdividing constipation in practice the observations will remain problematic to apply.

N. J. Talley, MD, PhD

Evidence for Pelvic Floor Dyssynergia in Patients With Irritable Bowel Syndrome

Suttor VP, Prott GM, Hansen RD, et al (Univ of Sydney, Australia)
Dis Colon Rectum 53:156-160, 2010

Purpose.—Although functional constipation is known to often manifest concomitant features of pelvic floor dyssynergia, the nature of pelvic floor symptoms and anorectal dysfunction in non-diarrhea predominant irritable bowel syndrome is less clear. This study aims to compare anorectal sensorimotor function and symptoms of patients who have non-diarrhea predominant irritable bowel syndrome with those who have functional constipation.

Methods.—We studied 50 consecutive female patients referred with constipation and 2 or more symptoms of pelvic floor dyssynergia, who also satisfied Rome II criteria for either non-diarrhea predominant irritable bowel syndrome (n = 25; mean age, 47 ± 3 y) or functional constipation (n = 25; 49 ± 3 y). Assessments included the Rome II Integrative Questionnaire, a validated constipation questionnaire, Hospital Anxiety and Depression scale, visual analog scores for satisfaction with bowel habit and for impact on quality of life, and a comprehensive anorectal physiology study.

Results.—Both groups displayed physiological evidence of pelvic floor dyssynergia; but patients with non-diarrhea predominant irritable bowel syndrome exhibited a higher prevalence of abnormal balloon expulsion ($P < .01$) and less paradoxical anal contraction with strain ($P = .045$) than patients with functional constipation. These patients with irritable bowel syndrome also reported more straining to defecate ($P = .04$), a higher total constipation score ($P = .02$), lower stool frequency ($P = .02$), a trend toward harder stools ($P = .06$), and less satisfaction with bowel habit ($P = .03$) than patients with functional constipation.

Conclusion.—Patients with non-diarrhea predominant irritable bowel syndrome with symptoms of pelvic floor dyssynergia exhibit overall pelvic floor dyssynergia physiology similar to that of patients with functional constipation. Certain features, however, such as abnormal balloon expulsion, may be more prominent in the patients with irritable bowel syndrome. Therapeutic modalities, such as biofeedback, that are effective in patients with functional constipation with pelvic floor dyssynergia

should therefore be considered in selected patients with irritable bowel syndrome with pelvic floor dyssynergia.

▶ Irritable bowel syndrome (IBS) is a very common problem and is defined by the Rome III diagnostic criteria; patients are further subdivided into subtypes including constipation-predominant IBS, all based on symptoms. A common cause of constipation often missed in clinical practice is pelvic floor dyssynergia or dysfunction, characterized by the inability to expel a rectal balloon because of learned abnormalities of the pelvic floor muscles (such as paradoxical contraction on straining, blocking defecation). Pelvic floor dysfunction can be cured by biofeedback in over 70% of cases.[1] Although constipation symptoms are common in patients with IBS, pelvic floor dysfunction is not considered to be a part of the spectrum of IBS based on current diagnostic criteria. In patients fulfilling criteria for constipation-predominant IBS, pelvic floor function testing (by anorectal manometry) has not been considered routine to rule out pelvic floor dyssynergia.

The results from this Australian study suggest that the current dogma needs to be revisited. This study was striking in that 56% of patients with IBS who did not have diarrhea had absent anal relaxation on straining while 44% had paradoxical anal contractions on straining. Furthermore, 56% with IBS had abnormal balloon expulsion times. These results suggest that pelvic floor dyssynergia is very common in patients fulfilling Rome III criteria for IBS, although admittedly the results might be skewed by some selection bias. Notably, some false-positive results can occur with pelvic floor function testing, and the absence of a healthy control group is a limitation of this work.

Overall, these important data suggest that in any patient with IBS and symptoms of constipation it is reasonable to consider pelvic floor function testing. While pelvic floor dyssynergia is potentially curable with biofeedback, how well this technique works in IBS with constipation is unknown.

N. J. Talley, MD, PhD

Reference

1. Koh CE, Young CJ, Young JM, et al. Systematic review of randomized controlled trials of the effectiveness of biofeedback for pelvic floor dysfunction. *Br J Surg.* 2008;95:1079-1087.

Familial Clustering of Habitual Constipation: A Prospective Study in Children From West Virginia

Ostwani W, Dolan J, Elitsur Y (Marshall Univ, Huntington, WV)

J Pediatr Gastroenterol Nutr 50:287-289, 2010

Objective.—To investigate familial clustering of habitual constipation in pediatric patients who attended our medical facilities.

Patients and Methods.—Children with the diagnosis of functional, habitual constipation or patients without constipation and their respective family members were prospectively recruited to our study. Constipation was established in all participants using a standard questionnaire (Rome criteria).

Results.—A total of 112 children and their families participated in the study, of which 37 were probands families (test) and 75 children and their respective family members constituted the control group. A total of 310 family members completed the questionnaire. No significant differences were found between the study and the control groups in age, sex, or family size. Siblings or parents from the study group (probands) had significantly higher rates of constipation compared with the control group (30% vs 7% and 42% vs 9%, respectively; $P = 0.001$).

Conclusions.—Habitual constipation in children seemed to cluster in families. The pathophysiology behind this phenomenon is yet unknown.

▶ It is now well established that familial clustering of common diseases such as gastroesophageal reflux disease occurs in children and adults. Furthermore, familial clustering of constipation has also been reported in adults from Hong Kong.[1] However, to date, familial clustering of constipation has not been studied in children. In this case-control study, nearly one-third of the siblings or parents of the proband (the affected case with constipation) also were constipated, and this was substantially higher than the 7% affected rate seen in controls. What remains unknown is whether familial clustering of constipation reflects a common environmental influence (eg, poor toilet training) or genetics or both. Furthermore, it is unknown whether familial clustering of constipation is due to pelvic floor dysfunction or slow colonic transit or both in children; this area definitely deserves further investigation. In adults, a family history of constipation has been associated with more complications such as hemorrhoids, fissures, or prolapse.[2] Clinicians should consider routinely asking about a family history of constipation in their patients with severe constipation and review toileting practices.

N. J. Talley, MD, PhD

Reference

1. Chan AO, Hui WM, Lam KF, et al. Familial aggregation in constipated subjects in a tertiary referral center. *Am J Gastroenterol.* 2007;102:149-152.
2. Chan AO, Lam KF, Hui WM, et al. Influence of positive family history on clinical characteristics of functional constipation. *Clin Gastroenterol Hepatol.* 2007;5:197-200.

Long-Term Outcome of Sacral Nerve Stimulation for Fecal Incontinence

Altomare DF, Ratto C, Ganio E, et al (Univ of Bari, Italy; Catholic Univ, Rome, Italy; S. Rita Hosp, Vercelli, Italy; et al)

Dis Colon Rectum 52:11-17, 2009

Purpose.—Sacral nerve stimulation is a safe and effective procedure for fecal incontinence. We investigated whether its efficacy is maintained long term.

Patients and Methods.—Sixty patients with fecal incontinence underwent permanent sacral nerve stimulation. Patients' data were prospectively recorded in the national registry of the Italian Group of sacral nerve stimulation. The severity of fecal incontinence was evaluated by the Wexner score, and data were collected in a bowel function diary. Quality of life was evaluated by the Italian version of the Medical Outcomes Survey Short Form (SF-36) questionnaire.

Results.—Fifty-two patients were available for long-term follow-up lasting at least 5 years. Compared with baseline, the Wexner score decreased significantly after definitive implantation (from 15 ± 4 to 5 ± 5, $P < 0.001$). At least 50 percent improvement in continence was achieved in 74 percent of the patients, and at least 70 percent improvement (median value) was achieved in 50 percent. The mean number of solid/liquid incontinence episodes decreased significantly from 0.5 (± 0.5) to 0.1 (± 0.3) per day ($P = 0.004$). Quality of life improved in all domains. The overall mean improvement in SF-36 scores was 39.8 percent. Both mean resting and squeeze anal pressures increased significantly, and maximum volume tolerated decreased significantly.

Conclusions.—Sacral nerve stimulation maintains its efficacy long term, not only in regard to control of symptoms but also regarding quality of life.

▶ Fecal incontinence is a common referral in our gastrointestinal practice. Besides antimotility medications and a colostomy, we have not had much to offer these patients. Sacral nerve stimulation (SNS) has now been recognized as a safe and perhaps effective procedure for treating fecal incontinence. In this prospective study of 60 patients, the outcome of SNS was evaluated. Clinical improvement was noted in most patients with a follow-up period of 5 years. Given these and other published results I believe SNS should be tried in those patients in which antimotility agents have not helped and before performing a colostomy in most patients.

J. S. Scolapia, MD

Miscellaneous

Proton-Pump Inhibitor Use Is Not Associated With Osteoporosis or Accelerated Bone Mineral Density Loss

Targownik LE, Lix LM, Leung S, et al (Univ of Manitoba, Winnipeg, Canada; Univ of Saskatchewan, Saskatoon, Canada; et al)

Gastroenterology 138:896-904, 2010

Backgrounds & Aims.—Recent studies have shown an association between proton-pump inhibitor use (PPI) and hip fracture. The mechanism by which PPI use promotes the development of hip fracture is uncharacterized. Therefore, we sought to determine whether PPI use is associated with osteoporosis or accelerated bone mineral density (BMD) loss.

Methods.—We used the Manitoba Bone Mineral Density Database to determine the relationship between chronic PPI use and osteoporosis on an initial assessment of BMD and on BMD loss between successive assessments of BMD. In the cross-sectional study, cases with osteoporosis at the hip or lumbar vertebrae (T-score ≤ -2.5) were matched to 3 controls with normal BMD (T-score ≥ -1.0). In the longitudinal analysis, the change in BMD among PPI users and nonusers between successive BMD assessments was assessed. Conditional logistic regression and multivariate linear regression were used to obtain estimates of the association between PPI use and osteoporosis and of the annualized change in BMD associated with PPI use.

Results.—PPI use was not associated with having osteoporosis at either the hip (OR, 0.84; 95% CI, 0.55–1.34) or the lumbar spine (OR, 0.79; 95% CI, 0.59–1.06) for PPI use >1500 doses over the previous 5 years. In the longitudinal study no significant decrease was observed in BMD at either site attributable to PPI use.

Conclusions.—PPI use does not appear to be associated with either the presence of osteoporosis or accelerated BMD loss. The association between PPI use and hip fracture is probably related to factors independent of osteoporosis.

▶ This is an important study that suggests that previous reports linking proton-pump inhibitors (PPIs) with osteopenia or osteoporosis may have been misleading. Both a cross-sectional and longitudinal study were done to investigate the association of PPI use with osteoporosis. In the cross-sectional study 2193 subjects with osteoporosis of the hip were matched to 5527 controls with normal hip measurements. In this analysis, PPI use was actually associated with a lower risk of osteoporosis of the lumbar spine and of the hip. A longitudinal study identified 2649 subjects who had 2 separate bone mineral assessments with a mean interval between assessments of 2.3 years. Again, there was no association between PPI use and osteoporosis. It is conceivable that previous studies of the association may have been biased by the presence of unmeasured confounders, but unfortunately, the jury must remain out regarding this association based on the conflicting data. At this stage, clinicians still need to plot a cautious course when advising patients about the pros and cons of long-term use of PPIs. However, the data here do provide some reassurance. It is not unreasonable to continue to ensure that patients on long-term PPIs are receiving adequate amounts of calcium and vitamin D.

N. J. Talley, MD, PhD

Ischemic Colitis and Complications of Constipation Associated With the Use of Alosetron Under a Risk Management Plan: Clinical Characteristics, Outcomes, and Incidences

Chang L, Tong K, Ameen V (David Geffen School of Medicine at UCLA, Los Angeles, CA; Prometheus Laboratories Inc, San Diego, CA)

Am J Gastroenterol 105:866-875, 2010

Objectives.—Alosetron is a potent, selective 5-HT_3 receptor antagonist prescribed for women with severe diarrhea-predominant irritable bowel syndrome (IBS-D) under a risk management plan (RMP). The RMP was implemented following cases of ischemic colitis (IC) and complications of constipation (CoC) associated with the use of alosetron. The Objectives of this study were to characterize IC and CoC clinical features, outcomes, and incidence rates in the new restricted patient population to evaluate the effectiveness of the RMP in the prevention of serious outcomes.

Methods.—Safety data from adverse event reporting from November 2002 through June 2008 were reviewed for probable and possible IC and CoC using the US Food and Drug Administration/sponsor-defined criteria and definitions. Evidence for IC included medical documentation, colonoscopy, and sigmoidoscopy ± biopsy. Evidence for CoC included medical history and confirmation from health-care professionals.

Results.—Within the inclusion dates, 29,072 patients received 203,939 alosetron prescriptions. Although the absolute numbers of IC and CoC cases have declined, the incidence rates for IC and CoC (0.95 and 0.36 cases per 1,000 patient-years, respectively) were similar to rates during the postmarketing cycle before alosetron withdrawal. In patients with severe IBS-D receiving alosetron ($n = 998$) or placebo ($n = 411$) in clinical trials since reintroduction, incidence rates for IC were 4 and 2 cases per 1,000 patients, respectively. Rates for CoC were 2 and 0 cases per 1,000 patients in the alosetron and placebo groups, respectively. No mesenteric ischemia, surgeries, transfusions, or deaths occurred in patients with IC and no cases of CoC were associated with toxic megacolon, perforation, surgeries, transfusions, or deaths. IC and CoC cases were typically of short duration and all improved on prompt withdrawal of alosetron.

Conclusions.—Serious outcomes associated with IC and CoC appear to be mitigated since introduction of alosetron under the RMP.

▶ This is a timely and very important clinical article that all gastroenterologists should review. Lotronex (alosetron hydrochloride) is a selective 5-HT_3 receptor antagonist that is used for the treatment of women with severe, diarrhea-predominant irritable bowel syndrome. This article reviews the safety data from adverse events reported from 2002-2008. Specifically, the data review cases of ischemic colitis and constipation. Over 29 000 patients were studied. The results of this study have shown that the incidence rates for ischemic colitis (IC) and complications of constipation (CoC) have remained stable in the first 5 years since the introduction of alosetron. Most patients with ulcerative colitis (UC) and CoC had comorbid conditions, and there were no cases of death reported. This is a very important article that clinicians and patients who may be treated should review.

J. S. Scolapio, MD

3 Pancreaticobiliary Disease

ERCP

Biliary stenting in the management of large or multiple common bile duct stones

Horiuchi A, Nakayama Y, Kajiyama M, et al (Showa Inan General Hosp, Komagane, Matsumoto, Japan; et al)
Gastrointest Endosc 71:1200-1203, 2010

Background.—Endoscopic biliary stenting with a plastic stent is often performed to prevent impaction of common bile duct (CBD) stones. The therapeutic effect of a plastic stent placement in terms of reduction in stone size and number has not been established.

Objective.—The aim of this study was to study the effect of biliary stenting as therapy for CBD stones.

Design.—Retrospective study.

Setting.—Municipal hospital outpatients.

Interventions.—Patients with large (≥20 mm) and/or multiple (≥3) stones had placement of a 7F double-pigtail plastic stent without stone extraction at the initial ERCP. Approximately 2 months later, stone removal was attempted. The number and size of CBD stones before and after stent placement, stone clearance, complications, and 180-day mortality were evaluated.

Results.—Forty patients were studied. Stent placement averaged 65 days (range, 50-82 days). The median number (interquartile range) of stones per patient fell after stent placement (4.0 [3.0] before vs. 2.0 [1.0] after; $P < .0001$). Characteristically, larger stones became smaller and small stones disappeared (ie, the median stone index decreased from 4.6 [3.0] to 2.0 [1.5]; $P < .0001$). Stone clearance at the second ERCP was achieved in 37 out of 40 patients (93%). Complications included cholangitis (13%) and pancreatitis (5%) after the second ERCP. No 180-day mortality occurred.

Limitations.—A retrospective, single-center study.

Conclusions.—Stent placement for 2 months was associated with large and/or multiple CBD stones becoming smaller and/or disappearing without any complications. Stenting followed by a wait period may assist in difficult CBD stone removal.

▶ Current clinical practice includes endoscopic sphincterotomy and attempt at stone extraction as the primary methods of management of common bile duct stones. Occasionally, when the stones are difficult to extract, temporary biliary stenting is used to prevent stone impaction and cholangitis, and a repeat endoscopic retrograde cholangiopancreatography (ERCP) is performed 2 months later. Anecdotally, it has been observed that the stones disappear or become smaller by the time the repeat ERCP is performed. This retrospective study of 40 patients confirms this anecdotal observation with a decrease in the mean stone index from 4.6 to 2.0.

The authors of this study recommend that biliary stenting could be used as the initial treatment in patients with common bile duct stones, particularly in elderly or high-risk patients, for example, those on anticoagulants or antiplatelet agents at the time of presentation.

This is a small retrospective study from a single center using a nonvalidated index to compare the groups. Therefore, we believe that further prospective randomized controlled trials are needed to confirm this observation and to validate the index in a larger group of patients. However, this study reaffirms current clinical practice of inserting a biliary stent where stone extraction is difficult or incomplete.

S. Bollipo, FRACP
V. Ambikaipaker, MB, ChB
N. J. Talley, MD, PhD

Early Laparoscopic Cholecystectomy Improves Outcomes After Endoscopic Sphincterotomy for Choledochocystolithiasis

Reinders JSK, Goud A, Timmer R, et al (St Antonius Hosp, Nieuwegein, The Netherlands; et al)

Gastroenterology 138:2315-2320, 2010

Background & Aims.—Patients with choledochocystolithiasis generally undergo endoscopic sphincterotomy (ES) followed by laparoscopic cholecystectomy (LC). However, many patients receive this surgery 6–8 weeks after ES. There is a high conversion rate of elective LC after ES, and patients can develop recurrent biliary events during the waiting period. We investigated whether the timing of surgery influences outcome.

Methods.—We performed a randomized trial of patients with choledochocystolithiasis who underwent successful ES. Patients were randomly assigned to groups that received early LC (within 72 hours after ES, n = 49) or delayed LC (after 6–8 weeks, n = 47), based on an expected difference in conversion rate of 25% vs 5%, respectively. Conversion rate, biliary events during follow-up, duration and difficulty of surgeries, postoperative morbidity, and hospital stay were scored. Intention-to-treat analyses were performed.

Results.—Groups were comparable in age, sex, and comorbidity. There was no difference between groups in conversion rate (4.3% in early vs 8.7% in delayed group) nor were there differences in operating times and/or difficulties or hospital stays. During the waiting period for LC, 17 patients in the delayed group (36.2%) developed recurrent biliary events compared with 1 patient in the early group ($P < .001$).

Conclusions.—In a randomized trial to evaluate timing of LC after ES, recurrent biliary events occurred in 36.2% of patients whose LC was delayed for 6–8 weeks. Early LC (within 72 hours) appears to be safe and might prevent the majority of biliary events in this period following sphincterotomy.

▶ Patients presenting with stones in common bile duct and gallbladder often are referred for an early laparoscopic cholecystectomy (LC) following endoscopic retrograde cholangiopancreatography (ERCP) and endoscopic sphincterotomy. However, most patients often wait up to 6 to 8 weeks for the operation. Some of these patients return to the hospital with further episodes of cholangitis during this time. Although this practice is common, it is not clear whether this is because of logistic reasons or the belief that late cholecystectomy is better. If it is because of the latter, the results of this study would certainly help change the clinical practice.

In this randomized study, patients who underwent early LC were compared with those who underwent a delayed LC. Conversion rates (laparoscopic to open cholecystectomy) were higher in the delayed group (8.7% vs 4.3%). Recurrent biliary events occurred in 36.2% of the patients whose LC was delayed for 6 to 8 weeks compared with 23.5% in early LC group.

This study once again confirms the benefits of an early LC, preferably during the same hospital admission after the ERCP and sphincterotomy procedures.

S. Bollipo, FRACP
V. Ambikaipaker, MB, ChB
N. J. Talley, MD, PhD

ERCP in the Very Elderly: Outcomes Among Patients Older than Eighty

Lukens FJ, Howell DA, Upender S, et al (UT Houston Med School, TX; Maine Med Ctr, Portland; et al)

Dig Dis Sci 55:847-851, 2010

Life expectancy is rising, which is increasing the demand for endoscopic retrograde cholangiopancreatography (ERCP) in the elderly. Little data, particularly on complex procedures, has been reported. In this study, we compare the differences in the success and complications in ERCP between patients older and younger than 80 years old. We used a large endoscopic database reviewing the ERCPs performed and 30-day complications addressing age, degree of difficulty of procedures, and complications. A total of 2,606 patients underwent 3,924 ERCPs. Six hundred and twenty-eight were octogenarians undergoing 728 procedures. Mean age was 83.5 years in the octogenarian group and 59.0 years in the younger group. The endoscopic success rate was lower in octogenarians (96.9 vs. 98.3%, $P = 0.004$). Overall, complication rates between both groups was significantly less in older compared to younger patients (1.64 vs. 3.50%, $P = 0.006$). Complication and failure rates were higher as procedure complexity increased in all patients. ERCP in the elderly carries a high degree of success with low complication rates. Elderly patients carry similar risks of bleeding and perforation and a lower risk of pancreatitis.

▶ There are limited data on the safety and effectiveness of endoscopic retrograde cholangiopancreatography (ERCP) in elderly patients older than 80 years. What is known, however, is that this group of patients, who also have multiple comorbidities, is increasing with the aging population. The mortality and morbidity for biliary tract surgery in octogenarians is as high as 9.5%, and the complication rate is as high as 62%, which makes endoscopic intervention a much preferred alternative.

In this review of a prospectively maintained database with 628 octogenarians and 1978 nonoctogenarians undergoing ERCP over a 10-year period, the success rate in octogenarians was high (96.9%) with a significantly lower complication rate than the younger patients. The risk of pancreatitis was lower, and the risk of perforation and bleeding was similar to the younger patients. Even the more difficult procedures were as successful and well tolerated in elderly patients.

This study adds to the safety and effectiveness data of ERCP in the elderly with a reassurance to the clinicians that age should not be a barrier for recommending an ERCP in those who need it. This is a required reading for all clinicians who are involved in performing or referring elderly patients for an ERCP.

S. Bollipo, FRACP
V. Ambikaipaker, MB, ChB
N. J. Talley, MD, PhD

Carbon dioxide insufflation during ERCP for reduction of postprocedure pain: a randomized, double-blind, controlled trial

Maple JT, Keswani RN, Hovis RM, et al (Univ of Oklahoma Health Sciences Ctr; Washington Univ School of Medicine, St Louis, MO)

Gastrointest Endosc 70:278-283, 2009

Background.—Abdominal pain after ERCP is common, and although it is frequently nonspecific and self-limited, it may provoke concern for complications and thus distress both patients and physicians. Carbon dioxide (CO_2) insufflation during ERCP may reduce abdominal distension in comparison to insufflation of air, resulting in less pain.

Objective.—To compare the incidence and severity of post-ERCP pain in patients receiving CO_2 versus air insufflation during ERCP.

Design.—Randomized, double-blind, controlled trial.

Setting.—University medical center.

Patients.—This study involved consecutive patients presenting for ERCP, excluding those with significant preprocedure pain or obstructive lung disease.

Intervention.—Randomization to insufflation with air or CO_2; all other care was identical.

Main Outcome Measurements.—Pre-ERCP and post-ERCP pain and nausea were assessed by using a 0 to 10 visual analogue scale. Patient waist circumferences were measured before and after procedures.

Results.—One hundred patients (82 outpatients, 51 women, mean age 54.4 years, 50 randomized to CO_2) completed the study. The CO_2 and air groups were similar in regard to demographics, indication for ERCP, and procedure duration. The mean pain score 1 hour post-ERCP was higher with air than with CO_2 insufflation (1.9 vs 0.7, $P = .01$). Similarly, the incidence of any pain at 1 hour post-ERCP was higher with air than with CO_2 (48% vs 28%, $P = .04$). The mean increase in waist circumference was greater with air than with CO_2 (2.1 cm vs 0.3 cm, $P = .003$). Adverse events were infrequent and did not differ by group. No serious cardiopulmonary complications occurred.

Limitations.—Single-center, selected patient population.

Conclusion.—Insufflation of CO_2 during ERCP reduces postprocedure pain and abdominal distension in comparison to insufflation of air. The use of CO_2 in deeply sedated, prone patients appears to be safe.

▶ This is a very interesting article with significant clinical application. In this randomized, double-blind controlled study of 100 patients the authors note that CO_2 insufflation instead of air insufflation reduces postprocedure pain following endoscopic retrograde cholangiopancreatography (ERCP). This appears to be the result of CO_2 being rapidly absorbed by the small bowel and is excreted through the lungs faster than air. The adverse events appear to be no greater in the CO_2 group compared with the air group. This is a recommended article to read for those clinicians that perform ERCPs.

J. S. Scolapio, MD

Sclerosing Mesenteritis Involving the Pancreas: A Mimicker of Pancreatic Cancer

Scudiere JR, Shi C, Hruban RH, et al (The Johns Hopkins Med Insts, Baltimore, MD)

Am J Surg Pathol 34:447-453, 2010

Sclerosing mesenteritis (SM), also known as mesenteric lipodystrophy, rarely involves the parenchyma of the pancreas. When SM does involve the pancreas, it can mimic pancreatic carcinoma both clinically and radiographically with pain, obstructive jaundice, a mass lesion, and even the appearance of vascular invasion. We report 6 patients with SM involving the pancreas (mean age 43.2 y, 5 female), and review their clinical presentation, radiographic findings, pathology, and outcome. Five of these 6 patients were originally thought to have a primary pancreatic neoplasm. Initial presenting clinical information was available for each patient: all 6 reported abdominal or epigastric pain, 3 reported weight loss, and 2 reported one or more of the following: back pain, fever, abdominal bloating/distention, nausea with/without vomiting, and anorexia. The lesions formed masses with an infiltrative pattern and all had 3 key histologic features: fibrosis, chronic inflammation, and fat necrosis—without a known etiology. The inflammatory infiltrate was composed of a mixture of lymphocytes, plasma cells, and scattered eosinophils. Of the 5 patients with post-treatment clinical information available, 4 had at least a partial response to treatment with steroids, tamoxifen, azathioprine, resection, or a combination of these, and 1 did not respond. A dramatic response to immunosuppressive therapy is illustrated by the case of a 46-year-old woman who presented with the presumptive diagnosis of an unresectable pancreatic cancer. Distinguishing SM from pancreatic carcinoma is crucial to appropriate management, as patients with SM may benefit from immunosuppressive therapy.

▶ This is an outstanding article of 6 patients with sclerosing mesenteritis involving the pancreas. This article has an excellent discussion on the diagnosis and management of sclerosing mesenteritis. This article makes the point that sclerosing mesenteritis of the pancreas may present with symptoms very similar to pancreatic cancer (ie, abdominal pain and weight loss). On CT scanning, findings may also appear very similar to pancreatic cancer as well. Sclerosing mesenteritis is a rare mass-forming lesion characterized by fibrosis, chronic inflammation, and fat necrosis. Although the small bowel mesentery is usually involved, this case series illustrates that other organs may be involved as well. Lymphocytes in the absence of cancer cells are the predominant inflammatory cell type noted. However, the diagnoses can be difficult to make with a biopsy alone. Surgical resection is required in many cases. Also this article points out that there is no current consensus as to the appropriate treatment. Some investigators have reported a response with corticosteroids and immunosuppressive therapy. I find this to be a very interesting case series with important clinical implications.

J. S. Scolapio, MD

Chronic Pancreatitis

IgG4 immunostaining of duodenal papillary biopsy specimens may be useful for supporting a diagnosis of autoimmune pancreatitis

Moon S-H, Kim M-H, Park DH, et al (Univ of Ulsan College of Medicine, Seoul, South Korea)

Gastrointest Endosc 71:960-966, 2010

Background.—Autoimmune pancreatitis (AIP) is now considered to be part of an immunoglobulin G4 (IgG4)-related systemic fibroinflammatory disease.

Objective.—We evaluated whether IgG4 immunostaining of duodenal papillary biopsy specimens is useful for supporting a diagnosis of AIP.

Design.—A prospective study.

Setting.—A tertiary academic center.

Patients/Interventions.—We obtained 2 forceps biopsy specimens from the major duodenal papilla (MDP) of 19 symptomatic AIP patients during ERCP before steroid administration. As a control, biopsy specimens were obtained from the MDP of patients with pancreatic cancer (n = 35), cholangiocarcinoma (n = 20), ampullary cancer (n = 11), ordinary chronic pancreatitis (n = 18), and AIP in remission (n = 16) and immunohistochemically examined.

Main Outcome Measurements.—Specimens were considered positive for IgG4 immunostaining if there were more than 10 IgG4-positive plasma cells per high-power field.

Results.—Positive IgG4 immunostaining of the MDP was found in 10 (53%) of 19 symptomatic AIP patients, but was absent in the control groups. Among symptomatic AIP patients (n = 19), 5 (83%) of 6 AIP patients with elevated serum IgG4 levels exhibited positive IgG4 staining of the MDP, whereas 5 (38%) of 13 AIP patients with normal serum IgG4 levels showed positive IgG4 staining of the MDP. Nine of 19 symptomatic AIP patients also underwent pancreatic biopsy, and positive IgG4 immunostaining of the MDP was observed in patients with positive pancreas IgG4 staining (4/6, 67%), but not in patients with negative pancreas IgG4 staining (0/3).

Limitations.—Small symptomatic AIP patient population.

Conclusions.—Positive IgG4 immunostaining of the MDP was an extremely specific and moderately sensitive tool for the diagnosis of AIP. IgG4 immunostaining of the MDP may be useful for supporting a diagnosis of AIP, especially when AIP is suspected clinically but serum IgG4 levels are normal or pancreatic tissue is not available.

▶ The diagnosis of autoimmune pancreatitis (AIP) is suspected on a combination of clinical features, imaging, and supported by laboratory features and histological findings of pancreatic tissue. The characteristic feature is the immunoglobulin G4 (IgG4) staining of the pancreatic tissue. However, obtaining a Tru-Cut biopsy of the pancreas is technically demanding and can only be done in limited centers with endoscopic ultrasound (EUS) expertise. As AIP is a systemic condition, extrapancreatic tissue such as kidney and retroperitoneum may also be involved, but obtaining a biopsy sample would be just as difficult. Thus, there is a need for a safer alternative to pancreatic biopsy.

In this study of 19 patients with known AIP, a biopsy of the major duodenal papilla (MDP) obtained safely during endoscopic retrograde cholangiopancreatography (ERCP) was shown to have useful diagnostic value. The IgG4 staining of the biopsy from MDP had a moderate sensitivity (51%) and 100% specificity. Although the IgG4 staining of MDP in AIP has been demonstrated in the past, this study adds more to our knowledge by having a large number of controls (100) who were all negative for IgG4 staining.

As ERCP is usually performed in patients with AIP either for a pancreatogram or for the treatment of obstructive jaundice, it would be possible to safely biopsy the MDP for supporting the diagnosis, thus avoiding the more invasive and less easily available EUS-guided Tru-Cut biopsy of the pancreas.

S. Bollipo, FRACP
V. Ambikaipaker, MB, ChB
N. J. Talley, MD, PhD

Long-term quality of life after surgery for chronic pancreatitis

van Loo ES, van Baal MCPM, Gooszen HG, et al (Univ of Groningen, The Netherlands; Univ of Utrecht, The Netherlands)

Br J Surg 97:1079-1086, 2010

Background.—Surgery for chronic pancreatitis is indicated for intractable pain or the treatment of complications. This retrospective cohort study evaluated the applicability of pain, coping and quality-of-life (QOL) scoring in patients with chronic pancreatitis.

Methods.—Between 1995 and 2008, 155 patients underwent surgery for chronic pancreatitis in two Dutch university hospitals. Medical charts were reviewed, and QOL and coping with pain were assessed by two validated questionnaires.

Results.—Median follow-up was 5·6 years. The aetiology was alcohol related in 48·3 per cent. Some 111 resections and 46 drainage procedures were performed. Fifty-seven patients had major complications and the hospital mortality rate was 1·3 per cent. After surgery the number of patients needing analgesics was reduced ($P < 0{\cdot}001$). Alcohol consumption significantly reduced pain coping mechanisms ($P = 0{\cdot}032$). Overall, QOL remained poor after surgery. Scores on three dimensions of the QOL questionnaire were significantly better after drainage than after resection, procedures.

Conclusion.—In general, QOL after surgery for chronic pancreatitis remains poor, owing to pre-existing lifestyle and co-morbidity. Patients selected for a pancreatic duct drainage procedure have a better postoperative QOL than those undergoing resectional procedures. Alcohol consumption is associated with poor ability to cope with pain after surgery and should be discouraged.

► Intractable abdominal pain is a frequent indication for surgical treatment of chronic pancreatitis. Surgical methods involve either resection of part of the pancreas or some form of a drainage procedure. The selection of surgical method varies widely owing to lack of any evidence-based guidelines. Given that pain is the key symptom here, any method should be evaluated for its outcome based on the pain relief and improvement in quality of life (QOL) after surgery.

In this retrospective cohort study involving 155 patients using a questionnaire (response rate of 42%), it appears that there is some improvement in QOL after surgery, especially for those who underwent a drainage procedure rather than a resection procedure. While it is good to know that surgery can offer pain relief (more than half of the patients no longer required analgesics), it should be noted that the QOL remained poor overall, even after surgery.

The most important take-home message from this study, however, is that alcohol plays a significant role in the outcome. Those who continue to drink alcohol even moderately have poor ability to cope with pain after surgery. Preoperative counseling to encourage permanent alcohol abstinence is needed to improve outcomes after surgery for chronic pancreatitis.

S. Bollipo, FRACP
V. Ambikaipaker, MB, ChB
N. J. Talley, MD, PhD

Imaging in Pancreatic and Biliary Disorders

Absence of a Dilated Duct Predicts Benign Disease in Suspected Pancreas Cancer: A Simple Clinical Rule

Rodriguez S, Faigel D (Oregon Health and Science Univ, Portland)
Dig Dis Sci 55:1161-1166, 2010

Background.—Pancreatic cancer can be difficult to diagnose. Fine-needle aspiration (FNA) biopsies may be negative even when malignancy is present.

Aims.—To identify endosonographic features predictive of malignancy that will separate patients into high- and low-risk groups, in whom a negative FNA effectively rules out malignancy.

Methods.—Patients presenting for endoscopic ultrasound (EUS) evaluation for suspected pancreatic mass were prospectively enrolled. If a mass or abnormal lymph nodes were present, sampling via fine-needle aspiration (FNA) was performed. The characteristics of patients with cancer were compared to the characteristics of patients without cancer using Chi-square testing and *t*-tests.

Results.—Seventy-three patients were enrolled. Thirty-three patients had cancer and 40 had benign disease. On multivariate analysis, only vascular or organ invasion and dilation of the pancreatic duct (PD) were significantly associated with cancer. PD dilation was examined as a stand-alone feature. The presence of a dilated PD placed patients into a group with a 65% prevalence of malignancy. In the non-dilated PD group, the prevalence of malignancy was only 17%, and in this group, the negative predictive value of FNA was 100%, compared to an NPV of 73% in the entire cohort.

Conclusions.—The most significant negative predictive endosonographic finding in patients with suspected pancreatic cancer is a non-dilated PD. If a patient with suspected pancreatic cancer does not have a dilated PD and the FNA is negative for malignancy, the likelihood of cancer is low.

▶ Despite advances in imaging and endoscopic ultrasound guided–fine-needle aspiration (EUS-FNA), the diagnosis of pancreatic cancer remains difficult, as the negative predictive value of EUS-FNA remains between 73% to 85%. Historically, 5% to 10% of Whipple procedures are done for patients who eventually are found to have no malignancy. Pancreatic surgery is associated with some morbidity, mortality, and cost. Hence, it would be useful to find a way to increase the negative predictive value of a negative FNA to be able to effectively rule out malignancy and avoid unnecessary surgery in those with benign disease.

In this prospective study of patients presenting for EUS for suspected pancreatic cancer, 8 of 31 patients with cancer had a negative FNA. FNA was negative in all 22 patients with no cancer. Following multivariate logistic regression analysis, the absence of pancreatic duct dilation predicted benign disease in those with a negative EUS-FNA, improving the negative predictive value from 53% to 100%.

The authors suggest a simple clinical rule that if the pancreatic duct is not dilated and the FNA is negative, the patient most likely does not have a pancreatic cancer. There are some limitations to this rule as early malignancy may not be associated with a dilated pancreatic duct, and similarly, a cancer involving the body or tail of the pancreas may not have a dilated pancreatic duct. The conclusions are based on very small numbers; nevertheless, the authors must be congratulated for attempting to develop a simple clinical rule for a complex problem.

S. Bollipo, FRACP
V. Ambikaipaker, MB, ChB
N. J. Talley, MD, PhD

Variability in measurements of pancreatic cyst size among EUS, CT, and magnetic resonance imaging modalities

Maimone S, Agrawal D, Pollack MJ, et al (Univ Hosps Case Med Ctr, Cleveland, OH)

Gastrointest Endosc 71:945-950, 2010

Background.—Cyst size is an important factor in the management of pancreatic cysts, both in predicting the need for surgery and the frequency of follow-up.

Objective.—To determine agreement and precision of EUS, CT, and magnetic resonance imaging (MRI) modalities in the evaluation of pancreatic cyst diameter.

Design.—Retrospective chart review.

Setting.—Tertiary-care center, January 2000 to June 2009.

Patients.—This study involved 175 patients presenting for EUS evaluation of pancreatic cysts, with size measured by at least two of the aforementioned imaging studies within a 90-day period.

Main Outcome Measurements.—Largest cyst diameter from EUS, CT, MRI/MRCP, and surgical pathology.

Results.—A total of 175 patients underwent EUS. Seventy-three had CT plus EUS, 33 had MRI/MRCP plus EUS, 23 had MRI/MRCP plus CT, and 15 had all imaging studies, occurring within 90 days of each other. Median size differences between studies: EUS and CT (ie, absolute value of size determined by EUS minus size determined by CT) = 4 mm (range 0-25 mm), EUS and MRI = 4 mm (range 0-17 mm), CT and MRI = 3 mm (range 2-20 mm). Median size differences for surgical pathology specimens compared with results of 12 EUS, 13 CT, and 8 MRI/MRCP studies were as follows: EUS and pathology = 9.5 mm (range 0-20 mm), CT and pathology = 5 mm (range 0-21 mm), MRI and pathology = 5.5 mm (range 2-44 mm).

Limitations.—Interobserver variability and small sample of surgical pathology cysts.

Conclusion.—There is considerable variation in size estimates of pancreatic cysts by different imaging modalities, which practitioners should take into account when making management decisions. Use of a single imaging modality is recommended during follow-up. The precision of imaging studies for measuring pancreatic cysts must be prospectively defined if change in size is to be reliably used for clinical management.

▶ The incidental finding of small pancreatic cyst is becoming increasingly common with frequent use of cross-sectional abdominal imaging. Once noted, these patients are often referred for further evaluation by endoscopic ultrasound (EUS). This retrospective study describes 175 such patients who underwent EUS and 1 or more other modalities, including a CT or an MRI.

Size does matter in the management of pancreatic cysts, as consensus guidelines recommend surgery for cysts > 30 mm. For cysts < 30 mm, observation is recommended with the understanding that one can never be sure whether they are benign. The frequency of follow-up imaging varies between once yearly for cysts <10 mm to once in 3 to 6 months for cysts >20 mm. If any increase in size is noted, the patient may need a more frequent follow-up or may be sent for surgery.

In this study, the authors warn that there was a wide variation of size of the same cysts as measured by different methods, sometimes by as much as a 10-mm difference. This could well lead to an unnecessary change in management, which may even include unnecessary surgery. Until we know more about the precision of different modalities of imaging in monitoring size from prospective studies, it seems prudent to follow at least a single method of imaging to follow up pancreatic cysts, especially as the clinical decision depends on the size of the lesion.

S. Bollipo, FRACP
V. Ambikaipaker, MB, ChB
N. J. Talley, MD, PhD

Miscellaneous

Endoscopic gallbladder drainage for management of acute cholecystitis

Itoi T, Coelho-Prabhu N, Baron TH (Tokyo Med Univ, Japan; Mayo Clinic, Rochester, MN)

Gastrointest Endosc 71:1038-1045, 2010

Background.—Nonoperative gallbladder drainage methods for acute cholecystitis include percutaneous transhepatic gallbladder drainage and percutaneous transhepatic gallbladder aspiration, endoscopic nasogallbladder drainage and gallbladder stenting via a transpapillary endoscopic approach, and EUS-guided nasogallbladder drainage and gallbladder stenting via a transmural endoscopic approach.

Objective.—A systematic review was performed to evaluate the current potential role of each gallbladder drainage technique for acute cholecystitis.

Design.—MEDLINE, EMBASE, and manual searches were performed to identify pertinent English-language articles.

Results.—The technical success rate, clinical success rate, and the frequency of adverse events in percutaneous transhepatic gallbladder aspiration (n = 122) and percutaneous transhepatic gallbladder drainage (n = 246) were 93% and 98%, 83% and 90%, and 0.8% and 3.7%, respectively. In contrast, the technical success rate, clinical success rate, and the frequency of adverse events in endoscopic nasogallbladder drainage (n = 194) and endoscopic gallbladder stenting (n = 127) were 81% and 96%, 75% and 88%, and 3.6% (n = 7) and 6.3% (n = 8), respectively. Although there have been 2 small case series of successful EUS-guided transmural nasogallbladder drainage (total n = 12), the procedure was technically and clinically successful in all of the patients with 2 adverse events. Only 1 case of successful EUS-guided gallbladder stent placement without any procedure-related adverse events has been reported.

Limitations.—Retrospective studies, small number of patients, and lack of randomized, controlled trials.

Conclusions.—Although prospective evaluation of the feasibility, safety, and efficacy of these various approaches will help identify the most suitable therapeutic modality for patients with acute cholecystitis, endoscopic gallbladder drainage may have a high potential as an alternative drainage method in acute cholecystitis.

▶ Acute cholecystitis is a fairly common problem with potential for significant morbidity. Current practice in managing this problem is dependent on the severity of the disease. There are a number of different operative and nonoperative techniques for gallbladder drainage. The authors of this study have undertaken a systematic review of all current literature evaluating the various techniques of gallbladder drainage with a special focus on various endoscopic methods of gallbladder drainage.

The option of which procedure is most appropriate for the individual patient still needs to be determined by taking into account the advantages and limitations of the various procedures. The new treatment modalities with endoscopic-guided approach are promising, but more prospective evaluation is needed to determine the optimal, minimally invasive, safe, and effective management of acute cholecystitis.

This is a literature review of a number of varying studies that included no randomized controlled trials. There was no formal meta-analysis of data but merely pooling of the raw numbers from each study. Nevertheless, this is a useful technical review of the various techniques of gallbladder drainage for management of acute cholecystitis.

S. Bollipo, FRACP
V. Ambikaipaker, MB, ChB
N. J. Talley, MD, PhD

Risk factors for portal venous thrombosis after splenectomy in patients with cirrhosis and portal hypertension

Kinjo N, Kawanaka H, Akahoshi T, et al (Kyushu Univ, Higashi-ku, Fukuoka, Japan)
Br J Surg 97:910-916, 2010

Background.—Portal venous thrombosis (PVT) is a potentially fatal complication following splenectomy. Its mechanisms and risk factors are poorly understood, especially in patients with cirrhosis and portal hypertension. This study investigated risk factors for PVT following splenectomy in such patients.

Methods.—All consecutive patients with cirrhosis who underwent splenectomy in Kyushu University Hospital between 1998 and 2004 were included in this retrospective study. They were divided into two groups based on the presence or absence of postoperative PVT. Preoperative and operative factors were compared, and the relationships between formation of PVT and its independent variables were analysed. In some cases, portal venous flow was measured before and after splenectomy using duplex Doppler ultrasonography.

Results.—PVT developed after surgery in 17 (24 per cent) of 70 patients studied. Multivariable analysis showed that increased splenic vein diameter and low white cell count were significant independent risk factors for PVT. Portal venous flow after splenectomy was greatly reduced in the PVT group, but not in patients without PVT.

Conclusion.—Large splenic vein diameter and low white cell count are independent risk factors for PVT after splenectomy in patients with cirrhosis and portal hypertension.

▶ Low platelet count due to hypersplenism interferes with the ability of cirrhotic patients to undergo surgical treatments such as shunt procedures, operations for hepatocellular carcinoma, and interferon treatment for hepatitis C. The platelet count in these patients can be improved by a splenectomy, but this can be occasionally complicated by postoperative portal vein thrombosis (PVT), which can be potentially fatal.

Although cirrhotic patients often have coagulopathy, PVT still occurs. Preventing this by anticoagulation in the first few days after the operation is hampered by the possibility of postoperative bleeding. This study attempts to identify the risk factors for postoperative PVT in cirrhotic patients undergoing splenectomy.

In this retrospective study of 70 cirrhotic patients undergoing splenectomy, 17 patients developed postoperative PVT. Using multiple logistic regression with selected variables, increased splenic vein diameter and low white cell count were identified as independent risk factors.

The study was retrospective and the numbers were small. However, it is useful to know that cirrhotic patients with a large splenic vein and a low white cell count are at higher risk of postoperative PVT after splenectomy. It may be worthwhile selecting these patients for postoperative anticoagulation. Prospective randomized studies with larger number of patients and noncirrhotic controls undergoing splenectomy are needed to confirm the findings from this study.

S. Bollipo, FRACP
V. Ambikaipaker, MB, ChB
N. J. Talley, MD, PhD

Validating a Simple Scoring System to Predict Malignancy and Invasiveness of Intraductal Papillary Mucinous Neoplasms of the Pancreas

Shin SH, Han DJ, Park KT, et al (Univ of Ulsan College of Medicine, Songpa-gu, Seoul, Korea; Korea Univ Med Ctr, Seongbuk-Gu, Seoul)

World J Surg 34:776-783, 2010

Background.—The objective of the present study was to identify reliable preoperative factors predicting malignancy or invasiveness of intraductal papillary mucinous neoplasm (IPMN) of the pancreas and the effectiveness of a diagnostic scoring system based on these factors.

Methods.—Between August 1994 and December 2007, 204 patients underwent pancreatic resection for IPMN at a single institute. Medical records were reviewed retrospectively, and a new diagnostic scoring system for predicting malignant IPMN preoperatively was designed.

Results.—Univariate analysis revealed nine significant predictors of both malignant and invasive IPMN: age ≥60 years, history of pancreatitis, presence of mural nodule(s), diameter of main pancreatic duct (MPD) >6 mm, main duct or mixed type, total bilirubin >1.2 mg/dl, CA-19-9 >37 U/ml, tumor location in the pancreatic head, and tumor size >30 mm. Multivariate analysis showed that age, pancreatitis, mural nodule(s), and MPD diameter were independent predictors of invasive IPMN, and that all these parameters, plus elevated carbohydrate antigen-19-9 (CA-19-9), were independent predictors of malignant IPMN. A scoring system based on these five factors, each assigned 1 point, and with a cut-off of 3 points, could predict malignant IPMN with a sensitivity of 50.7% and a specificity of 90.1%. The 5-year survival rates of patients with benign and malignant IPMN were 95.0% and 64.0%, respectively.

Conclusions.—Our scoring system using five independent factors (age ≥60 years, history of pancreatitis, presence of mural nodule(s), elevated level of CA-19-9, and MPD diameter >6 mm) may be helpful for predicting malignancy and postoperative survival.

▶ The management of intraductal papillary mucinous neoplasms of the pancreas varies depending on whether they are benign or malignant and invasive or noninvasive. The treatment strategies can vary from simple observation to extensive surgery. However, there is no simple way of predicting malignancy or invasiveness, although various predictive factors, such as the elevated level of carbohydrate antigen (CA)-19-9, have been identified.

The authors of this study have designed a very simple scoring system using 5 variables, giving each of them 1 point and having 3 points as a cutoff for predicting malignancy. The variables were identified using univariate and multivariate analysis. These include age > 60 years, history of pancreatitis, presence of mural nodules, elevated level of CA-19-9, and main pancreatic duct diameter of > 6 mm. Notably, the sensitivity for this score was only 51%, while the specificity was very good at 90%. Therefore, this scoring system may be helpful in identifying those low-risk patients who may be able to be managed conservatively while avoiding extensive surgery. However, prospective validation and more sensitive scoring systems are required.

S. Bollipo, FRACP
V. Ambikaipaker, MB, ChB
N. J. Talley, MD, PhD

4 Gastrointestinal Cancers and Benign Polyps

Colon Cancer

Calculation of Risk of Colorectal and Endometrial Cancer Among Patients With Lynch Syndrome

Stoffel E, Mukherjee B, Raymond VM, et al (Brigham and Women's Hosp, Boston, MA; Univ of Michigan Med School and School of Public Health, Ann Arbor; Univ of Michigan Med School; et al)
Gastroenterology 137:1621-1627, 2009

Background & Aims.—Lynch syndrome is the most common hereditary colorectal cancer (CRC) syndrome. Some previous estimates of lifetime risk for CRC and endometrial cancer (EC) did not control for ascertainment and were susceptible to bias toward overestimated risk.

Methods.—We studied 147 families with mismatch repair gene mutations (55 *MLH1*, 81 *MSH2*, and 11 *MSH6*) identified at 2 US cancer genetics clinics. Age-specific cumulative risks (penetrance) and hazard ratio (HR) estimates of CRC and EC risks were calculated and compared with the general population using modified segregation analysis. The likelihood for each pedigree was conditioned on the proband and first-degree relatives affected with CRC to reduce ascertainment bias and overestimation of penetrance.

Results.—We analyzed 628 cases of CRC, diagnosed at the median ages of 42 and 47 years for men and women, respectively. The cumulative risk of CRC was 66.08% (95% confidence interval [CI], 59.47%–76.17%) for men and 42.71% (95% CI, 36.57%–52.83%) for women, with overall HRs of 148.4 and 51.1, respectively. CRC risk was highest for males with mutations in *MLH1*. There were 155 cases of EC, diagnosed at a median age of 47.5 years. The cumulative risk of EC was 39.39% (95% CI, 30.78%–46.94%) with an overall HR of 39.0 (95% CI, 30.4–50.2). For women, the cumulative risk of CRC or EC was 73.42% (95% CI, 63.76%–80.54%).

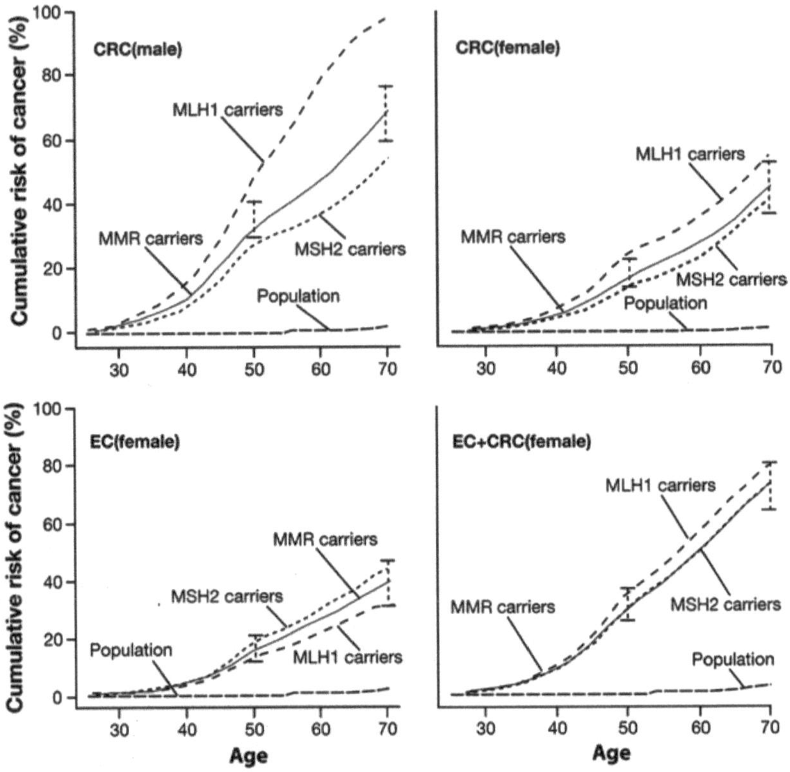

FIGURE 1.—Cumulative risk of CRC by sex in MMR gene mutation carriers compared with the SEER population (*top left*, males; *top right*, females). EC in females (*bottom left*) and either CRC or EC in females (*bottom right*) in MMR carriers and the population. The 95% CIs are reported at age 50 and at age 70. (Reprinted from Stoffel E, Mukherjee B, Raymond VM, et al. Calculation of risk of colorectal and endometrial cancer among patients with Lynch syndrome. *Gastroenterology.* 2009;137:1621-1627, with permission from AGA Institute.)

Conclusions.—Lifetime risks of CRC and EC in mismatch repair gene mutation carriers are high even after adjusting for ascertainment. These estimates are valuable for patients and providers; specialized cancer surveillance is necessary (Fig 1).

▶ Hereditary nonpolyposis colon cancer (HNPCC) or Lynch syndrome accounts for 3% to 5% of all cases of colorectal cancer (CRC) and is the result of germline mutations in DNA mismatch repair (MMR) genes. Tumors that develop in Lynch syndrome are the consequence of defective mutation repair associated with the biochemical phenotype of microsatellite instability. HNPCC is the most common gastrointestinal hereditary cancer syndrome, and although a variety of tumors have been observed, early age onset and rapidly progressive adenocarcinomas of the colorectum and endometrium are the most common.

Inherited in an autosomal dominant fashion with variable penetrance, germline mutations in 4 MMR genes (*MLH1*, *MSH2*, *MSH6*, and *PMS2*) have been linked to HNPCC. Prior to the recognition of these mutations, a diagnosis of Lynch syndrome was made clinically by comparing family history with the Amsterdam criteria, which required a family to have 3 individuals with CRC over 2 generations, with 1 case diagnosed before the age of 50. Recognition of other cancers associated with HNPCC led to the inclusion of endometrial cancer (EC) and transitional cell cancer of the bladder and renal pelvis in the more inclusive Bethesda criteria. Estimates of lifetime CRC approached 70% to 80%, and 40% to 60% for EC. Furthermore, because of the early age and aggressive nature of the cancers, aggressive screening and surveillance guidelines have been published.[1]

These estimates were often criticized as inflated because of ascertainment bias resulting from an over representation of families with unusually high numbers of affected individuals and for failure to correct for the cancers that defined the kindred using Amsterdam criteria. Recent studies controlling for ascertainment bias observed much lower risk estimates, calling into question the screening and surveillance recommendations.[2]

This large study from 2 cancer genetic clinics in the United States included 147 families with proven deleterious mutations in 1 of the MMR genes, and overall, a total of 6342 individuals were analyzed. Ascertainment bias was corrected by a statistical technique known as conditioning and then sensitivity analysis was conducted. For example, CRC diagnoses in the probands and first-degree relatives were excluded.

Fig 1 nicely summarizes the clinically relevant findings from this important study. Compared with the average-risk population calculated from Surveillance Epidemiology and End Results (SEER) trial, carriers of MMR gene mutations have a risk of CRC that is 2 times the population risk for males by the age of 30 and 4.5 times the population risk for women by age 40. The figure also shows that the risk continues to rise with increasing age for a cumulative absolute risk for CRC and EC of 70% at 70 years for men and women.

This study supports the current cancer screening recommendations for MMR gene mutation carriers that includes colonoscopy screening every 1 to 2 years beginning at age 20 to 25 (depending on the age of the youngest affected in the kindred) and uterine cancer screening for women beginning at age 30 to 35. For women, prophylactic hysterectomy once child bearing is complete is often recommended.

R. K. Pearson, MD

References

1. Lindo NM, Petersen GM, Hadley DW, et al. Recommendations for the care of individuals with an inherrited predisposition to Lynch syndrome: a systematic review. *JAMA*. 2006;296:1507-1517.
2. Alarcon F, Lasset C, Carayol J, et al. Estimating cancer risk in HNPCC by the GRL method. *Eur J Hum Genet*. 2007;15:831-836.

Colonoscopic surveillance improves survival after colorectal cancer diagnosis in inflammatory bowel disease

Lutgens MWMD, On behalf of the Initiative on Crohn and Colitis (ICC) (Univ Med Ctr, Utrecht, The Netherlands; et al)

Br J Cancer 101:1671-1675, 2009

Background.—Colonoscopic surveillance provides the best practical means for preventing colorectal cancer (CRC) in inflammatory bowel disease (IBD) patients. Strong evidence for improved survival from surveillance programmes is sparse.

Method.—The aim of this study was to compare tumour stage and survival of IBD patients with CRC who were a part of a surveillance programme with those who were not. A nationwide pathology database (PALGA (pathologisch anatomisch landelijk geautomatiseerd archief)) was consulted to identify IBD patients with CRC treated in all eight university hospitals in The Netherlands over a period of 15 years. Patients were assigned to the surveillance group when they had undergone one or more surveillance colonoscopies before a diagnosis of CRC. Patients who

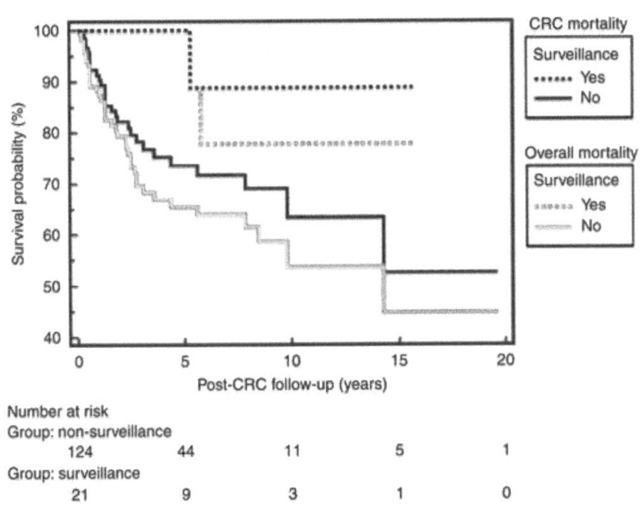

FIGURE 1.—Survival analysis for CRC-related and overall mortality. The Tarone–Ware test of equality of survival distribution was used to compare survival between the two groups. CRC-related mortality is presented by solid squares and line. Overall mortality is presented by outlined squares and line. For CRC-related mortality, the 5-year survival in the surveillance group (solid squares) was 100% compared with 74% in the nonsurveillance group (solid black line) ($P = 0.029$); the primary end point was date of death due to CRC; cases were censored for date of end of study, date of death related to any other primary malignancy, date of death related to colectomy, date of death by any other cause, and date of lost to follow-up. For overall mortality, the 5-year survival in the surveillance group (outlined squares) was 100% compared with 65% in the non-surveillance group (outlined line; $P = 0.042$); the primary end point was date of death; cases were censored for date of end of study period and date of lost to follow-up. CRC, colorectal cancer. (Reprinted from Lutgens MWMD, On behalf of the Initiative on Crohn and Colitis (ICC). Colonoscopic surveillance improves survival after colorectal cancer diagnosis in inflammatory bowel disease. *Br J Cancer.* 2009;101:1671-1675.)

had not undergone surveillance served as controls. Tumour stage and survival were compared between the two groups.

Results.—A total of 149 patients with IBD-associated CRC were identified. Twenty-three had had colonoscopic surveillance before CRC was discovered. The 5-year CRC-related survival rate of patients in the surveillance group was 100% compared with 74% in the non-surveillance group ($P = 0.042$). In the surveillance group, only one patient died as a consequence of CRC compared with 29 patients in the control group ($P = 0.047$). In addition, more early tumour stages were found in the surveillance group ($P = 0.004$).

Conclusions.—These results provide evidence for improved survival from colonoscopic surveillance in IBD patients by detecting CRC at a more favourable tumour stage (Fig 1).

▶ Inflammatory bowel disease (IBD) is a well-established risk factor for colorectal cancer (CRC). To detect dysplasia or early CRC, it is recommended that patients with IBD, especially chronic ulcerative colitis (CUC), enroll in a colonoscopy surveillance program. However, in spite of the expense and risk associated with this procedure, the level of evidence in support of this practice is considered low. A randomized controlled clinical trial would be ideal but is impractical and probably unethical.

This study is a retrospective analysis of a relatively large cohort of patients with IBD in the Netherlands. It included 149 patients with CRC complicating IBD. Importantly, both Crohn's colitis and CUC were included in the registry. To be considered in the surveillance cohort, colonoscopy with biopsies every 10 cm of colon had to be performed every 1 to 3 years. The aim was to compare tumor stage and survival between those enrolled in a surveillance program and those who were not.

As Fig 1 demonstrates, there was improved survival in patients with IBD who developed CRC in whom surveillance colonoscopy was performed. Of the cancers detected in the surveillance cohort, half were stage 0 or 1 reflecting the excellent (100%) 5-year survival.

While the authors acknowledge the deficiencies and biases inherent in retrospective registry studies, this study strengthens the standard clinical practice in the United States to offer colonoscopic surveillance for patients with longstanding IBD with high-risk profiles to reduce the risk of CRC mortality.

R. K. Pearson, MD

Inflammatory Bowel Disease Confers a Lower Risk of Colorectal Cancer to Females Than to Males

Söderlund S, Granath F, Broström O, et al (Stockholm Söder Hosp, Sweden; Karolinska Univ Hosp, Solna, Sweden)

Gastroenterology 138:1697-1703, 2010

Background & Aims.—Reported differences in cancer risk between male and female animals after chronic inflammation suggest that estrogen has inflammation-modifying properties. Little is known about these effects in human beings. Inflammatory bowel disease (IBD) is associated with an increased risk of colorectal cancer (CRC); we studied differences in inflammation-associated CRC between men and women patients with IBD.

Methods.—By using a large population-based cohort (n = 7607) of individuals diagnosed with IBD from 1954 to 1989, we assessed the sex-specific incidence of CRC from 1960 to 2004. Incidence was determined within the cohort (modeled using Poisson regression) and compared with the general population (assessed as standardized incidence ratios) using data from national Swedish health and census registers.

Results.—During 171,000 person-years of follow-up evaluation, 196 new cases of CRC were observed (123 in males, 73 in females). Males with IBD had a 60% higher risk of CRC (relative risk [RR], 1.6; 95% confidence interval [CI], 1.2–2.2) than females (cumulative incidence 40 years after IBD diagnosis, 8.3% vs 3.5%). Compared with the rate of CRC among the general population, in males with IBD the RR was 2.6 and the 95% CI was 2.2–3.1, whereas in females the RR was 1.9 and the 95% CI was 1.5–2.4. The effect of sex was limited to the period after 10 years of follow-up evaluation (RR, 0.8 before vs 2.2 after), and to patients diagnosed before age 45 (RR, 2.1 before vs 1.0 after).

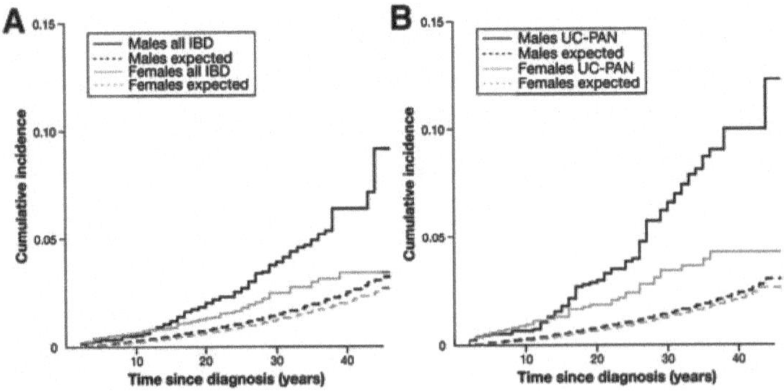

FIGURE 2.—(*A*) Sex-specific observed CRC incidence vs that expected in the general population for all cases of IBD. (*B*) Sex-specific observed CRC incidence vs that expected in the general population for patients with UC pan-colitis. (Reprinted from Söderlund S, Granath F, Broström O, et al. Inflammatory bowel disease confers a lower risk of colorectal cancer to females than to males. *Gastroenterology*. 2010;138:1697-1703, with permission from the AGA Institute.)

Conclusions.—IBD confers a lower risk of CRC to females than to males (Fig 2).

▶ The increased risk of neoplasia associated with chronic inflammation is a common theme in all fields of gastroenterology, and we routinely screen and survey patients with cirrhosis, Barrett's esophagus, and inflammatory bowel disease (IBD). The practice of surveillance colonoscopy for IBD, especially pancolonic chronic ulcerative colitis (CUC) dates back 30 years and has not changed significantly in 3 decades. Only a few clinical parameters alter the frequency of surveillance examinations, including duration and extent of colitis, the presence of primary sclerosing cholangitis, confirmed dysplasia on a previous examination, and dysplasia in a raised (mass) lesion. A family history of colorectal cancer (CRC) and the severity of histologic inflammation have also been reported to increase the risk of CRC complicating IBD.[1] This report from Sweden suggests that female gender also modifies (lowers) the risk for neoplasia in IBD.

This is a large-scale cohort study performed by experienced and respected epidemiologists from the Karolinska institute. Using 3 well-established IBD registries linked to national registries for death and cancer, the investigators were able to generate a large population-based cohort of >7000 patients with IBD and determine the sex-specific incidence of CRC for a 40-year time frame. As Fig 2 demonstrates, the differences in risk of CRC between the sexes occurs after 10 years and continues to diverge over time. As expected, the absolute risk of CRC is highest for pancolonic CUC; after 40 years of disease, there is an absolute higher risk of CRC in men of 5.4% (12.8% vs 7.4%).

The authors implicate estrogen in the protective effect from inflammation-associated cancer described for female sex. Indeed, other studies have shown a protective effect of female sex in the rate of CRC in the general population, an effect the investigators controlled for in this study of IBD-specific risk. Animal model and in vitro studies point to a direct effect of sex hormones on the inflammatory response and subsequent protection from neoplasia. The observation in this study that the entire protective effect for female sex was restricted to patients with the onset of disease before age 45 years (premenopausal) supports the estrogen hypothesis. In postmenopausal women, hormone replacement therapy has been associated with a protective effect on disease activity in 1 study.

However, the authors are quick to point out that other effects of female sex, including behavioral, could also be acting. For example, it has been shown in other studies that women are more likely to be compliant with prescription medications, including mesalamine that may be protective against CRC. Are women more likely compliant with colonoscopic and dysplasia surveillance? While the study did not address this question, both sexes had a colectomy rate of 20% over the duration of the study and had the same stage of cancer at diagnosis.

While this study should not be used as a clinical decision tree for surveillance intervals, it does suggest the need for additional studies, especially on the potential modification of cancer risk by sex hormones.

R. K. Pearson, MD

Reference

1. Rutter M, Saunders B, Wilkinson K, et al. Severity of Inflammation is a risk factor for colorectal neoplasia in ulcerative colitis. *Gastroenterology.* 2004;126:451-459.

Low Risk of Colorectal Cancer and Advanced Adenomas More Than 10 Years After Negative Colonoscopy

Brenner H, Haug U, Arndt V, et al (German Cancer Res Ctr, Heidelberg, Germany; et al)
Gastroenterology 138:870-876, 2010

Background & Aims.—Screening colonoscopy is an effective method to reduce the incidence of and mortality from colorectal cancer (CRC). There is little empirical evidence available about the optimal interval for screening, making this a subject of debate. We associated the prevalence of advanced colorectal neoplasms with time since negative colonoscopies.

Methods.—In a study of participants in the German colonoscopy screening program, we determined the prevalence of colorectal neoplasias detected at screening colonoscopy among subjects who had undergone a previous colonoscopy without detection of polyps (negative colonoscopy). Data were compared with that from subjects who had not received colonoscopies.

Results.—No CRCs were detected in participants who had a previous negative colonoscopy an average of 11.9 years previously (n = 553), compared with the 8.4 CRC cases expected based on age- and gender-specific prevalences among participants who had not received a colonoscopy (n = 2701; standardized prevalence ratio [SPR] = 0.00; 95% confidence interval [CI]: 0.00–0.55). Prevalence of advanced adenoma was also much lower among subjects who had previous colonoscopies (SPR = 0.42; 95% CI: 0.25–0.68). Adjusted prevalence ratios (95% CIs) for detecting an advanced adenoma were 0.38 (95% CI: 0.16–0.90), 0.34 (95% CI: 0.15–0.74), 0.38 (95% CI: 0.16–0.90), and 0.53 (95% CI: 0.27–1.04) among participants with a negative colonoscopy conducted 1–5, 6–10, 11–15, and >16 years ago, respectively, compared to participants with no previous colonoscopy.

Conclusions.—The low risk of CRC and advanced adenomas after a negative colonoscopy supports suggestions that screening intervals be extended to ≥10 years (Table 2).

▶ Colonoscopy is considered the gold standard for screening for colorectal cancer (CRC) because the removal of premalignant adenomatous polyps has

TABLE 2.—Findings at Screening Colonoscopy According to History of Previous Colonoscopy

	Most Advanced Finding at Screening Colonoscopy											
	Colorectal Cancer		Advanced Adenoma[a]		Other Adenoma		Hyperplastic Polyp		Unspecified polyp		None	
Previous Colonoscopy	n	%	n	%	n	%	n	%	n	%	n	%
No (n = 2701)	41	1.5	267	9.9	494	18.3	281	10.4	54	2.0	1564	57.9
Yes, no polyps detected												
1+ y ago (n = 533)	0	0.0	25	4.7	86	16.1	33	6.2	5	0.9	384	72.0
1–5 y ago (n = 115)	0	0.0	5	4.4	13	11.3	9	7.8	1	0.9	87	75.7
6–10 y ago (n = 166)	0	0.0	6	3.6	31	18.7	6	3.6	1	0.6	122	73.5
11–15 y ago (n = 117)	0	0.0	5	4.3	23	19.7	9	7.7	0	0.0	80	68.4
16+ y ago (n = 135)	0	0.0	9	6.7	19	14.1	9	6.7	3	2.2	95	70.4

[a]Defined as presence of at least 1 adenoma with at least 1 of the following features: >1 cm in size, tubulovillous or villous components, high-grade dysplasia.

been demonstrated to lower the risk of future CRC.[1] Considerable effort has been expended to establish the appropriate interval between surveillance colonoscopy procedures due to the expense and risk of this modality.

The National Polyp Study established high-risk cohorts needing surveillance examinations at 3 years. However, the timing of surveillance after a negative colonoscopy has been more problematic due to the lack of data. A recent prospective study of more than 1200 participants demonstrated very low rates of CRC or advanced neoplasia 5 years after a negative colonoscopy. However, there are few studies to help policy makers determine how far surveillance can be pushed beyond 5 years.

In this cohort study from a small state located in Germany, participants presenting for screening colonoscopy filled out a standardized questionnaire that included whether a previous examination had been performed and if polyps were identified. Outcomes of the colonoscopy were compared between those with a previous negative examination versus first-time examinees. This methodology had been previously validated as accurate in this population.

Table 2 shows that patients with a previous negative colonoscopy up to 16 years before had no cancers and a statistically and clinically significant reduction in advanced adenomas. Not surprisingly, the rate of small polyps was similar in the 2 groups. The authors conclude that surveillance intervals after a negative colonoscopy could be extended to 10 years and possibly beyond.

This well-designed but relatively small study (n = 533 subjects in the negative examination cohort) is unlikely to quell the controversy or need for prospective studies to address surveillance intervals. This is especially true in light of recent studies indicating a relative lack of protection in larger population studies from right-sided colon cancer.

R. K. Pearson, MD

Reference

1. Winawer SJ, Zauber AG, Ho MN, et al. Prevention of colorectal cancer by colonoscopic polypectomy. The National Polyp Study Workgroup. *N Engl J Med.* 1993;329:1977-1981.

Once-only flexible sigmoidoscopy screening in prevention of colorectal cancer: a multicentre randomised controlled trial

Atkin WS, UK Flexible Sigmoidoscopy Trial Investigators (Imperial College London, UK; et al)

Lancet 375:1624-1633, 2010

Background.—Colorectal cancer is the third most common cancer worldwide and has a high mortality rate. We tested the hypothesis that only one flexible sigmoidoscopy screening between 55 and 64 years of age can substantially reduce colorectal cancer incidence and mortality.

Methods.—This randomised controlled trial was undertaken in 14 UK centres. 170 432 eligible men and women, who had indicated on a previous questionnaire that they would accept an invitation for screening, were randomly allocated to the intervention group (offered flexible sigmoidoscopy screening) or the control group (not contacted). Randomisation by sequential number generation was done centrally in blocks of 12, with stratification by trial centre, general practice, and household type. The primary outcomes were the incidence of colorectal cancer, including prevalent cases detected at screening, and mortality from colorectal cancer. Analyses were intention to treat and per protocol. The trial is registered, number ISRCTN28352761.

Findings.—113 195 people were assigned to the control group and 57 237 to the intervention group, of whom 112 939 and 57 099, respectively, were included in the final analyses. 40 674 (71%) people underwent flexible sigmoidoscopy. During screening and median follow-up of 11·2 years (IQR 10·7–11·9), 2524 participants were diagnosed with colorectal cancer (1818 in control group *vs* 706 in intervention group) and 20 543 died (13 768 *vs* 6775; 727 certified from colorectal cancer [538 *vs* 189]). In intention-to-treat analyses, colorectal cancer incidence in the intervention group was reduced by 23% (hazard ratio 0·77, 95% CI 0·70–0·84) and mortality by 31% (0·69, 0·59–0·82). In per-protocol analyses, adjusting for self-selection bias in the intervention group, incidence of colorectal cancer in people attending screening was reduced by 33% (0·67, 0·60–0·76) and mortality by 43% (0·57, 0·45–0·72). Incidence of distal colorectal cancer (rectum and sigmoid colon) was reduced by 50% (0·50, 0·42–0·59; secondary outcome). The numbers needed to be screened to prevent one colorectal cancer diagnosis or death, by

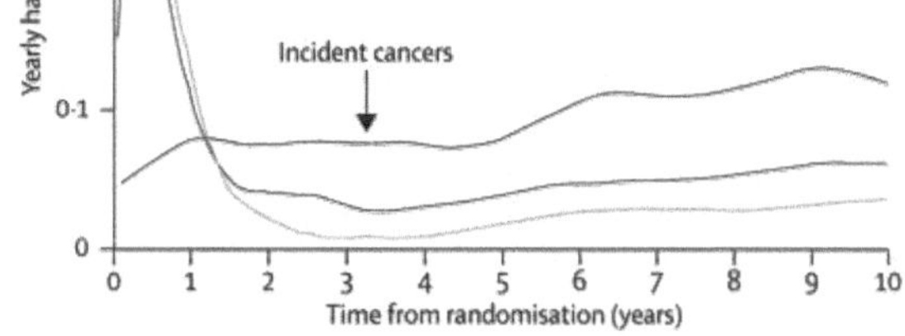

FIGURE 3.—Smoothed yearly hazard rates for distal cancer (rectum and sigmoid colon). Curves are truncated at 10 years of follow-up because of incomplete ascertainment of cancers in the final calendar year of the study. (Reprinted from Atkin WS, UK Flexible Sigmoidoscopy Trial Investigators. Once-only flexible sigmoidoscopy screening in prevention of colorectal cancer: a multicentre randomised controlled trial. *Lancet*. 2010;375:1624-1633, with permission from Elsevier.)

the end of the study period, were 191 (95% CI 145–277) and 489 (343–852), respectively.

Interpretation.—Flexible sigmoidoscopy is a safe and practical test and, when offered only once between ages 55 and 64 years, confers a substantial and longlasting benefit (Fig 3).

▶ While assumptions are made about the value of colonoscopy screening in reducing colorectal cancer (CRC) incidence and mortality, it is important to recognize the limitations of the evidence to date. The often-cited report by Atkin and colleagues[1] on 60% to 70% reduction of CRC incidence within the reach of sigmoidoscopy screening is based on a case-control study. The even higher protection afforded by colonoscopic polypectomy (76%-90%) reported in the National Polyp Study used historical controls.[2] Definitive evidence from a sufficiently powered randomized controlled trial has been lacking until this report in *The Lancet*.

Atkin and colleagues from the United Kingdom followed up their influential case-control study reported in the 1990s with this highly anticipated large-scale, randomized, multicenter trial of once-only flexible sigmoidoscopy in preventing CRC. Advocates of colonoscopy screening will be pleased with the results. Table 3 in the original article summarizes the important outcomes: a 50% reduction in incidence and a 43% reduction in mortality in patients receiving sigmoidoscopy compared with a control group. This result is large for any cancer screening test and compares favorably with mammography and prostate-specific antigen testing for prostate cancer.

This study used a prerandomization questionnaire to improve compliance in the sigmoidoscopy group; only potential participants indicating willingness to undergo sigmoidoscopy were enrolled in the intervention group. The 71% enrollment rate even with this prescreening methodology points out one of the challenges with endoscopic screening—patient acceptance.

One of the reasons for the less than 70% to 80% expected reduction of CRC incidence within the reach of sigmoidoscopy is the impact of the detection of prevalent cancers demonstrated in Fig 3. Prevalent CRCs dilute the impact of polypectomy on the reduction of incident cancers. While the follow-up of 11 years in this study is impressive, longer follow-up will likely continue to show additional benefits from the sigmoidoscopy and polyp removal. It is also important to acknowledge that this study was once only sigmoidoscopy; other large-scale trials that include serial examinations are underway.

Not surprisingly, the rate and mortality from right-sided cancer were not influenced by this study. This is particularly true given the restrictions placed on colonoscopy screening; only patients with advanced or multiple (>3) adenomas were referred. This represented only 5% of the subjects. A randomized trial of colonoscopy has been started in Europe, but there is concern that in the current climate of enthusiasm for CRC screening, enrollment will suffer.

In the meantime, this important study provides the first-tier[1] evidence that endoscopic screening with polypectomy protects against CRC.

R. K. Pearson, MD

References

1. Atkin W, Morson B, Cuzick J. Long-term risk of colorectal cancer after excision of rectosigmoid adenomas. *N Engl J Med.* 1992;326:658-662.
2. Winawer SJ, Zauber AG, Ho MN, et al. Prevention of colorectal cancer by colonoscopic polypectomy. The National Polyp Study Workgroup. *N Engl J Med.* 1993;329:1977-1981.

Postpolypectomy bleeding in patients undergoing colonoscopy on uninterrupted clopidogrel therapy

Singh M, Mehta N, Murthy UK, et al (VA Med Ctr, Syracuse, NY; et al)
Gastrointest Endosc 71:998-1005, 2010

Background.—The risk of postpolypectomy bleeding (PPB) in patients undergoing colonoscopy on uninterrupted clopidogrel therapy has not been established.

Objective.—To assess the PPB rate and outcome and identify risk factors associated with PPB in patients taking clopidogrel.

Design.—Single-center, retrospective study. Demographics, clinical parameters, polyp characteristics, polypectomy techniques, and postpolypectomy events in the groups were compared by univariate analysis. Stepwise logistic regression analyses identified independent risk factors associated with PPB.

Setting.—Veterans Affairs Medical Center.

Patients.—A total of 142 patients (375 polypectomies) taking clopidogrel (cases) and 1243 patients (3226 polypectomies) not taking clopidogrel (controls).

Interventions.—None.

Main Outcome Measurements.—Postpolypectomy bleeding, hospitalization, and mortality.

Results.—The immediate (intraprocedural) bleeding rate was similar in the 2 groups (2.1% vs 2.1%). Delayed (postprocedural) PPB rate was higher in the group taking clopidogrel (3.5% vs 1.0%, $P = .02$). Delayed bleeding of significance requiring hospitalization and transfusion/intervention was also higher in patients taking clopidogrel (2.1% vs 0.4%, $P = .04$). The length of hospital stay and interventions for PPB were comparable between the 2 groups. There was no mortality. Concomitant use of clopidogrel and aspirin/other nonsteroidal anti-inflammatory drugs (odds ratio 3.7; 95% CI, 1.6-8.5) and the number of polyps removed (OR 1.3; 95% CI, 1.2-1.4) were the only significant risk factors associated with PPB. Clopidogrel alone was not an independent risk factor for PPB.

Limitations.—Retrospective study and small number of patients with PPB.

Conclusions.—The PPB rate is significantly higher in patients undergoing polypectomy while taking clopidogrel and concomitant aspirin/nonsteroidal anti-inflammatory drugs; however, the risk is small and the

TABLE 3.—Postpolypectomy Bleeding with and without Clopidogrel Therapy

	Group A (On Clopidogrel) (n = 142)	Group B (Not On Clopidogrel) (n = 1243)	*P* Value
Overall PPB	8 (5.6%)*	38 (3.0%)*	.1
Immediate PPB (intraprocedural)	3 (2.1%)	26 (2.1%)	1.0
Delayed PPB (postprocedural)	5 (3.5%)	12 (1%)	.02
Significant PPB† (all delayed)	3 (2.1%)	5 (0.4%)	.04

PPB, Postpolypectomy bleeding.
*Eight of 8 PPB patients in group A and 16 of 38 PPB patients in group B were taking aspirin ($P = .002$).
†Significant bleeding: patients requiring transfusions, other interventions, or hospitalization.

outcome is favorable. Routine cessation of clopidogrel in patients before colonoscopy/polypectomy is not necessary (Table 3).

▶ The cornerstone of colonoscopic screening is the reduction in colorectal cancer incidence and mortality associated with polypectomy. Bleeding is the most common complication associated with this intervention and ranges from 0.3% to 3.6% per patient and up to 6.1% per polyp.[1] There are both polyp factors (size and method of removal) and patient factors (comorbidities) that influence the rate of bleeding after polypectomy. Anticoagulation increases the risk substantially, while antiplatelet agents like aspirin and other anti-inflammatory drugs do not.

Newer, more potent antiplatelet agents, including clopidogrel, present a new challenge for endoscopists. Increasingly, cardiologists are recommending these agents for 1 year (or more) of uninterrupted therapy, especially in patients with drug eluting coronary stents. These patients are often referred for colonoscopy, and how to handle the clopidogrel therapy is an unanswered question. Stopping clopidogrel in these individuals predisposes them to serious ischemic events. While acknowledging the lack of published data on the safety of high-risk endoscopic procedures, including polypectomy in the setting of this therapy, the American Society of Gastrointestinal Endoscopy guidelines suggested the discontinuation of clopidogrel for 7 to 10 days before high-risk procedures.[2]

At the Syracuse Veterans Affairs Medical Center, clopidogrel was not routinely held prior to colonoscopy and polypectomy. This retrospective review reports on the experience with 142 patients undergoing polypectomy on uninterrupted clopidogrel therapy.

As Table 3 illustrates, the results are reassuring for performing polypectomy in this setting. The overall bleeding rate was similar between subjects on clopidogrel and a randomly selected control group not on the drug. Furthermore, the bleeding rate of 5.6% was similar to controls. While the delayed bleeding rate was statistically increased over controls, only 3 patients (2.1%) had significant bleeding requiring transfusion, hospitalization, or other interventions.

While limited by the relatively small number of patients and its retrospective design, this study calls into question the routine practice of insisting on cessation of clopidogrel therapy before colonoscopic polypectomy. The authors suggest that a better strategy based on this study would be to halt therapy only after the removal of large or multiple polyps. Given the almost certain increase in patients on these potent antiplatelet therapies, larger, prospective (likely multicenter) studies are needed.

R. K. Pearson, MD

References

1. Kim HS, Kim TI, Kim WH, et al. Risk factors for immediate postpolypectomy bleeding of the colon: a multicenter study. *Am J Gastroenterol.* 2006;101: 1333-1341.
2. Zuckerman MJ, Hirota WK, Adler DG, et al. Standards of practice committee of the American Society for Gastrointestinal Endoscopy. ASGE guideline: the management of low-molecular-weight heparain and non-aspirin antiplatelet agents for endoscopic procedures. *Gastrointest Endosc.* 2005;61:189-194.

Utilization of Surveillance Colonoscopy in Community Practice

Schoen RE, Pinsky PF, Weissfeld JL, et al (Univ of Pittsburgh Med Ctr, PA; Natl Cancer Inst, Bethesda, MD; et al)
Gastroenterology 138:73-81, 2010

Background & Aims.—The recommended timing of surveillance colonoscopy for individuals with adenomatous polyps is based on adenoma histology, size, and number. The burden and cost of surveillance colonoscopy are significant. The aim of this study was to examine the use of surveillance colonoscopy on a community-wide basis.

Methods.—We retrospectively queried participants in the Prostate, Lung, Colorectal, and Ovarian Cancer screening trial in 9 US communities about use of surveillance colonoscopy. Subjects whose initial colonoscopy showed advanced adenoma (AA), nonadvanced adenoma (NAA), or no adenoma (NA) findings were included. Colonoscopy examinations were confirmed by reviewing colonoscopy reports.

Results.—Of 3876 subjects selected for inquiry, 3627 (93.6%) responded. The cumulative probability of a surveillance colonoscopy within 5 years was 58.4% (n = 1342) in the AA group, 57.5% in those with ≥3 NAAs (n = 117), 46.7% in those with 1–2 NAAs (n = 905), and 26.5% (n = 1263) in subjects with NAs. Within 7 years, 33.2% of subjects with AAs received ≥2 surveillance examinations versus 26.9% for those with ≥3 NAAs, 18.2% for those with 1 or 2 NAAs, and 10.4% for those with NAs. Incomplete colonoscopy, family history of colorectal cancer, or interval adenomatous findings could explain only a minority of surveillance colonoscopy in low-risk subjects.

Conclusions.—In community practice, there is substantial overuse of surveillance colonoscopy among low-risk subjects and underuse among

TABLE 2.—Cumulative Kaplan–Meier Estimates of Probability of Surveillance Colonoscopy

	Baseline Colonoscopy Result			
		NAA (n = 1022)		
	AA (n = 1342)	≥3 NAAs (n = 177)	1–2 NAAs (n = 905)	NA (n = 1263)
Year		%		
1	5.3	2.3	1.0	1.0
2	20.3	13.5	7.0	4.2
3	30.7	19.5	15.1	8.8
4	50.2	45.8	33.6	17.3
5[a]	58.4	57.5	46.7	26.5
6	67.9	67.0	59.2	35.7
7	72.2	74.7	66.6	45.1
8	76.5	77.2	69.8	52.5
9	79.3	81.9	74.2	57.9

[a]Pairwise comparisons at year 5: AA vs 1–2 NAAs, $P < .0001$; AA vs NA, $P < .0001$; ≥3 NAAs vs NA, $P < .0001$; 1–2 NAAs vs NA, $P < .0001$; ≥3 NAAs vs 1–2 NAAs, $P = .03$; ≥3 NAAs vs AA, $P = .8$ (not significant).

subjects with AAs. Interventions to better align use of surveillance colonoscopy with risk for advanced lesions are needed (Table 2).

▶ Colorectal cancer (CRC) screening with colonoscopy is widely endorsed because the identification and removal of adenomatous polyps can reduce the incidence and mortality of CRC. Surveillance colonoscopy is recommended because of the risk of recurrent adenomas and interval cancers. The burden of surveillance colonoscopy is substantial, accounting for at least 25% of all colonoscopies performed. Because of the high costs associated with colonoscopy, guidelines have emphasized risk stratification of additional neoplasia for the surveillance interval based on the number, size, and histology of the adenomas found at the index procedure. Surveillance is recommended at 3 years for advanced adenomas (AA) (> 1 cm or villous histology) or > 3 adenomas, and less frequent examinations are advised for subjects with nonadvanced adenomas (NAA; 5-10 years) or no adenomas (NA; every 10 years). These guidelines have been available for several years and are generally accepted.[1]

The authors of this article made use of the multicenter Prostate, Lung, Colorectal, ,and Ovarian (PLCO) screening trial that is a community-based study of cancer screening and included flexible sigmoidoscopy. Polypoid abnormalities found at flexible sigmoidoscopy had a baseline diagnostic colonoscopy, but the decision for subsequent surveillance was managed by local care providers and not the study design. Through telephone interviews, study subjects in the colonoscopy cohort were queried; the frequency of surveillance examinations and findings were corroborated by reviewing the colonoscopy reports. Individuals with AA, NAA, and NA were included, and the yield of surveillance has been previously reported.[2] This study addressed the relationship between utilization and risk stratification.

Similar to previous studies and as summarized in Table 2, this study shows substantial overuse of surveillance colonoscopy in low-risk patients and significant underuse in high-risk subjects with AA. The implications for overuse are a substantial underestimation of the costs associated with colonoscopy screening programs. Patients with AA are known to have a higher rate of recurrent neoplasia, and the guidelines for a 3-year examination have been in place for several years. Nevertheless, less than one third underwent the surveillance examination within the timeframe.

This study confirms most practicing gastroenterologists' suspicion that published surveillance guidelines are often not followed in an era of open-access colonoscopy. Further research to strengthen the evidence supporting the guidelines and efforts to educate referring physicians to align surveillance intervals with risk of advanced neoplasia are needed.

R. K. Pearson, MD

References

1. Winawer SJ, Zauber AG, Fletcher RH, et al. US Multi-Society Task Force on Colorectal Cancer, American Cancer Society. Guidelines for colonscopy surveillance after polypectomy: a consensus update by the US Multi Society Task Force on Colorectal Cancer and the American Cancer Society. *Gastroenterology.* 2006; 130:1872-1885.
2. Pinsky PF, Schoen RE, Weissfeld JL, et al. The yield of surveillance colonoscopy by adenoma history and time to examination. *Clin Gastroenterol Hepatol.* 2009;7: 86-92.

Cetuximab and Chemotherapy as Initial Treatment for Metastatic Colorectal Cancer

Van Cutsem E, Köhne C-H, Hitre E, et al (Univ Hosp Gasthuisberg, Leuven, Belgium; Klinikum Oldenburg; Országos Onkológiai Intézet, Budapest; et al)

N Engl J Med 360:1408-1417, 2009

Background.—We investigated the efficacy of cetuximab plus irinotecan, fluorouracil, and leucovorin (FOLFIRI) as first-line treatment for metastatic colorectal cancer and sought associations between the mutation status of the *KRAS* gene in tumors and clinical response to cetuximab.

Methods.—We randomly assigned patients with epidermal growth factor receptor–positive colorectal cancer with unresectable metastases to receive FOLFIRI either alone or in combination with cetuximab. The primary end point was progression-free survival.

Results.—A total of 599 patients received cetuximab plus FOLFIRI, and 599 received FOLFIRI alone. The hazard ratio for progression-free survival in the cetuximab–FOLFIRI group as compared with the FOLFIRI group was 0.85 (95% confidence interval [CI], 0.72 to 0.99; $P = 0.048$). There was no significant difference in the overall survival between the two treatment groups (hazard ratio, 0.93; 95% CI, 0.81 to 1.07; $P = 0.31$). There was a significant interaction between treatment group and *KRAS* mutation status for tumor response ($P = 0.03$) but not for progression-free survival ($P = 0.07$) or overall survival ($P = 0.44$). The hazard ratio for progression-free survival among patients with wild-type–*KRAS* tumors was 0.68 (95% CI, 0.50 to 0.94), in favor of the cetuximab–FOLFIRI group. The following grade 3 or 4 adverse events were more frequent with cetuximab plus FOLFIRI than with FOLFIRI alone: skin reactions (which were grade 3 only) (in 19.7% vs. 0.2% of patients, $P < 0.001$), infusion-related reactions (in 2.5% vs. 0%, $P < 0.001$), and diarrhea (in 15.7% vs. 10.5%, $P = 0.008$).

Conclusions.—First-line treatment with cetuximab plus FOLFIRI, as compared with FOLFIRI alone, reduced the risk of progression of metastatic colorectal cancer. The benefit of cetuximab was limited to patients with *KRAS* wild-type tumors. (ClinicalTrials.gov number, NCT00154102.)

▶ Colorectal cancer (CRC) ranks third in frequency and mortality in the United States. Approximately 25% of patients present with metastatic disease and overall 40% to 50% develop metastases in spite of attempts at curative resection and adjuvant therapy. While progress with first-line combination chemotherapy (for example, irinotecan, fluorouracil, and leucovorin [FOLFIRI]) has been made, long-term survival remains uncommon. The epidermal growth factor receptor (EGFR) is growth promoting and is expressed on many colorectal

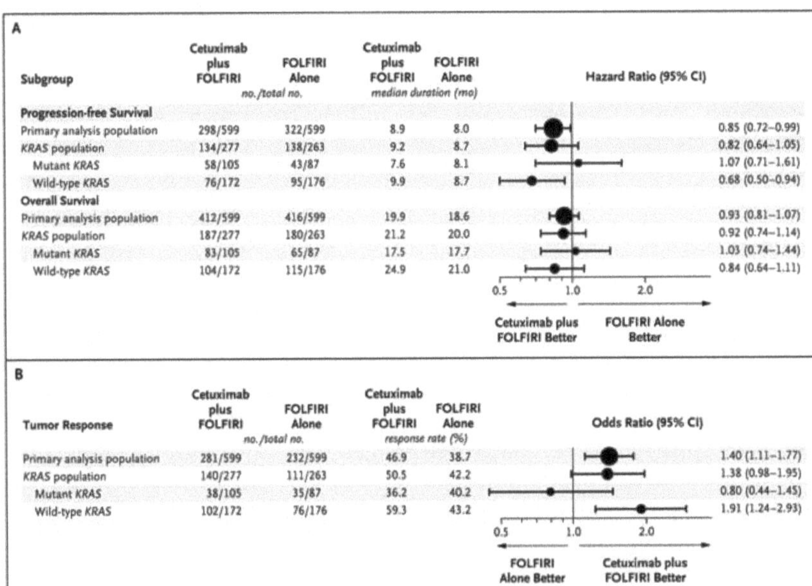

FIGURE 2.—Hazard Ratios for Progression-free and Overall Survival and Odds Ratios with Tumor Response, According to the Mutation Status of *KRAS* in the Tumor. For the primary analysis population, the hazard ratio for progression-free survival with cetuximab plus FOLFIRI as compared with FOLFIRI alone was significant ($P = 0.048$) (Panel A), as was the odds ratio for tumor response with cetuximab plus FOLFIRI ($P = 0.004$) (Panel B). The interaction between treatment group and *KRAS* mutation status was not significant for progression-free survival ($P = 0.07$) or overall survival ($P = 0.44$) (Panel A) but was significant for response ($P = 0.03$) (Panel B). In both panels, the sizes of the circles are proportional to the numbers of patients. (Reprinted from Van Cutsem E, Köhne C-H, Hitre E, et al. Cetuximab and chemotherapy as initial treatment for metastatic colorectal cancer. *N Engl J Med.* 2009;360:1408-1417.)

cancers. Cetuximab is a monoclonal antibody against EGFR that inhibits growth of many cancer cell lines in vitro and is shown to be effective clinically in several cancers, including phase 1 and 2 studies in CRC.

This large scale, international, multicenter phase III study randomized nearly 1200 patients with an initial diagnosis of metastatic CRC to standard FOLFIRI and FOLFIRI plus cetuximab. Fig 2 demonstrates that cetuximab reduced the risk of disease progression by 15% and increased the response rate by nearly 10%. Furthermore, subgroup analysis shows that the efficacy of cetuximab can be predicted by the status of *KRAS* in the tumor. *KRAS* is a proto-oncogene that is a key intracellular regulator of the growth-promoting effects of EGFR. Activating mutations of *KRAS* occur in approximately one third of colon cancer (36% in this study). Cancers with mutant *KRAS* would be predicted to be unresponsive to EGFR antagonism because the stimulatory pathway is constitutively activated downstream from the receptor. The results from this study support this hypothesis. In Fig 2 tumor response and progression-free survival improvement with cetuximab is confined to the subgroup with wild-type *KRAS*. Tumor *KRAS* mutation analysis is recommended as standard of care for patients with colon cancer requiring chemotherapy. It is likely that other gastrointestinal malignancies with frequent *KRAS* mutations (eg, pancreatic cancer) will also be tested to guide the clinical use of EGFR antagonism.

R. K. Pearson, MD

Gastric Cancer

Diagnostic utility of EUS-guided FNA in patients with gastric submucosal tumors

Mekky MA, Yamao K, Sawaki A, et al (Assiut Univ, Egypt; et al)
Gastrointest Endosc 71:913-919, 2010

Background.—Submucosal tumors (SMTs) comprise both benign and malignant lesions, and most of the gastric lesions tend to be malignant. The addition of EUS-guided FNA (EUS-FNA) has the potential to improve this distinction, but published series are limited.

Objective.—To evaluate the yield of EUS-FNA in gastric SMTs with referral to a criterion standard final diagnosis.

Design.—Retrospective study.

Setting.—Tertiary-care referral center.

Patients.—This study involved 141 consecutive patients with gastric SMTs, who underwent EUS-FNA from January 2000 to December 2008. Immunohistochemical staining with c-kit, CD34, actin, and S-100 antibodies was done if a spindle cell tumor was found. Based on FNA sample adequacy, and whether a specific diagnosis could be established, EUS-FNA results were categorized as diagnostic, suggestive, or nondiagnostic. The criterion standards for final diagnosis were the surgical histopathological results or the follow-up course for malignant, inoperable cases.

Intervention.—EUS-FNA.

TABLE 2.—Diagnostic Yield of EUS-FNA and its Presumptive Pathological Diagnosis in Patients with Gastric Submucosal Tumors (n = 141)

	Sufficient Samples (n = 117; 83%)					Insufficient Samples (n = 24; 17%)	
	IHC Stained (n = 64)			IHC not Stained (n = 53)			
Diagnostic Category	GIST	Leiomyoma	Schwannoma	Spindle Cell Tumor	Misc	Unknown	Total, No. (%)
Diagnostic	37	9	2	0	13	0	61 (43.3)
Suggestive	9	7	0	29	10	0	55 (39)
Nondiagnostic	0	0	0	0	1	24	25 (17.7)
Total, no. (%)	46 (32.6)	16 (11.3)	2 (1.4)	29 (20.6)	24 (17)	24 (17)	141 (100)

EUS-FNA, EUS-guided FNA; *IHC*, immunohistochemical; *GIST*, GI stromal tumor; *misc*, miscellaneous tumor; *CI*, confidence interval.
EUS-FNA was classified as *diagnostic* in 61 cases (43.3%; 95% CI, 35%-51%), *suggestive* in 55 cases (39%; 95% CI, 31%-47%), and *nondiagnostic* in 25 cases (17.7%; 95% CI, 12.5%-25%).

Main Outcome Measurements.—Diagnostic yield of EUS-FNA and factors related to sampling adequacy for cytological and immunohistochemical evaluation.

Results.—A total of 141 patients (52% female, mean age 56.7 years) underwent EUS-FNA (range 1-5 passes). The overall results of EUS-FNA were diagnostic, suggestive, and nondiagnostic in 43.3%, 39%, and 17.7% of cases, respectively. Adequate specimens were obtained in 83% of cases, and 69 cases (48.9%) had a definitive final diagnosis. The most common gastric SMT was GI stromal tumor (59.5%). EUS-FNA results were 95.6% accurate (95% confidence interval [CI], 87.5%-99%) for the final diagnosis and 94.2% (95% CI, 85.6%-98.1%) accurate for differentiating potentially malignant lesions. A heterogeneous echo pattern was the only independent predictor for sampling adequacy (adjusted odds ratio 6.15; $P = .002$). There were no procedure-related complications.

Limitations.—Possibility of selection bias.

Conclusion.—EUS-FNA is an accurate method for diagnosis of gastric SMTs and for differentiating malignant lesions (Table 2).

▶ Gastric submucosal tumors are typically observed incidentally at the time of upper endoscopy. The clinician is faced with the challenge of differentiating the type and malignant potential of the submucosal lesion. They have been reported with a frequency of 1 in every 100 to 300 upper endoscopies. Most of these will be asymptomatic; selecting the appropriate patient for resection based on the malignant risk is of paramount importance.

Endoscopic ultrasound (EUS) has the capacity to image the lesion, but imaging characteristics alone are not capable of determining the malignant potential. The role of fine-needle aspiration (FNA), directed by EUS, can provide material for cytological examination and immunohistochemical staining to improve the diagnostic accuracy. The latter is particularly important in the approach to gastrointestinal stromal tumors (GISTs). However, previous studies suffered from small numbers of patients and limited types of tumors sampled.

This is a large but retrospective series from an endoscopic center in Japan that touts the diagnostic use of EUS-guided FNA. As the authors demonstrate in Table 2, adequate samples were obtained by FNA to provide blocks of cells for immunohistochemistry to allow the accurate differentiation of GIST from its benign counterparts: leiomyoma and schwannoma. Essentially all of the non-diagnostic cases were because of inadequate samples. The authors make reference to the growing interest in EUS-directed trucut biopsies that provide a core that would increase the diagnostic use. While this intervention has higher risks, it is increasingly reported as safe and effective.

While limited by its retrospective and potential tertiary care center biases, this study supports the use of EUS in the evaluation of submucosal masses in the stomach and to select appropriate patients for surgical resection.

R. K. Pearson, MD

Pancreaticobiliary Cancer

Cisplatin plus Gemcitabine versus Gemcitabine for Biliary Tract Cancer

Valle J, for the ABC-02 Trial Investigators (Christie Hosp, Manchester, UK; et al)

N Engl J Med 362:1273-1281, 2010

Background.—There is no established standard chemotherapy for patients with locally advanced or metastatic biliary tract cancer. We initially conducted a randomized, phase 2 study involving 86 patients to compare cisplatin plus gemcitabine with gemcitabine alone. After we found an improvement in progression-free survival, the trial was extended to the phase 3 trial reported here.

Methods.—We randomly assigned 410 patients with locally advanced or metastatic cholangiocarcinoma, gallbladder cancer, or ampullary cancer to receive either cisplatin (25 mg per square meter of body-surface area) followed by gemcitabine (1000 mg per square meter on days 1 and 8, every 3 weeks for eight cycles) or gemcitabine alone (1000 mg per square meter on days 1, 8, and 15, every 4 weeks for six cycles) for up to 24 weeks. The primary end point was overall survival.

Results.—After a median follow-up of 8.2 months and 327 deaths, the median overall survival was 11.7 months among the 204 patients in the cisplatin–gemcitabine group and 8.1 months among the 206 patients in the gemcitabine group (hazard ratio, 0.64; 95% confidence interval, 0.52 to 0.80; $P<0.001$). The median progression-free survival was 8.0 months in the cisplatin–gemcitabine group and 5.0 months in the gemcitabine-only group ($P<0.001$). In addition, the rate of tumor control among patients in the cisplatin–gemcitabine group was significantly increased (81.4% vs. 71.8%, $P=0.049$). Adverse events were similar in the two groups, with the exception of more neutropenia in the cisplatin–gemcitabine group; the number of neutropenia-associated infections was similar in the two groups.

Conclusions.—As compared with gemcitabine alone, cisplatin plus gemcitabine was associated with a significant survival advantage without the addition of substantial toxicity. Cisplatin plus gemcitabine is an appropriate option for the treatment of patients with advanced biliary cancer. (ClinicalTrials.gov numbers, NCT00262769).

▶ Cancer of the biliary tract (cholangiocarcinoma) is a relatively uncommon malignancy, accounting for approximately 9000 new cases annually in the United States. Most patients present with advanced disease and even if initially operable will relapse after resection. This grim prognosis is in part because of the lack of any established, effective chemotherapy regimen. While response to a variety of agents for biliary cancer has been reported, the studies were too small to provide enough evidence for a standard-of-care chemotherapy approach. This includes gemcitabine, often used as a single agent in gastrointestinal cancers (including pancreatic cancer), and cisplatin.

This report is a large, phase 3, multicenter trial from the United Kingdom involving over 200 patients in each arm. As shown in Fig 2 in the original article, overall survival and progression-free survival were statistically and clinically significantly improved by combination therapy with gemcitabine and cisplatin. For example, the absolute rate of progression-free survival was increased by nearly 20% by the combination chemotherapy (59.3% vs 42.5%).

With combination therapy, one would expect toxicity and adverse events to be increased; neutropenia was observed more often. However, serious infections were similar. Furthermore, the liver function abnormalities were less common with combination therapy. The authors speculate that the tumor response seen in combination therapy patients may have led to improved maintenance of biliary drainage. Management of the obstructed biliary tree associated with cholangiocarcinoma can be especially challenging. These patients benefit from management in a center with multidisciplinary care teams, including endoscopists, interventional radiologists, oncologists, oncologic surgeons, and radiotherapists. Now clinicians caring for these patients have a standard chemotherapeutic program that has been shown to improve survival and possibly improve management of the morbidity of duct obstruction. It is likely that these agents will be tested in the adjuvant setting in the select patients who qualify for resection.

R. K. Pearson, MD

Frequency of Extrapancreatic Neoplasms in Intraductal Papillary Mucinous Neoplasm of the Pancreas: Implications for Management

Reid-Lombardo KM, Mathis KL, Wood CM, et al (Mayo Clinic, Rochester, MN)

Ann Surg 251:64-69, 2010

Objective.—To estimate the frequency of extrapancreatic neoplasms in patients with IPMN compared with those with ductal pancreatic cancer and a general referral population.

Summary Background Data.—Several studies have reported an increased risk of extrapancreatic neoplasms in patients with IPMN, but these studies focused only on those patients who underwent resection and excluded those patients treated nonoperatively.

Methods.—All patients diagnosed with IPMN at Mayo Clinic from 1994 to 2006 were identified. Two control groups consisting of Group 1–patients with a diagnosis of ductal pancreatic adenocarcinoma (1:1) and Group 2–a general referral population (3:1) were matched for gender and age at diagnosis, year of registration, and residence. Logistic regression was used to assess the risk of a diagnosis of extrapancreatic neoplasms among cases versus controls.

Results.—There were 471 cases, 471 patients in Group 1, and 1413 patients in Group 2. The proportion of IPMN patients having any extrapancreatic neoplasm diagnosed before or coincident to the index date was 52% (95% CI, 47%–56%), compared with 36% (95% CI, 32%–41%) in Group 1 ($P < 0.001$), and 43% (95% CI, 41%–46%) in Group 2

($P = 0.002$). Benign neoplasms most frequent in the IPMN group were colonic polyps (n = 114) and Barrett's neoplasia (n = 18). The most common malignant neoplasms were nonmelanoma skin (n = 35), breast (n = 24), prostate (n = 24), colorectal cancers (n = 19), and carcinoid neoplasms (n = 6).

Conclusions.—Patients with IPMN have increased risk of harboring extrapancreatic neoplasms. Based on the frequency of colonic polyps, screening colonoscopy should be considered in all patients with IPMN.

▶ Intraductal papillary mucinous neoplasm (IPMN) of the pancreas is being recognized with increasing frequency due to the increased utilization of cross-sectional imaging. There is a clear risk of malignant transformation of this dysplastic epithelium lining the main pancreatic duct or its side branches. In addition, several studies from Asia have suggested that patients harboring IPMN have an increased risk of extrapancreatic neoplasms compared with the general population or patients with other pancreatic disorders. However, these studies have not been reproduced in the West and involved only patients undergoing operative therapy for IPMN. Many branch duct IPMN lesions are found incidentally and appear to have a low potential for malignancy and undergo nonoperative management with surveillance imaging.

Investigators at the Mayo Clinic used a retrospective case-control methodology capturing all subjects with IPMN diagnosed by histology (about half) and by clinical criteria undergoing surveillance. The observation that 52% of patients with IPMN were found to have an extrapancreatic neoplasm confirms previous observations utilizing the largest cohort published to date. Of particular interest to gastroenterologists following these patients was the finding of a high rate of colorectal cancer and polyps and Barrett's esophagus. Fully acknowledging the limitations of the retrospective nature of the study, the authors nevertheless recommended that all patients with a new diagnosis of IPMN undergo screening colonoscopy and, for subjects with sufficient symptoms of gastroesophageal reflux, an upper endoscopy.

R. K. Pearson, MD

Preoperative Biliary Drainage for Cancer of the Head of the Pancreas

van der Gaag NA, Rauws EAJ, van Eijck CHJ, et al (Academic Med Ctr, Amsterdam, the Netherlands; Erasmus Med Ctr, Rotterdam, the Netherlands; et al)

N Engl J Med 362:129-137, 2010

Background.—The benefits of preoperative biliary drainage, which was introduced to improve the postoperative outcome in patients with obstructive jaundice caused by a tumor of the pancreatic head, are unclear.

Methods.—In this multicenter, randomized trial, we compared preoperative biliary drainage with surgery alone for patients with cancer of the pancreatic head. Patients with obstructive jaundice and a bilirubin level of 40 to 250 μmol per liter (2.3 to 14.6 mg per deciliter) were randomly assigned to undergo either preoperative biliary drainage for 4 to 6 weeks, followed by surgery, or surgery alone within 1 week after diagnosis. Preoperative biliary drainage was attempted primarily with the placement of an endoprosthesis by means of endoscopic retrograde cholangiopancreatography. The primary outcome was the rate of serious complications within 120 days after randomization.

Results.—We enrolled 202 patients; 96 were assigned to undergo early surgery and 106 to undergo preoperative biliary drainage; 6 patients were excluded from the analysis. The rates of serious complications were 39% (37 patients) in the early-surgery group and 74% (75 patients) in the biliary-drainage group (relative risk in the early-surgery group, 0.54; 95% confidence interval [CI], 0.41 to 0.71; P<0.001). Preoperative biliary drainage was successful in 96 patients (94%) after one or more attempts, with complications in 47 patients (46%). Surgery-related complications occurred in 35 patients (37%) in the early-surgery group and in 48 patients (47%) in the biliary-drainage group (relative risk, 0.79; 95% CI, 0.57 to 1.11; P = 0.14). Mortality and the length of hospital stay did not differ significantly between the two groups.

Conclusions.—Routine preoperative biliary drainage in patients undergoing surgery for cancer of the pancreatic head increases the rate of

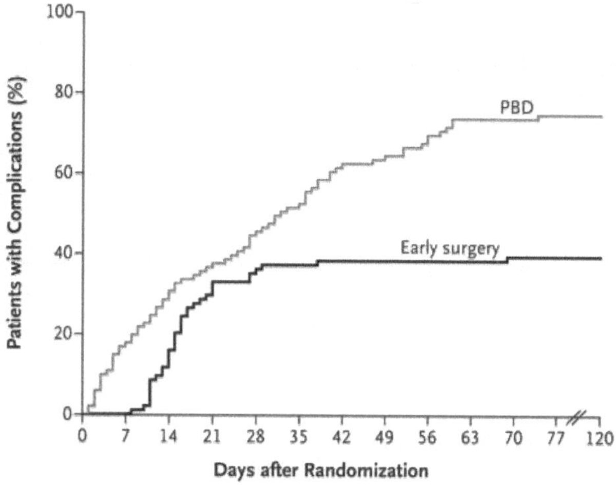

No. at Risk													
PBD	102	84	72	64	56	49	38	36	32	26	25	24	23
Early surgery		94	83	66	61	59	58	58	58	57	55	55	54

FIGURE 2.—Proportion of patients with complications. The primary outcome — the rate of serious complications within 120 days after randomization — occurred in 37 patients (39%) who underwent early surgery alone and 75 patients (74%) who underwent preoperative biliary drainage (PBD) followed by surgery (relative risk in the early-surgery group, 0.54; 95% confidence interval [CI], 0.41 to 0.71; P<0.001). (Reprinted from van der Gaag NA, Rauws EAJ, van Eijck CHJ, et al. Preoperative biliary drainage for cancer of the head of the pancreas. *N Engl J Med.* 2010;362:129-137. Copyright 2010 Massachusetts Medical Society. All rights reserved.)

complications. (Current Controlled Trials number, ISRCTN31939699.) (Fig 2).

▶ Obstructive jaundice is the most common presenting symptom in patients with periampullary or pancreatic head cancer. For pancreatic cancer, these patients account for the majority of those few patients (10%-15%) found to be candidates for surgical resection. Pancreaticoduodenectomy (Whipple resection) is the only option for cure but carries a high risk for perioperative morbidity (at least 20%).[1] Perioperative mortality rates approach 5% even in high-volume centers and have been documented to be as high as 20% in community hospitals.

Experimental and clinical evidence from retrospective series suggested that the metabolic mucosal intestinal barrier and hepatic synthetic perturbations associated with obstructive jaundice contributed to the high rate of complications associated with pancreatic head resection. Relieving obstructive jaundice before surgery has been suggested to reduce surgical complications and mortality. Several randomized controlled trials have been performed but differed in the method of biliary drainage (percutaneous vs endoscopic) and duration of drainage before surgery. A meta-analysis of the 5 randomized trials and a systematic review of the case series indicated increased complications in the preoperative biliary drainage (PBD) cohorts.[2] Nevertheless, PBD has been touted as beneficial by several prominent academic surgical centers.

For these reasons and because many of the trials used percutaneous drainage that usually increases hospital stay and does not reestablish the enterohepatic circulation, investigators from the Netherlands conducted this multicenter randomized controlled trial of endoscopic PBD for 4 to 6 weeks followed by surgical resection versus early surgery. The study was powered to detect a 10% absolute difference in complications. Technically, 94% of the experimental group had successful drainage. Plastic stents were placed at endoscopic retrograde cholangiopancreatography (ERCP) in the majority with percutaneous drainage only after failure of 2 endoscopic attempts. Importantly, the study excluded patients with a bilirubin level greater than 14.6 mg/dL.

Fig 2 from the article shows that the complication rate in the PBD groups was nearly double the rate in the early surgery cohort. The excess complications were related to the drainage procedure itself; cholangitis and pancreatitis accounted for the majority, and nearly one third of the patients required a stent exchange in the preoperative period. The theoretical advantage of relieving obstruction before surgery was not realized; surgery-related complications were increased in the PBD cohort, and there was no difference in mortality or hospital stay.

This study supports the clinical practice patterns at our and many other high-volume pancreatic resection centers. If surgery can be performed in a timely fashion, cholangitis is uncommon if the biliary tree has not been instrumented (2% in this study). Furthermore, the risks of a preoperative ERCP with stent placement outweigh the benefits.

R. K. Pearson, MD

References

1. Trede M, Schwall G. The complications of pancreatectomy. *Ann Surg*. 1988;207: 39-47.
2. Wang Q, Gurusamy KS, Lin H, et al. Preoperative biliary drainage for obstructive jaundice. *Cochrane Database Syst Rev*. 2008;3:CD00544.

Miscellaneous

Antidiabetic Therapies Affect Risk of Pancreatic Cancer

Li D, Yeung S–CJ, Hassan MM, et al (The Univ of Texas M. D. Anderson Cancer Ctr, Houston)

Gastroenterology 137:482-488, 2009

Background & Aims.—Antidiabetic drugs have been found to have various effects on cancer in experimental systems and in epidemiologic studies, although the association between these therapeutics and the risk of human pancreatic cancer has not been explored. We investigated the effect of antidiabetic therapies on the risk of pancreatic cancer.

Methods.—A hospital-based case-control study was conducted at M. D. Anderson Cancer Center from 2004 to 2008 involving 973 patients with pancreatic adenocarcinoma (including 259 diabetic patients) and 863 controls (including 109 diabetic patients). Information on diabetes history and other risk factors was collected by personal interview. The frequencies of use of insulin, insulin secretagogues, metformin, and other antidiabetic medications among diabetic patients were compared between cases and controls. The risk of pancreatic cancer was estimated using unconditional logistic regression analysis.

Results.—Diabetic patients who had taken metformin had a significantly lower risk of pancreatic cancer compared with those who had not taken metformin (odds ratio, 0.38; 95% confidence interval, 0.22–0.69; $P = .001$), with adjustments for potential confounders. This difference remained statistically significant when the analysis was restricted to patients with a duration of diabetes >2 years or those who never used insulin. In contrast, diabetic patients who had taken insulin or insulin secretagogues had a significantly higher risk of pancreatic cancer compared with diabetic patients who had not taken these drugs.

Conclusions.—Metformin use was associated with reduced risk, and insulin or insulin secretagogue use was associated with increased risk of pancreatic cancer in diabetic patients.

► Pancreatic cancer (PC) has the poorest prognosis among primary gastrointestinal (GI) malignancies and is the fourth leading cause of cancer death. Established risk factors for PC include smoking, obesity, chronic pancreatitis, and a family history. The relationship between type 2 diabetes mellitus (DM2) and PC is a complex one. Recent evidence indicates that even early, subclinical PC induces diabetes, probably through a mechanism of insulin resistance.[1,2] In these studies, PC appears to be the cause of new onset glucose

TABLE 4.—Duration of Antidiabetic Therapy and Risk of Pancreatic Cancer

	All Subjects		Diabetes Duration >2 Years	
Duration of Use (y)	No. of Cases/ No. of Controls	OR (95% CI)[a]/ *P* Value	No. of Cases/ No. of Controls	OR (95% CI)[a]/ *P* Value
Insulin				
Never use	147/88	1.0	58/63	1.0
≤2	70/4	11.3 (3.86–33.3)/<.001	36/1	33.5 (4.26–264)/.001
3–5	9/0	—	9/0	—
>5	17/9	1.30 (0.52–3.23)/.572	17/9	2.78 (1.00–7.73)/.049
Metformin				
Never use	138/32	1.0	62/24	1.0
≤2	63/35	0.34 (0.18–0.63)/.001	11/14	0.26 (0.09–0.74)/.012
3–5	23/10	0.44 (0.18–1.09)/.076	23/10	0.89 (0.33–2.42)/.816
>5	29/27	0.18 (0.09–0.38)/<.001	29/27	0.30 (0.13–0.69)/.005
Insulin secretagogues				
Never use	171/84	1.0	78/57	1.0
≤2	50/6	4.94 (1.90–12.8)/.001	14/4	1.91 (0.54–6.76)/.314
3–5	16/7	1.05 (0.40–2.77)/.924	16/7	1.68 (0.61–4.67)/.317
>5	16/8	0.71 (0.27–1.90)/.498	16/8	1.01 (0.35–2.93)/.987

[a]OR was adjusted for age, sex, race, smoking, alcohol, BMI, and family history of cancer.

intolerance in adults approximately 1% of the time (1 in 125).[1] Alternatively, long-standing DM2 has been associated with an increased risk of PC. Furthermore, hyperinsulinemia associated with the metabolic syndrome can be proposed as a mechanism for the observed increased risk of PC and other malignancies in obesity.

Insulin is a growth-promoting hormone and the exocrine pancreas could be chronically exposed to high local concentrations of this mitogenic factor in hyperinsulinemic states. Therapies for DM2 include agents that both increase circulating insulin (eg, exogenous insulin, sulfonylureas) or reduce insulin resistance (biguanides, including metformin). Recent epidemiological studies showed that long-term use of metformin was associated with a reduction in the risk of dying from cancer.[3]

To further explore this provocative hypothesis, this well-designed case-control study from M. D. Anderson examined the relationship between antidiabetic therapies and risk of PC. Metformin use was associated with a significant reduction in PC risk and as shown in Table 4, using the agent for more than 5 years resulted in an 80% risk reduction. The study also suggests that therapies associated with higher insulin levels have a higher-than-average risk of PC. The authors openly acknowledge the potential limitations of this case-control study, including recall bias, limited sample size (973 PC subjects), and the single, tertiary referral hospital sample. These observations require confirmation from other centers and in larger populations. However, this remarkable study suggests that this strategy may provide primary chemoprevention for patients with DM2 against this dreadful disease.

R. K. Pearson, MD

References

1. Chari ST, Leibson CL, Rabe KG, et al. Pancreatic cancer-associated diabetes mellitus: prevalence and temporal association with diagnosis of cancer. *Gastroenterology.* 2008;134:95-101.
2. Pannala R, Leiness JB, Bamlet WR, Basu A, Petersen GM, Chari ST. Prevalence and clinical profile of pancreatic cancer-associated diabetes mellitus. *Gastroenterology.* 2008;134:981-987.
3. Evans JMM, Donnelly LA, Emslie-Smith AM, Alessi DR, Morris AD. Metformin and reduce risk of cancer in diabetic patients. *BMJ.* 2005;330:1304-1305.

Capsule Endoscopy versus Colonoscopy for the Detection of Polyps and Cancer

Van Gossum A, Navas MM, Fernandez-Urien I, et al (Université Libre de Bruxelles, Brussels, Belgium; Univ of Navarra, Pamplona, Spain; et al)

N Engl J Med 361:264-270, 2009

Background.—An ingestible capsule consisting of an endoscope equipped with a video camera at both ends was designed to explore the colon. This study compared capsule endoscopy with optical colonoscopy for the detection of colorectal polyps and cancer.

Methods.—We performed a prospective, multicenter study comparing capsule endoscopy with optical colonoscopy (the standard for comparison) in a cohort of patients with known or suspected colonic disease for the detection of colorectal polyps or cancer. Patients underwent an adapted colon preparation, and colon cleanliness was graded from poor to excellent. We computed the sensitivity and specificity of capsule endoscopy for polyps, advanced adenoma, and cancer.

Results.—A total of 328 patients (mean age, 58.6 years) were included in the study. The capsule was excreted within 10 hours after ingestion and before the end of the lifetime of the battery in 92.8% of the patients. The sensitivity and specificity of capsule endoscopy for detecting polyps that were 6 mm in size or bigger were 64% (95% confidence interval [CI], 59 to 72) and 84% (95% CI, 81 to 87), respectively, and for detecting advanced adenoma, the sensitivity and specificity were 73% (95% CI, 61 to 83) and 79% (95% CI, 77 to 81), respectively. Of 19 cancers detected by colonoscopy, 14 were detected by capsule endoscopy (sensitivity, 74%; 95% CI, 52 to 88). For all lesions, the sensitivity of capsule endoscopy was higher in patients with good or excellent colon cleanliness than in those with fair or poor colon cleanliness. Mild-to-moderate adverse events were reported in 26 patients (7.9%) and were mostly related to the colon preparation.

Conclusions.—The use of capsule endoscopy of the colon allows visualization of the colonic mucosa in most patients, but its sensitivity for

TABLE 2.—The Prevalence of Lesions Detected by Colonoscopy in the 320 Patients in the Accuracy Analysis, and the Sensitivity and Specificity of Capsule Endoscopy for the Detection of These Lesions

Variable	Colonoscopy* Prevalence No. of Patients (%)	Capsule Endoscopy† Sensitivity	Specificity
		% (95% CI)	
Polyp			
Any size	212 (66.2)	72 (68–75)	78 (71–84)
<6 mm	188 (58.8)	61 (57–64)	82 (76–87)
≥6 mm	87 (27.2)	64 (59–72)	84 (81–87)
≥10 mm	50 (15.6)	60 (51–66)	98 (96–99)
Adenoma			
≥6 mm	71 (22.2)	68 (58–76)	82 (79–84)
≥10 mm	45 (14.1)	64 (54–72)	97 (96–99)
Advanced adenoma‡			
Any size	52 (16.2)	85 (73–93)	50 (48–51)§
≥6 mm	49 (15.3)	73 (61–83)	79 (77–81)
≥10 mm	45 (14.1)	64 (54–72)	97 (96–99)
Colorectal cancer¶	19 (5.9)	74 (52–88)	74 (72–75)

*Patients could be included in more than one size category.
†Per-patient data are listed. Colonoscopy was the standard criterion.
‡Advanced adenoma was defined as an adenoma 1 cm or larger or an adenoma with villous features or high-grade dysplasia.
§A high prevalence of polyps less than 6 mm in size, combined with a low likelihood of histologic features of advanced adenoma, decreased the specificity.
¶All colorectal cancers were 6 mm or larger (19 were ≥6 mm, and 18 of these were ≥10 mm).

detecting colonic lesions is low as compared with the use of optical colonoscopy. (ClinicalTrials.gov number, NCT00604162.)

▶ Colonoscopy remains the standard procedure for colorectal polyp and cancer screening in spite of its expense, invasiveness, risk, need for sedation, and recent recognition of its less-than-optimal performance for cancer risk reduction, especially in the right colon. Furthermore, despite reimbursement from virtually all payors, including Medicare, compliance with the recommendation for colonoscopy screening remains not much over 50%. For these reasons, alternatives to colonoscopy, including stool-based assays and CT colonography, compete for the screening population.

Entering the screening arena is the PillCam COLON capsule, an ingestible capsule with imaging capacity on both ends that builds on the success of the PillCam SB for imaging the small intestine (capsule endoscopy). Cleverly programmed, the device switches off for 1 hour 45 minutes during transit through the small bowel to save battery life. Successful application of the PillCam COLON in 2 pilot studies prompted this prospective, large scale ($n = 328$ patients) head-to-head comparison with colonoscopy for polyp and cancer detection from Europe.

Importantly, the device functioned well technically; 93% of the time images of the entire colorectal were obtained. To maximize the colon preparation and optimize performance, subjects took extra bowel preparation (phosphate based) for the capsule portion of the examination. However, as Table 2 demonstrates, colonoscopy outperformed the capsule significantly in all aspects, especially in the all important cancer and advanced adenoma detection rates. Furthermore, reading the capsule video requires, on average, 45 minutes, approximating the time to perform a screening colonoscopy.

Unless improvements are made in the technology, it seems unlikely that capsule colonoscopy will replace the real thing for most colon cancer screenings.

R. K. Pearson, MD

Endoscopic and Surgical Treatment of Mucosal (T1a) Esophageal Adenocarcinoma in Barrett's Esophagus

Prasad GA, Wu TT, Wigle DA, et al (Mayo Clinic College of Medicine, Rochester, MN)

Gastroenterology 137:815-823, 2009

Background & Aims.—Endoscopic therapy is emerging as an alternative to surgical therapy in patients with mucosal (T1a) esophageal adenocarcinoma (EAC) given the low likelihood of lymph node metastases. Long-term outcomes of patients treated endoscopically and surgically for mucosal EAC are unknown. We compared long term outcomes of patients with mucosal EAC treated endoscopically and surgically.

Methods.—Patients treated for mucosal EAC between 1998 and 2007 were included. Patients were divided into an endoscopically treated group (ENDO group) and a surgically treated group (SURG group). Vital status information was queried using an institutionally approved internet research and location service. Statistical analysis was performed using Kaplan–Meier curves and Cox proportional hazard ratios.

Results.—A total of 178 patients were included, of whom 132 (74%) were in the ENDO group and 46 (26%) were in the SURG group. The mean follow-up period was 64 months (standard error of the mean, 4.8 mo) in the SURG group and 43 months (standard error of the mean, 2.8 mo) in the ENDO group. Cumulative mortality in the ENDO group (17%) was comparable with the SURG group (20%) ($P = .75$). Overall survival also was comparable using the Kaplan–Meier method. Treatment modality was not a significant predictor of survival on multivariable analysis. Recurrent carcinoma was detected in 12% of patients in the ENDO group, all successfully retreated without impact on overall survival.

Conclusions.—Overall survival in patients with mucosal EAC when treated endoscopically appears to be comparable with that of patients treated surgically. Recurrent carcinoma occurs in a limited proportion of patients, but can be managed endoscopically.

► In the United States, the incidence of esophageal adenocarcinoma (EAC) is rising faster than any other malignancy and has an overall 5-year survival of less than 20%. For early stage disease, esophagectomy remains the treatment of choice but is associated with mortality rates up to 8% and morbidity of 30%

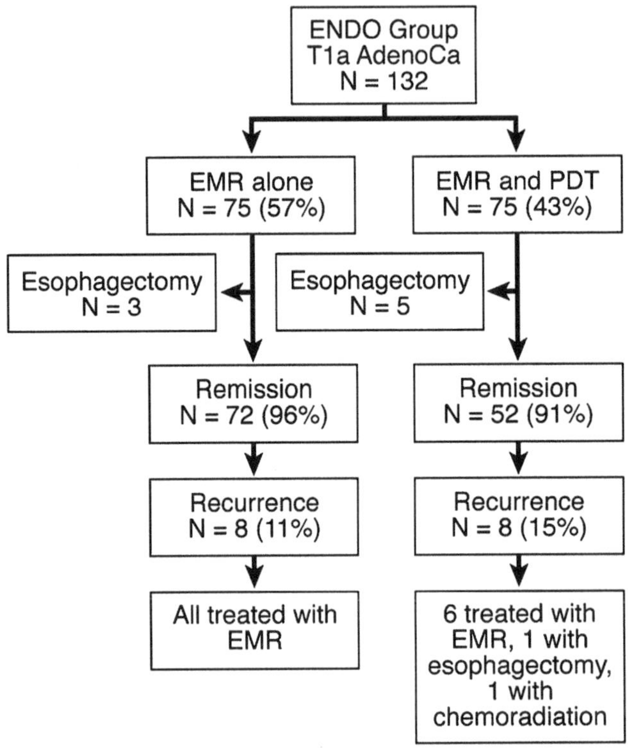

FIGURE 1.—Flowsheet of patients treated with endoscopic therapy. (Reprinted from Prasad GA, Wu TT, Wigle DA, et al. Endoscopic and surgical treatment of mucosal (T1a) esophageal adenocarcinoma in Barrett's esophagus. *Gastroenterology.* 2009;137:815-823, with permission from the AGA Institute.)

to 40%. Average hospital stay after esophagectomy is 20 days as reported recently from the surveillance epidemiology and end results (SEER) database.[1]

Early stage EAC (T1a confined to the mucosa or submucosa) accounts for approximately 20% with a much better long-term prognosis (survival at 5 years approaching 80%) and would be potentially amenable to endoscopic therapy, including endoscopic mucosal resection (EMR) and ablative therapies. Randomized, controlled trials comparing endoscopic management with surgical resection are lacking and would be challenging given the relative infrequency of early-stage EAC.

Led by Dr Kenneth Wang, the Mayo Clinic group reports their experience with EMR and photodynamic therapy compared with surgical resection in this large, retrospective cohort study. Champions of surgical resection can point to very low mortality in high-volume surgical centers (4%: 1 in 46) and excellent cancer free survival (97% at 5 years). However, in spite of the cohort treated endoscopically being older with more comorbidities, overall survival was comparable between the 2 groups. Fig 1 from the article outlines what happened to the patients treated with endoscopic therapy; local cancer recurrence could be managed with photodynamic therapy (PDT) ablation in the majority.

While acknowledging the limitations of this retrospective analysis and in the absence of controlled trials, the authors propose that EMR supplemented with ablative therapy is a viable alternative to esophagectomy for early-stage EAC. It is important to point out that the outcomes with endoscopic therapy in this study were associated with aggressive acid suppression (twice daily proton-pump inhibitor therapy) and endoscopic surveillance (every 3 months for 2 years).

R. K. Pearson, MD

Reference

1. Chang AC, Ji H, Birkmeyer NJ, Orringer MB, Birkmeyer JD. Outcomes after transhiatal and transthoracic esophagectomy for cancer. *Ann Thorac Surg.* 2008;85:424-429.

Age- and sex-specific yield of Barrett's esophagus by endoscopy indication

Rubenstein JH, Mattek N, Eisen G (Veterans Affairs Ctr for Clinical Management Res, Ann Arbor, MI; Oregon Health & Science Univ, Portland)

Gastrointest Endosc 71:21-27, 2010

Background.—Barrett's esophagus is a precursor of esophageal adenocarcinoma, both of which are associated with GERD. Screening GERD patients for Barrett's esophagus has been suggested, but it is not known which patients should be screened and at what age.

Objective.—To determine the age-specific yield of endoscopy for Barrett's esophagus stratified by sex and indication for endoscopy.

Design.—Retrospective cross-sectional study.

Setting.—National Endoscopic Database of the Clinical Outcomes Research Initiative (CORI).

Patients.—A total of 155,641 patients undergoing their first endoscopy at one of the CORI sites for clinical indications.

Main Outcome Measurements.—Age-specific yield of Barrett's esophagus.

Results.—Among white men with GERD, the yield of Barrett's esophagus increases steeply from early adulthood (2.1% in the third decade of life) to middle adulthood (9.3% in the sixth decade) and then plateaus (the difference for the eighth decade minus the sixth decade is −1.1%; 95% CI, −3.9% to 1.7%). There is no difference in the yield of Barrett's esophagus between middle-aged white women with GERD and white men without GERD (difference is −0.46%; 95% CI, −1.23% to 0.31%).

Limitations.—Possible bias by selection for endoscopy and the potential for misclassification of GERD status.

Conclusions.—The yield of upper endoscopy for the diagnosis of Barrett's esophagus increases rapidly among white men with GERD

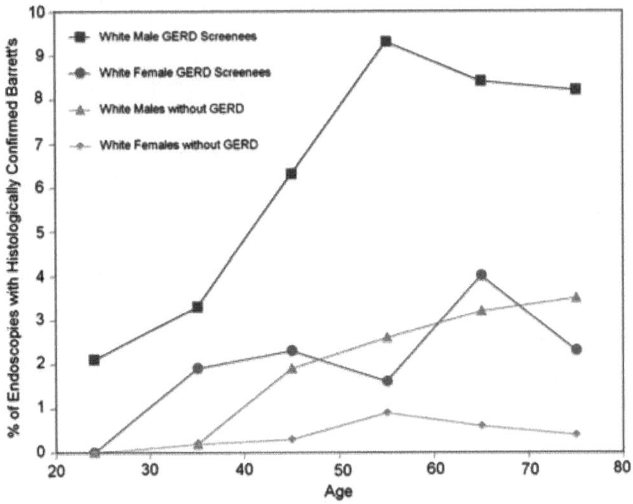

FIGURE 1.—Yield for upper endoscopy for histologically confirmed Barrett's esophagus. The x-axis represents age at the time of endoscopy. Patients were categorized by decade of age, and the proportion of endoscopies with histologically confirmed Barrett's esophagus for each decade is shown at the midpoint of that age category. Each line represents the yield of each sex with and without an indication of evaluation of GERD or screening for Barrett's esophagus (GERD screenees or without GERD). Data were obtained from the subcohort with pathology reports available. (Reprinted from Rubenstein JH, Mattek N, Eisen G. Age- and sex-specific yield of Barrett's esophagus by endoscopy indication. *Gastrointest Endosc.* 2010;71:21-27, with permission from American Society for Gastrointestinal Endoscopy.)

until approximately age 50 and then reaches a plateau. White women with GERD are at no increased risk compared with white men without GERD (Fig 1).

▶ To screen or not to screen for Barrett's esophagus remains an unanswered dilemma. The relatively low prevalence of the finding and the expense of endoscopy with biopsy to confirm the diagnosis are cited as rationale against the practice. However, Barrett's esophagus is the accepted precursor lesion for esophageal adenocarcinoma, a cancer with a rapid increase in incidence and poor survival. The development of endoscopic techniques to ablate the dysplastic epithelium of Barrett's esophagus has rekindled interest in screening. However, there remains no consensus on who should be screened.[1]

It is known that long-standing symptoms of gastroesophageal reflux disease (GERD), advancing age, male sex, and white race increase the relative risk of Barrett's esophagus. This multicenter study made use of a large endoscopic database to try to establish the absolute risk. Of the total study cohort of 155 000 patients undergoing a first time endoscopy, 31% listed GERD or screening for Barrett's esophagus as the primary indication. Overall, 9% of patients were suspected of having Barrett's esophagus. A smaller subset of centers linked pathological findings to endoscopy, and the primary analysis was restricted to this smaller cohort that included >25 000 subjects.

Fig 1 shows the primary finding of this study. The rate for Barrett's esophagus in white men with GERD increases steeply until age 50, while the rate for women is never greater than the rate in men without GERD. Acknowledging the limitations of this retrospective cohort study, the authors propose that if screening is shown to reduce mortality from esophageal adenocarcinoma, it should focus on white men older than 50 years with GERD.

R. K. Pearson, MD

Reference

1. Sharma P, McQuaid K, Dent J, et al. A critical review of the diagnosis and management of Barrett's esophagus: the AGA Chicago Workshop. *Gastroenterology.* 2004;127:310-330.

Complete Barrett's Eradication Endoscopic Mucosal Resection: An Effective Treatment Modality for High-Grade Dysplasia and Intramucosal Carcinoma—An American Single-Center Experience

Chennat J, Konda VJA, Ross AS, et al (Univ of Chicago Med Ctr, IL)
Am J Gastroenterol 104:2684-2692, 2009

Objectives.—Complete Barrett's eradication endoscopic mucosal resection (CBE-EMR) is the endoscopic removal of all Barrett's epithelium with the curative intent of eliminating high-grade dysplasia (HGD)/intramucosal carcinoma (IMC) and reducing the risk of metachronous lesion development. We report our single tertiary referral center's long-term clinical experience using this modality in HGD/IMC management.

Methods.—In this study, we retrospectively reviewed all patients who had CBE-EMR for Barrett's esophagus (BE) with HGD/IMC who had been entered into our center's prospectively collected database. High-definition white-light and narrow-band imaging examinations were used according to the protocol. Staging endoscopic ultrasound was done before CBE-EMR to exclude invasive disease or suspicious lymphadenopathy. High-dose proton pump inhibition was instituted after initial treatment, and Seattle-type surveillance biopsies were performed on follow-up every 6 months once the CBE-EMR procedure was completed.

Results.—A total of 49 patients (mean age 67 years, median 65, s.d. 11; 75% men) with histologically confirmed BE and HGD (33), IMC (16), underwent CBE-EMR from August 2003 to August 2008. The mean BE segment length was 3.2 cm (median 2, s.d. 2.2); 26 patients had short-segment BE, and 30 had visible lesions. A total of 106 EMR procedures were performed. On initial EMR, two patients had superficial submucosal carcinoma invasion (sm1) and two had IMC with lymphatic channel invasion. All four patients were referred for esophagectomy, but one opted for continued endoscopic management, without evidence of residual or recurrent carcinoma. A total of 14 patients await completion of EMR (9) or first follow-up endoscopy (5). CBE-EMR therapy was completed in 32 patients

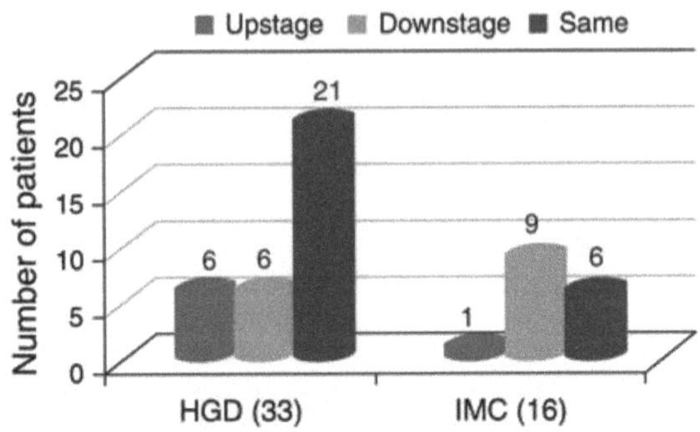

FIGURE 2.—Effect of initial endoscopic mucosal resection (EMR) results on final pathology diagnosis of total 49 patients. The *x* axis depicts highest-grade pathology on pre-EMR biopsies with the number of patients in each subgroup indicated in parentheses. HGD, high-grade dysplasia; IMC, intramucosal carcinoma. Numbers of patients who had upstaging, downstaging, or same diagnosis after initial EMR are labeled above respective columns. (Reprinted from Chennat J, Konda VJA, Ross AS, et al. Complete Barrett's eradication endoscopic mucosal resection: an effective treatment modality for high-grade dysplasia and intramucosal carcinoma—an American single-center experience. *Am J Gastroenterol.* 2009;104:2684-2692. Reprinted by permission from Macmillan Publishers Ltd: American Journal of Gastroenterology, copyright 2009.

by an average of 2.1 sessions (median 2, s.d. 0.9). Surveillance biopsies showed normal squamous epithelium in 31 of 32 (96.9%) patients (mean remission time 22.9 months, median 17, s.d. 16.7, interquartile range 11–38). In all, 10 of 46 patients who continued in the endoscopic protocol had subsquamous Barrett's epithelium on EMR specimens and/or treatment endoscopy biopsies. Overall, 1 of these 10 patients had Barrett's underneath squamous mucosa on most recent surveillance biopsies. CBE-EMR upstaged pre-EMR pathology results in 7 of 49 (14%) of patients and downstaged pathology in 15 of 49 (31%) patients. In all, 18 of 49 (37%) patients developed symptomatic esophageal stenosis after a mean of 24.4 days (median 13.5, s.d. 27.8); all were successfully managed by endoscopic treatment. No perforations or uncontrollable bleeding occurred.

Conclusions.—To our knowledge, this is the largest American single-center experience demonstrating that CBE-EMR with close endoscopic surveillance is an effective treatment modality for BE with HGD/IMC. Although the rate of stenosis development is significant, it is easily treated by endoscopic dilation. Patients considering endoscopic ablation should be counseled appropriately. The role of CBE-EMR in patients with lymphatic invasion or superficial submucosal invasion remains to be defined (Fig 2).

▶ With the well-described and marked increased (6-fold) incidence of esophageal adenocarcinoma in the United States, there is increasing interest in the management of the precursor Barrett's epithelium. Particularly challenging for clinicians is the management of Barrett's esophagus with high-grade dysplasia or early intramucosal carcinoma. Esophagectomy was the treatment of choice but carries a 3% mortality rate and serious morbidity of 40% to 50%. For this reason, endoscopic treatment of these conditions was introduced approximately 10 years ago and has become increasingly important.

Endoscopic techniques have evolved to meet this clinical challenge and consist of either ablating Barrett's epithelium with a variety of techniques or endoscopic mucosal resection (EMR). Definitive treatment is highly dependent on accurate staging of the disease; submucosal, vascular, or lymphatic invasion are candidates for radical surgery. Resection allows for very accurate staging and referral of patients at risk for recurrence and metastases to more aggressive surgical management. Even state-of-the-art endoscopic ultrasound techniques do not eliminate this understaging.

High recurrence rates with either technique, if only the dysplastic epithelium is treated, have led to the concept of complete Barrett's resection followed by ablative techniques to mop up the residual for curative intent. This study represents a retrospective report of all patients (n = 49) at the University of Chicago who underwent EMR for early neoplasia complicating Barrett's esophagus. Residual disease at the margin of the resection was treated with argon plasma coagulation, while islands of Barrett's esophagus were treated with radiofrequency ablation.

In this specialized center, this combination of treatment was highly effective; in the 32 patients completing treatment, 31 remain free of any evidence of Barrett's in surveillance endoscopy. Fig 2 shows the importance of pathological assessment of the resected specimen with nearly half of the patients having their stage of disease changed. Four patients were referred for surgical resection based on the tissue analysis. Strictures were the most common complication but were all managed with routine endoscopic dilation.

This and other reports from around the world have led to the position that endoscopic resection followed by thermal ablation should be considered the treatment of choice for early neoplasia complicating Barrett's esophagus.

R. K. Pearson, MD

Medications (NSAIDs, Statins, Proton Pump Inhibitors) and the Risk of Esophageal Adenocarcinoma in Patients With Barrett's Esophagus

Nguyen DM, Richardson P, El-Serag HB (Veterans Affairs Med Ctr, Houston, TX)

Gastroenterology 138:2260-2266, 2010

Background & Aims.—Limited evidence suggests that proton pump inhibitors (PPI), nonsteroidal anti-inflammatory drugs (NSAID)/aspirin, and statins may be associated with a low risk of esophageal neoplasia. However, the possible effect these medications may have on the risk of esophageal adenocarcinoma (EAC) in patients with existing Barrett's esophagus (BE) is unclear.

Methods.—We conducted a nested case-control study in a cohort of patients with BE identified in the national Department of Veterans' Affairs computerized databases. Cases with incident EAC were matched by incidence density sampling to controls with BE who remained without EAC

TABLE 3.—The Association Between Duration of Filled Prescriptions and the Risk of EAC

Duration of Filled Prescriptions, mo	Cases n (%)	Controls n (%)	Incidence Density Ratio (95% CI)	Cochrane–Armitage Trend Test, *P* Value
Number of patients	116	696		
PPI				
0	6 (5.2)	43 (6.2)	Reference	
>0 to 12	62 (53.5)	328 (47.1)	1.39 (0.33–3.41)	
>12 to 24	31 (26.7)	219 (31.5)	0.89 (0.33–2.36)	
>24	17 (14.7)	106 (15.2)	1.00 (0.33–3.00)	
NSAIDs/aspirin[a]				.30
0	59 (50.9)	285 (41.0)	Reference	
>0 to 12	43 (37.1)	295 (42.4)	0.70 (0.46–1.07)	
>12	14 (12.1)	116 (16.6)	0.55 (0.29–1.06)	
Statins[a]				.02
0	75 (64.7)	360 (51.7)	Reference	
>0 to 12	23 (19.8)	175 (25.1)	0.63 (0.38–1.06)	
>12	18 (15.5)	161 (23.2)	0.52 (0.30–0.91)	

NOTE. Cases were patients with BE and EAC, and controls were patients with BE and no EAC at the time of diagnosis or corresponding case.

[a]More than 24 months was not examined because <5% of patients were in this category.

at the date of the EAC diagnosis for the corresponding case. We identified prescriptions for PPI, NSAIDs/aspirin, and statins that were filled between BE diagnosis and EAC diagnosis. Incidence density ratios were calculated using conditional logistic regression models that adjusted for race, outpatient encounters, a disease comorbidity index, and socioeconomic status.

Results.—In a cohort of 11,823 patients with first-time BE diagnosis, we examined 116 EAC cases and 696 matched controls. Most cases and controls had at least one filled PPI prescription (95% vs 94%; $P = .5$). In this setting of almost universal PPI use, filled NSAID/aspirin prescriptions were associated with a reduced risk of EAC (adjusted incidence density ratio, 0.64; 95% confidence interval, 0.42–0.97). Filled statin prescriptions also were associated with a reduction in EAC risk (0.55; 95% confidence interval, 0.36–0.86), with a significant trend toward greater risk reduction with longer duration of statin use. However, the strong inverse associations with even short periods of use raise concerns of uncontrolled confounding.

Conclusions.—This observational study indicates that in patients with BE using PPI, NSAID/aspirin, or statin therapy might reduce the risk of developing EAC (Table 3).

▶ The Veterans Affairs (VA) system of health care delivery is a national integrated system that approximates the national databases that Canadian and European investigators exploit for large-scale epidemiological studies. The VA system largely included male patients and has limitations. However, Barrett's esophagus (BE) and the risk of esophageal adenocarcinoma (EAC) is predominantly a disease of older men, making this database an acceptable resource for this association.

Chemoprevention for BE would be an attractive development, given that EAC has increased by 6-fold over the past 3 decades.[1] Aspirin or nonsteroidal anti-inflammatory drug (NSAID) is a recognized protective agent for colorectal cancer, and observational studies have suggested a protective effect in EAC. These studies have been limited by the lack of information on the presence or the absence of BE in the control groups. Thus, it's not clear whether the protective effect is because of the prevention of BE or the progression of BE to EAC. Several studies have also suggested that inhibitors of 3-hydroxy-3-methylgluaryl coenzyme A reductase (statins) used commonly in patients with coronary artery disease protect against the development of cancer; studies specific for EAC complicating BE are lacking.

In this large-scale (11 823 patients with a first-time BE diagnosis) study, 116 cases of EAC complicating this large cohort were compared (1:6) with controls without a cancer diagnosis for the use of proton pump inhibitors, aspirin/NSAIDs, and statins. The strengths of the study are the large cohort and the accuracy of the database that measures prescriptions filled or dispensed (not prescribed), increasing the likelihood that the data represent drug usage. As Table 3 demonstrates, NSAIDs/aspirin and statin usage was protective against the development of EAC in a linear dose-dependent fashion, strengthening the possibility of a true chemopreventive effect of these agents.

There are several limitations to this study, including the restricted population studied (VA health care system) and prescriptions abstracted from the VA Pharmacy Benefit Management database; prescriptions filled outside this system would have escaped capture. However, previous studies have shown a 64% capture rate among Medicare-covered veterans. Similar to most nested case-control studies involving prescription medications, lifestyle habits linked to the use of preventive medication could not be accounted for. Statin and NSAID/aspirin use could be functioning as a surrogate for these behaviors (eg, tobacco, alcohol use, obesity).

Cohort studies such as these often generate hypotheses that lead to clinical trials, the cyclooxygenase inhibitor trials in colorectal cancer prevention being 1 important example. While the authors recommend caution when interpreting an observational study such as this, these findings warrant additional studies to evaluate the potential for statins in the prevention of esophageal cancer.

R. K. Pearson, MD

Reference

1. Pera M. Trends in incidence and prevalence of specialized intestinal metaplasia, Barrett's esophagus, and adenocarcinoma of the gastroesophageal junction. *World J Surg*. 2003;27:999-1008.

Smoking and Colorectal Cancer in Lynch Syndrome: Results from the Colon Cancer Family Registry and The University of Texas M.D. Anderson Cancer Center

Pande M, Lynch PM, Hopper JL, et al (The Univ of Texas M.D. Anderson Cancer Ctr, Houston; Univ of Melbourne, Victoria, Australia; et al)

Clin Cancer Res 16:1331-1339, 2010

Purpose.—Lynch syndrome family members with inherited germline mutations in DNA mismatch repair (MMR) genes have a high risk of colorectal cancer (CRC), and cases typically have tumors that exhibit a high level of microsatellite instability (MSI). There is some evidence that smoking is a risk factor for CRCs with high MSI; however, the association of smoking with CRC among those with Lynch syndrome is unknown.

Experimental Design.—A multicentered retrospective cohort of 752 carriers of pathogenic MMR gene mutations was analyzed, using a weighted Cox regression analysis, adjusting for sex, ascertainment source, the specific mutated gene, year of birth, and familial clustering.

Results.—Compared with never smokers, current smokers had a significantly increased CRC risk [adjusted hazard ratio (HR), 1.62; 95% confidence interval (95% CI), 1.01-2.57] and former smokers who had quit smoking for 2 or more years were at decreased risk (HR, 0.53; 95% CI, 0.35-0.82). CRC risk did not vary according to age at starting. However, light smoking (<10 cigarettes per day) and shorter duration of smoking (<10 years) were associated with decreased CRC risk (HR, 0.51; 95% CI, 0.29-0.91 and HR, 0.52; 95% CI, 0.30-0.89, respectively). For former smokers, CRC risk decreased with years since quitting (*P* trend < 0.01).

Conclusions.—People with Lynch syndrome may be at increased risk of CRC if they smoke regularly. Although our data suggest that former smokers, short-term smokers, and light smokers are at decreased CRC risk, these findings need further confirmation, preferably using prospective designs.

▶ Up to 20% of colorectal cancers in the United States may be caused in part by the usage of tobacco.[1] Patients with the Lynch syndrome (attenuated colonic polyposis) with inherited germline mutations in DNA mismatch repair (MMR) genes are at increased risk for developing colorectal cancer (CRC) when compared with normal populations. Whether cigarette smoking is associated with increased CRC in patients with Lynch syndrome is not known.

Pande and colleagues performed a multicenter, retrospective cohort analysis of 752 patient carriers of the pathogenic MMR gene mutation to determine whether a history of smoking was associated with an increased risk of CRC. They concluded that people with Lynch syndrome are at increased risk for developing CRC if they smoked regularly.

A clinically relevant finding in the study was an observed dose-response effect of smoking. Former smokers, short-term smokers, and light smokers were proportionately at decreased risk for developing CRC, whereas individuals who continued to smoke regularly were at the highest risk. These data provide strong support for implementing antismoking programs, particularly among patients with genetic risks for CRC. It is not known whether continued provision of nicotine, such as supplied in the patches, negates the benefits of stopping smoking.

The retrospective design and reliance upon questionnaires to assess smoking habits are limitations to this study. Despite these concerns, the results are persuasive. The statistical analyses are sound, and the results provide compelling new information to help patients and their families. Most importantly, the younger the patients were when they quit smoking, the less likely they were to develop CRC.

J. L. Rombeau, MD

Reference

1. Giovannucci E. An updated review of the epidemiological evidence that cigarette smoking increases risk of colorectal cancer. *Cancer Epidemiol Biomarkers Prev.* 2001;10:725-731.

Locally Recurrent Rectal Cancer: Prognostic Factors and Long-Term Outcomes of Multimodal Therapy

Pacelli F, Tortorelli AP, Rosa F, et al (Catholic Univ of Rome, Italy)
Ann Surg Oncol 17:152-162, 2010

Background.—Pelvic recurrent rectal cancer is still a challenging clinical problem, and patients generally have a dismal prognosis and a poor quality of life. Surgical resection represents the only potentially curative treatment; neoadjuvant treatments are presently being taken into consideration to increase the resectability rate and to improve long-term survival.

Methods.—Among 157 patients observed with recurrent rectal cancer, a series of 58 patients who underwent surgical exploration with curative intent for isolated local recurrence at a single referral institution was retrospectively analyzed. Demographic, pathologic, and therapeutic factors were evaluated to assess long-term prognosis and local control.

Results.—Forty-four (75.9%) of 58 patients underwent surgical resection. The overall 5-year survival rate for patients who underwent surgical resection was 54.2%, whereas none of the unresected patients lived 5 years ($P < 0.001$). Patients with R0 resection showed a statistically higher 5-year overall survival and local control rate (72.4 and 70.2%, respectively) compared to R1 patients (37.5 and 31.2%, respectively). At multivariate survival analysis, feasibility of a surgical resection and radicality of excision proved to be independent positive prognostic factors. In contrast, increased presalvage carcinoembryonic antigen serum levels, back pain at diagnosis, and an increasing degree of fixation of recurrent disease to the pelvic wall at preoperative computed tomographic scan were statistically significantly linked to decreased overall survival. Preoperative chemoradiation and radicality of the surgical excision independently influenced the local control among surgically resected patients.

Conclusions.—Surgical resection still remains the most important therapeutic and prognostic factor for patients with locally recurrent rectal cancer. Multimodal treatments can be safely performed by an experienced team in referral tertiary centers and can result in a safer outcome, better local disease control, and even long-term survival in carefully selected patients.

▶ The treatment of locally recurrent rectal cancer is controversial. Most patients receive initial preoperative neoadjuvant therapy (chemotherapy-enhanced radiation), thus, either negating or reducing the option for further radiation therapy. Despite optimal staging, re-operative patients may have an unresectable tumor, thus, in retrospect, the patient is subjected to an unnecessary operation. Nonoperative patients with locally recurrent rectal cancer may occasionally have unrelenting pain due to neoplastic infiltration of pelvic nerves. This untoward effect can occur despite optimal adjuvant therapy.

Pacelli and colleagues retrospectively reviewed the outcomes of 58 patients with locally recurrent rectal cancer who underwent surgical exploration with curative intent. They concluded that surgical resection remains the most important therapeutic and prognostic factor in this clinical condition.

The importance of this report is the identification of those factors that either increased or decreased the favorability of postoperative outcome. Factors for a potential curative resection are not universally agreed upon. CT evidence of fixation of the tumor to the pelvic wall and inordinately high CEA levels were adverse predictors of resectability, whereas preoperative chemoradiation and radicality of the surgical excision independently influenced the local control. The overall 5-year survival for the surgical group was 54%, whereas none of the unresected group lived 5 years.

It is concluded that surgery can be performed in patients with locally resectable rectal cancer with reasonable benefit if appropriate preoperative criteria are met.

J. L. Rombeau, MD

Risk factors for sexual dysfunction after rectal cancer treatment

Lange MM, Cooperative clinical investigators of the Dutch. Total mesorectal excision trial (Leiden Univ Med Ctr, The Netherlands; et al)
Eur J Cancer 45:1578-1588, 2009

This study aimed to identify risk factors for long-term sexual dysfunction (SD) after rectal cancer treatment.

Patients with resectable rectal cancer were randomised to total mesorectal excision with or without preoperative radiotherapy (PRT). Preoperatively and at 3, 6, 12, 18 and 24 months postoperatively, SD scores were filled out in questionnaires. Possible risk factors for postoperative deterioration of sexual functioning, including patients' demographics, tumour-specific factors and treatment-related variables, were investigated with univariate and multivariable regression analyses.

Increase in general SD, erectile dysfunction and ejaculatory problems were reported by 76.4, 79.8 and 72.2 percent of the male patients, respectively. Risk factors were nerve damage, blood loss, anastomotic leakage, PRT and the presence of a stoma. In female patients, increase in general SD, dyspareunia and vaginal dryness were reported by 61.5, 59.1 and 56.6 percent, respectively. This was associated with PRT and the presence of a stoma.

SD occurs frequently after rectal cancer treatment and is caused by surgical (nerve) damage with an additional effect of PRT. Patients should be informed preoperatively, and education of surgeons in neuroanatomy may provide the key to the improvement of functional outcome.

▶ Operative treatment of rectal cancer is associated with sexual dysfunction in both men and women. This is characterized by erectile dysfunction, ejaculatory problems, dyspareunia, and vaginal dryness. Causes of these problems include pelvic nerve damage due to extensive pelvic dissection performed with total mesoexcision. Most patients operated upon for T2 and T3 rectal cancers receive preoperative radiation therapy (PRT), which decreases the size of the tumor but obliterates tissue planes and impairs wound healing. Whether PRT is associated with postproctectomy sexual dysfunction continues to be investigated.

Lange and colleagues from the Netherlands investigated the effect of PRT in a prospective randomized trial in patients undergoing proctectomy for nonmetastatic rectal cancer. In addition to other causative factors, PRT significantly enhanced sexual dysfunction in both genders.

This report has both weaknesses and strengths. Postoperative questionnaires are always of concern as to the accuracy of patient interpretation when compared with more objective measures. Although the first 5 operations performed by each surgeon were scrutinized by a more experienced surgeon, the question arises as to whether further training might decrease adverse postoperative sequelae. These operations are often difficult and successes are strongly associated with the experience of the surgeon. The prospective design of this study elevates it above the numerous retrospective reviews, which comprise the bulk of the literature on this subject.

This report is of interest to gastroenterologists, radiation oncologists, and surgeons. Most patients with rectal cancer are initially diagnosed by colonoscopy performed by gastroenterologists who are also responsible for informing the patient as to treatment risks and recommending a surgeon experienced in proctectomy. As the result of nerve injury being an important cause of sexual dysfunction, it is incumbent upon the surgeon to be well versed in pelvic neuroanatomy. Finally, PRT has not been shown to improve survival. Preoperative staging of possible node-negative patients may identify individuals who may not need to undergo PRT, thus reducing their risks of sexual dysfunction.

J. L. Rombeau, MD

5 Inflammatory Bowel Disease

Crohn's Disease

Adjunctive Antibiotic Therapy with Rifaximin May Help Reduce Crohn's Disease Activity

Shafran I, Burgunder P (Shafran Gastroenterology Ctr, Winter Park, FL)

Dig Dis Sci 55:1079-1084, 2010

Aims.—Enteric bacteria are thought to contribute to the pathogenesis of Crohn's disease, and antibiotics may be an effective therapy. This study examines the efficacy of the nonsystemic (<0.4% absorbed) antibiotic rifaximin for inducing remission in patients with Crohn's disease.

Methods.—Data from charts of patients with Crohn's disease who received rifaximin between 2001 and 2005 and had a Crohn's disease activity index score ≥220 at the time of rifaximin initiation were analyzed. The use of concomitant medications (e.g., steroids, anti-inflammatory agents) was allowed.

Results.—In the 68 patient charts analyzed, the median duration of rifaximin treatment was 16.6 weeks, and the majority of patients (94%) received rifaximin 600 mg/day. Eighteen patients (26%) received rifaximin monotherapy, and 31 patients (46%) received concomitant steroids. The median baseline Crohn's disease activity index score at the time of rifaximin initiation was 265 (range, 220–460), and the mean duration of Crohn's disease was 17 years (range, 1–50 years). Crohn's disease remission occurred in 65% of patients. A 70% remission rate was achieved in patients who did not receive steroids, versus 58% in patients who received steroids. Clinical improvements continued 4 months after rifaximin initiation. Remission was achieved in 67% of patients who received rifaximin monotherapy.

Conclusions.—Rifaximin therapy was associated with clinical improvement in patients with Crohn's disease and may be a useful treatment option to consider for inducing and maintaining remission.

▶ Antibiotic therapies have long been studied as treatments for Crohn's disease (CD). Metronidazole and ciprofloxacin have received the most attention and have had variable results. There may be a role for antibiotics in patients with colonic or ileocolonic disease, especially after surgery to prevent recurrence. Metronidazole has been the most studied and, while showing some efficacy, is often poorly tolerated by patients because of significant side effects. Rifaximin is an attractive alternative given its broad spectrum of activity and minimal systemic absorption. In this article, the authors suggest that rifaximin may be a treatment option among patients with active CD. Unfortunately, significant problems exist with the study that limited any conclusions that were made. The study was retrospective, and while all patients had a CD activity index score suggesting moderate disease, there may be other factors that influence treatment assignment with rifaximin that cannot be determined. Unfortunately, one cannot understand the impact of rifaximin because of a lack of a comparison group. We cannot determine the effect of other therapies on reported remission rates. Patient characteristics seemingly did not influence remission rates, and while a higher rate of remission was seen in those who did not receive steroids, the difference was small and, given the sample size, unlikely to be statistically significant. If this difference were significant, it might simply reflect a higher disease severity among those taking corticosteroids. High placebo rates in other studies among patients with IBD and the retrospective open-label study design further limit conclusions regarding the use of rifaximin as monotherapy in this article. The limited experience reported by the authors is of value in that it suggests the need to perform randomized clinical studies testing this nonabsorbable antibiotic in the management of CD.

M. F. Picco, MD, PhD

Capsule endoscopy in patients with Crohn's disease: diagnostic yield and safety

Mehdizadeh S, Chen GC, Barkodar L, et al (Cedars-Sinai Med Ctr, Los Angeles, CA)

Gastrointest Endosc 71:121-127, 2010

Background.—Capsule endoscopy (CE) is increasingly used in patients with suspected or known Crohn's disease (CD).

Objective.—To determine the diagnostic yield of CE and the distribution of small-bowel (SB) lesions in symptomatic patients with known CD.

Design and Setting.—Retrospective review of CE procedures performed in patients with CD between 2001 and 2005 in a tertiary care center.

Patients.—One hundred thirty-four patients with an established diagnosis of CD and symptoms suggestive of active disease.

Interventions.—Swallowing the capsule.

Main Outcome Measurements.—Diagnostic yield of CE and distribution of SB lesions in patients with CD.

Results.—One hundred forty-six CE procedures were performed on 134 CD patients. Fifty-two (39%) of 134 patients had CE findings diagnostic of active CD (>3 ulcerations), and 17 (13%) had findings suggestive of active CD (≤3 ulcerations). Fifty-seven (42%) patients had normal findings, and 6% had normal but incomplete studies. The distribution of SB lesions was 32% in the duodenum, 53% in the jejunum, 67% in the proximal ileum, and 85% in the distal ileum. CE was comparable to ileoscopy in detecting ileal ulcerations (55% vs 48%), but superior to SB follow-through in detecting CD lesions in the SB (incremental yield of 32%; 95% CI, 9%-54%; $P = .0017$).

Limitations.—Retrospective study from a single center.

Conclusions.—CE identified SB lesions in approximately half of symptomatic CD patients. Large-scale prospective studies are needed to evaluate whether positive CE findings may affect disease outcomes.

▶ In this interesting study, capsule endoscopy (CE) is performed in patients with Crohn's disease (CD) who have active signs and symptoms but minimal or no evidence for activity in the colon. The most striking finding was the high proportion of negative studies. This may have been related to selecting out a population with negative radiographic and endoscopic evaluations. However, the study was retrospective so that evaluation prior to CE was not the same in all patients, with only 41 patients having had small bowel follow-through and only 31 patients having had colonoscopy with ileoscopy within 90 days of the CE procedure. The overall yields may have been lower if all patients had these procedures resulting in some not requiring CE because of positive findings. Yield was clearly related to the indication for the CE procedure, but even among patients with diarrhea, the diagnostic yield was only 73%. That being said, patients presenting with symptoms consistent with active CD (without obstructive symptoms or findings) should be considered for CE since findings may alter therapy. Patients with negative studies may be spared more aggressive therapies. However, in this article, patient outcomes were not specifically studied, so it is not clear whether CE findings lead to better patient care. As the authors point out, more studies are needed.

M. F. Picco, MD, PhD

Clinical, Endoscopic, and Histological Differentiations Between Crohn's Disease and Intestinal Tuberculosis

Makharia GK, Srivastava S, Das P, et al (All India Inst of Med Sciences, New Delhi)

Am J Gastroenterol 105:642-651, 2010

Objectives.—The clinical, endoscopic, and histological features of Crohn's disease (CD) and intestinal tuberculosis mimic each other so much that it becomes difficult to differentiate between them. The aim was to find out clinical, endoscopic, and histological predictor features for differentiation between CD and intestinal tuberculosis.

Methods.—We recruited 106 patients, 53 each with CD and intestinal tuberculosis, in this study. The clinical, histological, and endoscopic features were subjected to univariate, bivariate, and multivariate analyses.

On the basis of regression coefficients of the final multivariate logistic model, a score to discriminate between CD and intestinal tuberculosis was devised. For the validation of the score, the same model was tested on 20 new patients, each with CD and intestinal tuberculosis.

Results.—On univariate analysis, although longer duration of disease, chronic diarrhea, blood in stool, perianal disease, extra-intestinal manifestations, involvement of left colon, skip lesions, aphthous ulcers, cobblestoning, longitudinal ulcers, focally enhanced colitis, and microgranulomas were significantly more common in CD, partial intestinal obstruction, constipation, presence of nodular lesions, higher number, and larger granulomas were significantly more common in intestinal tuberculosis. On multivariate analysis, blood in stool (odds ratio (OR) 0.1 (confidence interval (CI) 0.04–0.5)), weight loss (OR 9.8 (CI 2.2–43.9)), histologically focally enhanced colitis (OR 0.1 (CI 0.03–0.5)), and involvement of sigmoid colon (OR 0.07(0.01–0.3)) were independent predictors of intestinal tuberculosis. On the basis of regression coefficients of the final multivariate logistic model, a score that varied from 0.3 to 9.3 was devised. Higher score predicted more likelihood of intestinal tuberculosis. Once the cutoff was set at 5.1, then the sensitivity, specificity, and ability to correctly classify the two diseases were 83.0, 79.2, and 81.1%, respectively. Area under the curve for receiver-operating characteristic (ROC) to assess the ability of these features to discriminate between CD and intestinal tuberculosis was 0.9089. The area under ROC in the validation data set was 89.2% (95% CI 0.79–0.99). With a similar cutoff score of 5.1, sensitivity and specificity in the validation model were 90% (95% CI 66.9–98.2) and 60% (95% CI 36.4–80.0), respectively.

Conclusions.—Blood in stool, weight loss, focally enhanced colitis, and involvement of the sigmoid colon were the most important features in differentiating CD from intestinal tuberculosis.

▶ Intestinal tuberculosis can easily be confused with Crohn's disease (CD). The diagnosis remains difficult because no diagnostic test is completely sensitive. Acid-fast staining, culture, and PCR techniques may fail to identify many patients who are infected. An incorrect diagnosis of CD leading to corticosteroid and/or biologic/immunomodulator therapy may have disastrous consequences leading to miliary tuberculosis. In this article, the authors identify clinical, endoscopic, and histological criteria that suggest the diagnosis of intestinal tuberculosis. In a multivariate analysis they identified predictors that taken together were suggestive of the diagnosis. These data were then validated in a different series of patients. Unfortunately, while useful, these criteria remain nonspecific, and accurate diagnosis depends on a clinician with a high index of suspicion. In Western countries, tuberculosis is becoming more common because of immigrant populations from endemic areas. Clinicians must consider the diagnosis in all new patients with findings of CD, particularly ileal disease. A positive p-phenylenediamine and/or chest X-ray with typical findings should alert the physician to the possibility of tuberculosis, but these tests may be negative in elderly or immunosuppressed patients. This article does present important disease characteristics to consider when trying to distinguish between these 2 conditions. Where the likelihood is high and testing is negative, empiric antituberculosis therapy has been advocated, and surgical biopsy may be required.

M. F. Picco, MD, PhD

Early Crohn disease: a proposed definition for use in disease-modification trials

Peyrin-Biroulet L, Loftus EV Jr, Colombel J-F, et al (Mayo Clinic, Rochester, MN; Hopital Claude Huriez, Lille, France)
Gut 59:141-147, 2010

Crohn disease is a chronic condition characterised by intestinal inflammation and progressive bowel damage associated with impaired functioning.

In rheumatoid arthritis, which shares some common aetiological pathways and treatments with Crohn disease, treatment goals no longer include symptom control alone, but also alteration of the biological processes underlying synovial inflammation and progressive structural destruction, thereby preventing structural joint damage and functional decline. Analogous disease-modifying treatment goals for Crohn disease are currently being conceptualised and may include prevention of structural bowel damage (stricture, fistula, abscess) and impaired gastrointestinal physiology (ie, maintaining normal gastrointestinal physiology).

In order to achieve disease modification, an effective intervention must occur at the right time, that is, before the development of bowel damage and impaired functioning. While it has been said in this context 'the earlier, the better', there is no formal definition of early Crohn disease. This article will review the rationale for defining early Crohn disease and the rationale for specifically targeting early Crohn disease from both immunopathological and clinical points of view, using rheumatoid arthritis (another chronic, progressive, destructive disease), as an example. We will then propose a definition of early Crohn disease and briefly discuss its potential application in future clinical trials.

▶ Medication therapy for Crohn's disease (CD) has moved beyond induction of remission to disease modification. Early intervention (a top down approach) with biologic and/or immunomodulator therapy may alter the natural history of this disease in select patients. Identification of patients who are most likely to benefit is paramount, given the potential toxicity of these agents. In this article, the authors propose a definition of early CD drawing a comparison with rheumatoid arthritis (RA). In RA, aggressive early intervention with biologic therapies has been shown to prevent disability and joint damage. In CD, limited data are available but suggest that patients with early disease benefit from aggressive intervention. Central to the proposed definition of early CD is no history of fistula (including perianal fistula), abscess, or fibrotic stricture. Also, patients with early disease should not have taken immunomodulators (azathioprine, 6-mercaptopurine, and methotrexate), biologics, been steroid dependent, or received intravenous steroids in the past. Patients may not have had any CD-related surgery. While age at diagnosis is not included in the definition, duration should be 2 years or less. Finally, there should be no requirement for nutrition or vitamin supplementation indicating normal bowel function. As the authors admit, this definition is not a consensus statement and may require modification. The prognosis in early CD may vary based on other disease characteristics, including location, age at diagnosis, and genetic characteristics. These factors are not considered in the early disease definition. Patients with disease confined to the colon or who have onset after age 40 may have a better prognosis. Those with early onset disease or with a strong genetic predisposition (nucleotide-binding oligomerization domain 2 [NOD2]) are likely to have a worse prognosis. The presence of perianal fistula excludes a patient from the early disease group, yet perianal fistulae are classified as different from internal fistulae in the currently accepted Montreal Classification of CD. Perianal fistulae are also much more responsive to biologic therapy. The early disease definition does identify patients who would probably benefit for early aggressive therapy. It may be too restrictive but is a framework for discussion, modification, and future studies on early disease intervention.

M. F. Picco, MD, PhD

Fecal Calprotectin Correlates More Closely With the Simple Endoscopic Score for Crohn's Disease (SES-CD) than CRP, Blood Leukocytes, and the CDAI

Schoepfer AM, Beglinger C, Straumann A, et al (McMaster Univ, Hamilton, Ontario, Canada; Univ Hosp Basel, Switzerland; et al)
Am J Gastroenterol 105:162-169, 2010

Objectives.—Studies evaluating the correlation between the widely used Simple Endoscopic Score for Crohn's disease (SES-CD) and noninvasive markers are scarce. The aim of this study was to evaluate the correlation between the SES-CD and fecal calprotectin, C-reactive protein (CRP), blood leukocytes, and the Crohn's disease activity index (CDAI).

Methods.—Crohn's disease patients undergoing complete ileocolonoscopy were prospectively enrolled and scored independently according to the SES-CD and the CDAI. SES-CD was defined as follows: inactive 0–3; mild 4–10; moderate 11–19; and high ≥20.

Results.—Values in CD patients ($n = 140$ ileocolonoscopies) compared with controls ($n = 43$) are as follows: calprotectin, 334 ± 322 vs. 18 ± 5 μg/g; CRP, 26 ± 29 vs. 3 ± 2 mg/l; and blood leukocytes, 9.1 ± 3.4 vs. 5.4 ± 1.9 g/l (all $P < 0.001$). The SES-CD correlated closest with calprotectin (Spearman's rank correlation coefficient $r = 0.75$), followed by CRP ($r = 0.53$), blood leukocytes ($r = 0.42$), and the CDAI ($r = 0.38$). Calprotectin was the only marker that could discriminate inactive endoscopic disease from mild activity (104 ± 138 vs. 231 ± 244 μg/g, $P < 0.001$), mild from moderate activity (231 ± 244 vs. 395 ± 256 μg/g, $P < 0.008$), and moderate from high activity (395 ± 256 vs. 718 ± 320 μg/g, $P < 0.001$). The overall accuracy for the detection of endoscopically active disease was 87% for calprotectin (cutoff 70 μg/g), 66% for elevated CRP, 54% for blood leukocytosis, and 40% for the CDAI ≥150.

Conclusions.—Fecal calprotectin correlated closest with SES-CD, followed by CRP, blood leukocytes, and the CDAI. Furthermore, fecal calprotectin was the only marker that reliably discriminated inactive from mild, moderate, and highly active disease, which underlines its usefulness for activity monitoring.

▶ A reliable noninvasive method to assess activity in Crohn's disease (CD) is sorely needed. Endoscopy is costly and invasive. Fecal calprotectin has been shown in some studies to correlate with disease activity in CD. However, the appropriate use of fecal calprotectin in the management of patients with CD remains unsettled. In this study, the authors show a significant correlation of this marker with endoscopic disease severity among a population of patients with CD involving the colon, ileum, or both. Unfortunately, the study does suffer from problems that limit the application of this test for the assessment of disease activity in practice. It is not clear why patients with CD were compared with healthy controls except to provide data of specificity for the fecal calprotectin. The best group of patients to test specificity would be patients with CD with endoscopic quiescent disease who would likely be from a surveillance population. This would establish a fecal calprotectin level for true endoscopically negative patients. A larger population of these patients would lead to better comparisons, especially with patients with mildly active disease. While accuracy is important, sensitivity and specificity should also have been reported with a receiver operator characteristic curve. As threshold levels of fecal calprotectin increase, sensitivity is likely to go down and specificity likely to increase. This relationship is important to assess the validity of the test. It is not surprising that predictive values for the test were high, given the high prevalence of active disease in the patients tested. The accuracy reported is for distinction between active and inactive disease only. Most patients with active disease had moderate or high disease activity. Patients with moderate or high activity are probably less likely to be confused with irritable bowel syndrome. The role of fecal calprotectin in distinguishing mild from quiescent disease is not addressed in the study. Furthermore, endoscopic activity may not correlate with clinical improvement. Overall, the study does provide useful information on the correlation of endoscopic findings with fecal calprotectin, but more studies are needed to identify the role of this test in practice.

M. F. Picco, MD, PhD

Immunomodulators Are Associated With a Lower Risk of First Surgery Among Patients With Non-Penetrating Non-Stricturing Crohn's Disease

Picco MF, Zubiaurre I, Adluni M, et al (Mayo Clinic, Jacksonville, FL)

Am J Gastroenterol 104:2754-2759, 2009

Objectives.—Early immunomodulator therapy may alter the natural history of Crohn's disease in certain patients. We determined whether immunomodulator use was associated with a lower risk of first surgery among patients with non-stricturing non-penetrating Crohn's disease.

Methods.—A total of 159 consecutive patients with non-penetrating non-stricturing Crohn's disease from 1994 to 2005 were retrospectively identified and followed from diagnosis to either first surgery (surgery group) or last clinic follow-up (medication group) in a historical cohort analysis. Immunomodulator use, duration, disease location, age at diagnosis, smoking, family history, and decade of diagnosis were compared. Cox proportional hazards models were adjusted for propensity score to determine whether immunomodulator use lasting >6 months decreased the risk of first surgery and whether duration of therapy affected risk.

Results.—The median duration of follow-up was similar (6.0 vs. 5.5 years), age at diagnosis 10 years earlier, and isolated colonic disease three times less common (18 vs. 49%) in the surgery group as compared with the medication group. Immunomodulator use increased with time but overall was less common in the surgical group (24 vs. 48%). In the multivariate Cox proportional hazards model immunomodulator use was associated with a lower risk of surgery (hazard ratio, 0.41; 95% confidence interval 0.21–0.81) after adjustment for propensity score. Similarly, risk of surgery declined with duration of use.

Conclusions.—Immunomodulator use is associated with a decreased risk of first surgery among patients with non-stricturing non-penetrating CD. Early immunomodulator therapy may be beneficial in preventing first surgery in this population that has yet to develop penetrating or fistulizing complications.

▶ Current therapeutic goals in Crohn's disease (CD) have gone beyond induction or remission and now focus on altering natural history. Biologic therapies have been shown to reduce long-term complications. Unfortunately, despite their wide use, there is little evidence that immunomodulator therapies alter the course of CD. In fact, the evidence is conflicting. In this study from our group, we confined our analysis to patients with nonstricturing, nonpenetrating CD. These patients had yet to develop more aggressive behavior and might benefit most from immunomodulator therapy. In our analysis we showed that immunomodulator use (azathioprine or 6-mercaptopurine) did reduce the risk of first surgery. A drawback of the study is that while it was a cohort study, it was a retrospective or historical cohort. While we were careful to account for potential factors that might influence immunomodulator use or surgery leading to a biased result, the potential does remain. We used the propensity score method to adjust for these other factors that may have been associated with immunomodulator therapy independent of the need for surgery and showed that immunomodulator therapy still resulted in a lower risk. Ideally, a prospective randomized trial would answer the question as to whether these agents alter natural history. Unfortunately, such a trial would require significant time and cost, making it unlikely. This study supports the role of immunomodulator therapy in nonstricturing, nonpenetrating CD to alter natural history by reducing the risk of first surgery.

M. F. Picco, MD, PhD

Long-term outcome of endoscopic dilatation in patients with Crohn's disease is not affected by disease activity or medical therapy

Van Assche G, Thienpont C, D'Hoore A, et al (Univ Hosp Gasthuisberg, Leuven, Belgium)

Gut 59:320-324, 2010

Background.—Endoscopic dilatation of Crohn's disease-related strictures is an alternative to surgical resection in selected patients. The influence of disease activity and concomitant medical therapy on long-term outcomes is largely unknown.

Aim and Methods.—To study the long-term safety and efficacy of stricture dilatation in a single centre cohort.

Results.—Between 1995 and 2006, 237 dilatations where performed in 138 patients (mean age 50.6 ± 13.4, 56% female) for a clinically obstructive stricture (<5 cm, 84% anastomotic). Immediate success of a first dilatation was 97% with a 5% serious complication rate. After a median follow-up of 5.8 years (IQR 3.0–8.4), recurrent obstructive symptoms led to a new dilatation in 46% or surgery in 24%. Niether elevated levels of C-reactive protein nor endoscopic disease activity predicted the need for new intervention. None of the concomitant therapies influenced the outcome.

Conclusion.—This largest series ever reported confirms that long term efficacy of endoscopic dilatation of Crohn's disease outweighs the complication risk. Neither active disease at the time of dilatation nor medical therapy afterwards predict recurrent dilatation or surgery.

▶ In this article, endoscopic dilatation was both effective and safe among a large series of patients with clinically obstructive symptoms and strictures. However, this is a retrospective series with carefully selected patients and not a randomized trial. Patients had obstructive symptoms and a documented stricture less than 5 cm long. While disease activity at the site of the stricture did not alter dilatation results, a breakdown as to what proportion had significant endoscopic disease activity is not given. Since this procedure is typically reserved for patients with fibrostenotic strictures, most likely the proportion with active inflammation was low. Medication usage did not influence the results probably because the strictures were the result of fibrostenotic disease. Medication usage was only recorded at the time of dilatation so that the impact of medications on need for further therapy could not be assessed. The complication rate from this and other very experienced centers was high even in these carefully selected patients. However, the procedure may be justified in some patients in an attempt to prevent or delay surgery. Patient selection and physician experience are the most important factors influencing outcome. Only experienced physicians should perform the procedure on patients with short (< 5 cm) uncomplicated strictures without significant endoscopic disease activity.

M. F. Picco, MD, PhD

Outcome of surgery for rectovaginal fistula due to Crohn's disease

Ruffolo C, Penninckx F, Van Assche G, et al (Univ Hosp Gasthuisberg, Leuven, Belgium)

Br J Surg 96:1190-1195, 2009

Background.—This study examined the outcome of surgery for symptomatic Crohn's rectovaginal fistula (RVF) and assessed the effect of therapy with antibody against tumour necrosis factor (TNF) on healing.

Methods.—Fifty-six patients with Crohn's disease underwent surgery for a RVF between January 1993 and December 2006. Outcome analysis was performed in February 2008 in relation to the surgical procedures used and the effect of anti-TNF treatment.

Results.—Four patients with a healed fistula still had a stoma at final follow-up for other reasons and were excluded from the analysis. Fistula closure was achieved in 81 per cent of the remaining 52 patients. Primary and secondary surgical success rates were 56 and 57 per cent respectively. The primary healing rate was similar in patients who received anti-TNF treatment before the first operation (12 of 18 patients) and those who did not (19 of 34). In univariable analysis, duration of Crohn's disease ($P = 0.037$) and previous extended colonic resection ($P < 0.001$) were significantly related to failure of primary surgery, but only the latter remained significant in multivariable analysis ($P < 0.001$). Late recurrence developed in four patients.

Conclusion.—Fistula closure was achieved in most patients, but more than one operation was often required.

▶ Rectovaginal fistulas are a debilitating problem among women with Crohn's disease. Infliximab therapy has led to closure in up to 50% of the patients. Unfortunately, in the remaining patients, surgery remains the best option. The best chance to maintain surgical closure rests in treating luminal inflammation that fuels the fistula. In this study, the authors report surgical success rates for rectovaginal fistula closure. Surprisingly, they found no relationship of surgical success to active rectal disease at operation. While infliximab did not seem to influence surgical success rates, no information is provided as to whether patients had response to these agents (resolution of intestinal inflammation) and/or continued these agents after therapy. Inflixmab use was associated with active small/large intestinal and rectal disease, which might be because patients referred for surgery were infliximab failures. The description that "23 (44 percent) had received anti-TNF up to 12 weeks before and/or at some stage after surgical closure..." is not specific. One might expect different success rates among those who had clearly failed infliximab and those who had a clinical response but without fistula closure. If they did not continue infliximab postoperatively, the repair would probably be more likely to fail. This cannot be determined probably because of the relatively small sample size. Overall, high success rates reported for fistula closure are encouraging. The role of infliximab on surgical outcomes requires further study.

M. F. Picco, MD, PhD

Suspected Anastomotic Recurrence of Crohn Disease after Ileocolic Resection: Evaluation with CT Enteroclysis

Soyer P, Boudiaf M, Sirol M, et al (Hôpital Lariboisière-AP-HP-GHU Nord and Diderot-Paris 7 Univ, France)

Radiology 254:755-764, 2010

Purpose.—To determine the utility of computed tomographic (CT) enteroclysis for characterization of the status of the anastomotic site in patients with Crohn disease who had previously undergone ileocolic resection.

Materials and Methods.—Written informed consent was prospectively obtained from all patients, and the institutional review board approved the study protocol. CT enteroclysis findings in 40 patients with Crohn disease who had previously undergone ileocolic resection were evaluated independently by two readers. Endoscopic findings, histopathologic findings, and/or the Crohn disease activity index was the reference standard. Interobserver agreement between the two readers was calculated with κ statistics. Associations between CT enteroclysis findings and anastomotic site status were assessed at univariate analysis. The sensitivity, specificity, and accuracy of CT enteroclysis, with corresponding 95% confidence intervals (CIs), for the diagnosis of normal versus abnormal anastomosis and the diagnosis of anastomotic recurrence versus fibrostenosis were estimated.

Results.—Interobserver agreement regarding CT enteroclysis criteria was good to perfect ($\kappa = 0.72–1.00$). At univariate analysis, stratification and anastomotic wall thickening were the two most discriminating variables in the differentiation between normal and abnormal anastomoses ($P < .001$). Stratification ($P < .001$) and the comb sign ($P = .026$) were the two most discriminating variables in the differentiation between anastomotic recurrence and fibrostenosis. In the diagnosis of anastomotic recurrence, severe anastomotic stenosis was the most sensitive finding (95% [20 of 21 patients]; 95% CI: 76.18%, 99.88%), both comb sign and stratification had 95% specificity (18 of 19 patients; 95% CI: 73.97%, 99.87%), and stratification was the most accurate finding (92% [37 of 40 patients]; 95% CI: 79.61%, 98.43%). In the diagnosis of fibrostenosis, both severe anastomotic stenosis and anastomotic wall thickening were 100% sensitive (eight of eight patients; 95% CI: 63.06%, 100.00%), and using an association among five categorical variables, including severe anastomotic stenosis, anastomotic wall thickening with normal or mild mucosal enhancement, absence of comb sign, and absence of fistula, yielded 88% sensitivity (seven of eight patients; 95% CI: 47.35%, 99.68%), 97% specificity (31 of 32 patients; 95% CI: 83.78%, 99.92%), and 95% accuracy (38 of 40 patients; 95% CI: 83.08%, 99.39%).

Conclusion.—CT enteroclysis yields objective and relatively specific morphologic criteria that help differentiate between recurrent disease and fibrostenosis at the anastomotic site after ileocolic resection for Crohn disease.

▶ A reliable noninvasive assessment of Crohn's disease (CD) activity would allow patients to avoid colonoscopy. Colonoscopy, in addition to being performed for active symptoms, is often done several months after surgery to assess likelihood of disease recurrence at the anastomosis among patients who have had ileocolonic resection. Advances in radiology techniques, including CT enteroclysis enterography and MRI enterography have provided better assessments of CD activity and behavior. In this study, the authors use CT enteroclysis to attempt to distinguish between active inflammation and scarring (stenosis) among patients who previously had ileocolonic resection. Forty patients, 24 with clinical symptoms and 16 without symptoms (for assessment of anastomotic recurrence) who had ileocolonic resection were compared with 143 patients with CD who had not had this surgery. All underwent CT enteroclysis and had colonoscopy as part of routine clinical care. Enteroclysis results were compared with disease assessment (active vs fibrostenotic disease) that was obtained primarily through endoscopic score (Rutgeert score) and CD activity index (CDAI). Radiologists were blinded to clinical assessment and several criteria were analyzed and agreement between the 2 radiologists was excellent. They could distinguish between a normal and abnormal anastomosis with great sensitivity. They also did find criteria that distinguished active disease from stenosis that may be useful. However, these results do not mean that colonoscopy should be abandoned in this setting. CD symptoms are quite heterogeneous and active inflammation may exist with degrees of stenosis. The combination of CT and endoscopy is usually required to make a treatment decision. The excellent agreement of the radiologists regarding the findings needs to be confirmed in other studies. Finally, the frequent CT scans performed on these patients does expose them to high levels of radiation, which may have long-term consequences. MRI enterography may replace CT in the future as a more acceptable alternative.

M. F. Picco, MD, PhD

Magnetic resonance for assessment of disease activity and severity in ileocolonic Crohn's disease

Rimola J, Rodriguez S, García-Bosch O, et al (Hosp Clínic de Barcelona, Spain)

Gut 58:1113-1120, 2009

Objective.—Assessment of disease extension and activity is crucial to guide treatment in Crohn's disease. The objective of the current cross-sectional study was to determine the accuracy of MR for this assessment.

Design.—50 patients with clinically active ($n = 35$) or inactive ($n = 15$) Crohn's disease underwent ileocolonoscopy (reference standard) and MR. T2-weighted and precontrast and postcontrast-enhanced T1-weighted sequences were acquired. Endoscopic activity was evaluated by CDEIS (Crohn's Disease Endoscopic Index of Severity); in addition endoscopic lesions were classified as absent, mild (inflammation without ulcers) or severe (presence of ulceration).

Results.—The comparison of intestinal segments with absent, mild and severe inflammation demonstrated a progressive and significant ($p < 0.001$) increase in the following MR parameters: wall thickness, post-contrast wall signal intensity, relative contrast enhancement, presence of oedema, ulcers, pseudopolyps and lymph node enlargement. Independent predictors for CDEIS in a segment were wall thickness ($p = 0.007$), relative contrast enhancement ($p = 0.01$), presence of oedema ($p = 0.02$) and presence of ulcers at MR ($p = 0.003$). There was a significant correlation ($r = 0.82$, $p < 0.001$) between the CDEIS of the segment and the MR index calculated according to the logistic regression analysis coefficients. The MR index had a high accuracy for the detection of disease activity (area under the receiver operating characteristic (ROC) curve 0.891, sensitivity 0.81, specificity 0.89) and for the detection of ulcerative lesions (area under the ROC curve 0.978, sensitivity 0.95, specificity 0.91) in the colon and terminal ileum.

Conclusion.—The accuracy of MR for detecting disease activity and assessing severity brings about the possibility of using MR as an alternative to endoscopy in the evaluation of ileocolonic Crohn's disease.

▶ Assessment of disease activity is crucial in the management of patients with Crohn's disease (CD). Current testing methods have significant drawbacks. Colonoscopy is invasive, requires sedation but is generally safe and may rarely lead to complications. CT scanning leads to significant radiation exposure because of the need for repeated assessments over time. Magnetic resonance (MR) techniques have generated significant excitement because they are not invasive and do not expose the patient to radiation. In this study, MR is compared with colonoscopy for the assessment of disease activity among a population of patients with ileocolonic CD. MR proved reasonably accurate in detecting mucosal inflammation in these patients. However, combining MR findings (MR Index of Activity) had a sensitivity of 81% resulting in 19% with clear active mucosal disease being missed by this technique. The more important measure would be the likelihood of disease activity if the MRI findings were positive. This is the predictive value of MR and would be affected by the clinician's suspicion for active disease. For patients with clearly active disease, the predictive value would be high, but many clinicians would treat their disease with minimal testing. For those who present with unclear disease activity, testing is often performed. The pretest probability may be lower resulting in a lower predictive value of the test. For patients with small bowel disease out of the reach of the endoscope, lower sensitivity may be acceptable because the gold standard is far more invasive (double-balloon endoscopy or surgical biopsy). Only 50 patients participated in this study, and the authors' MR technique needs to be validated in many more patients and at different centers. Unfortunately, application of this technology to the assessment of patients with inflammatory bowel disease (IBD) is in its infancy with significant differences in its application, methods used, and results. Early findings with MR enterography have shown promise and MR has a clear role in the assessment of perianal CD and is an important alternative to CT. While the results of this study are interesting, the role of MR in the determination of activity in ileocolonic CD disease remains to be adequately defined.

M. F. Picco, MD, PhD

Ulcerative Colitis

Appendicectomy as a Therapy for Ulcerative Proctitis

Bolin TD, Wong S, Crouch R, et al (The Prince of Wales Hosp, Sydney, New South Wales, Australia; et al)

Am J Gastroenterol 104:2476-2482, 2009

Objectives.—Available data regarding whether appendicectomy performed after the onset of ulcerative colitis can modulate its clinical course are currently limited. This study aimed at addressing this issue.

Methods.—In this study, we report a prospective case series of 30 adult patients (median age 35 years, range 17–70 years; male/female: 11/19) with ulcerative proctitis (median duration of symptoms 5 years, range 8 months to 30 years; median Simple Clinical Colitis Activity Index score 9, range 7–12), who underwent appendicectomy in the absence of any history suggestive of previous appendicitis. Patients were subsequently followed up clinically with the assessment of the Simple Clinical Colitis Activity Index for a median of 14 months (range 9–32 months).

Results.—After appendicectomy, the clinical activity index improved significantly to a median score of 2 (range 0–12) ($P < 0.0005$). The improvement in the clinical activity index occurred in 27 of 30 (90%) patients, whereas the index remained unchanged in the remaining 3 of 30 (10%) patients. Furthermore, 12 of 30 (40%) patients experienced a complete resolution of symptoms (clinical activity index score of 0) by 12 months, such that all pharmacological treatments could be withdrawn, and have remained in remission off all previous treatments for a median 9 months (range 6–25 months). The time required for a complete resolution of symptoms post appendicectomy ranged from 1 to 12 months (median 3 months) (Kaplan–Meier analysis). None of the clinical or histological factors analyzed were significantly associated with post-appendicectomy outcome.

Conclusions.—This case series, the largest reported so far, provides rationale for controlled trials to properly evaluate the possible role of appendicectomy in the treatment of ulcerative proctitis.

▶ Appendectomy has long been associated with a lower risk for developing ulcerative colitis (UC). Controversy exists as to whether the benefit is among only those who had confirmed appendicitis who have yet to develop UC. Among those who develop UC, previous appendectomy may have resulted in a milder clinical course. This study is a case series of 30 patients with established active ulcerative proctitis who undergo appendectomy without history of previous appendicitis. The findings were striking, with 90% of the patients showing significant clinical improvement and 40% showing complete resolution of symptoms of their UC. The findings are provocative, but the conclusions drawn are limited by the study design and measurement of outcomes after appendectomy. Patients were not randomized or blinded to their treatment assignment (appendectomy). Previous trials on therapies for UC have demonstrated high placebo response rates. This is very important because only 2 patients had postappendectomy endoscopic assessment. We also were not told if self-limited enteric infections (particularly *Clostridium dificile*) before appendectomy were excluded. Length of follow-up was reasonable. The selection of patients with severe refractory symptoms was appropriate given the aggressive treatment of appendectomy. Patients with such severe symptoms may also be less likely to have a placebo response. The authors' conclusion that controlled trials are warranted is justified but should be reserved for patients with severe symptoms who are refractory to conventional therapy. Appendectomy, while a benign procedure, is not without risk, and such a trial may be justified for those with severe symptoms where this minor risk is outweighed by the potential benefit.

M. F. Picco, MD, PhD

Clinical outcomes of ileorectal anastomosis for ulcerative colitis

da Luz Moreira A, Kiran RP, Lavery I (Cleveland Clinic, OH)

Br J Surg 97:65-69, 2010

Background.—The aim of this study was to determine the fate of the rectum, functional results and quality of life after ileorectal anastomosis (IRA) in ulcerative colitis.

Methods.—Patients with ulcerative colitis and indeterminate colitis who underwent IRA from 1971 to 2006 were evaluated retrospectively. Twenty-two patients with an IRA were matched by age, sex and follow-up duration with 66 patients with an ileal pouch–anal anastomosis (IPAA) and compared for functional outcomes and quality of life.

Results.—Eighty-six patients with an IRA were included. Median follow-up was 9 (range 1–36) years. Rectal dysplasia and cancer rates were 17 and 8 per cent respectively. The rectum was resected in 46 patients (53 per cent) because of refractory proctitis in 24, rectal dysplasia in 15 and rectal cancer in seven. The cumulative probability of having a functioning IRA at 10 and 20 years was 74 and 46 per cent respectively. Patients with an IRA had fewer bowel movements ($P = 0{\cdot}020$) and less night-time seepage ($P = 0{\cdot}020$) but increased urgency ($P < 0{\cdot}001$) compared with patients with an IPAA, whereas quality of life was similar.

Conclusion.—In selected patients with ulcerative colitis IRA gives an acceptable quality of life and functional outcome that are comparable to those in patients with an IPAA. Owing to the risk of cancer, surveillance of the rectum is mandatory.

▶ Complete proctocolectomy with ileal pouch-anal anastomosis (IPAA) remains the procedure of choice for patients with ulcerative colitis who require surgery. Unfortunately, this procedure is associated with complications, including very high infertility rates in women. An attractive option to decrease the likelihood of complications would be to leave the rectum in place and create an ileorectal anastomosis. In this retrospective analysis, the authors observed a small cohort of patients who had this procedure for a median of 11 years. Not surprisingly, compared with IPAA, patients with ileorectal anastomosis had better quality of life. Nearly half retained their rectum during the follow-up period. Unfortunately, this strategy was not without adverse consequences, the most concerning of which was rectal dysplasia or rectal cancer in 25%, but the rates of advanced cancer were low. These results need to be interpreted with extreme caution. In this small retrospective study, conclusions regarding safety are limited. Prospective larger studies are needed. Frequent surveillance of the rectum is mandatory. If this procedure is applied to young patients, overall risk of dysplasia/cancer will likely be higher, given the expected long duration of disease. One option would be apply this procedure to young patients as a temporary or interim treatment with eventual completion colectomy and IPAA. The safety and efficacy of this approach remains to be determined but is a very important question for our patients with ulcerative colitis.

M. F. Picco, MD, PhD

Clinical Outcomes of Patients with Ulcerative Colitis and Co-existing *Clostridium difficile* Infection

Jodorkovsky D, Young Y, Abreu MT (Inflammatory Bowel Disease Ctr, NY)
Dig Dis Sci 55:415-420, 2010

Background.—The incidence of *Clostridium difficile* infection is increasing in the United States. The aim of our investigation is to compare short-term and long-term outcomes of patients admitted with an ulcerative colitis (UC) flare and co-existent *C. difficile* infection to those of non-infected patients.

Methods.—A historical cohort study was undertaken examining admissions at Mount Sinai Hospital between June 2004 and June 2005 using ICD-9 criteria for UC. Charts were abstracted for those patients for whom *C. difficile* testing was performed.

Results.—Of 288 admissions, 99 charts met the inclusion criteria. Fifty-two patients were *C. difficile*-negative and 47 were positive. Demographic data and laboratory values upon admission did not differ between the two groups. Patients who were *C. difficile*-positive had significantly more UC-related hospitalizations and emergency room visits in the year following initial admission (58 visits vs. 27, $P = 0.001$ and eight visits vs. 1 visit ($P = 0.012$), respectively). One year following the index admission, *C. difficile* patients had significantly higher rates of colectomy compared to *C. difficile*-negative patients (44.6% vs. 25%, $P = 0.04$). Length of hospitalization (11.7 vs. 11 days), use of cyclosporine therapy during index admission (48% vs. 47% of patients), and percentage requiring colectomy at initial admission (23.4% vs. 13.5%) did not reach statistical significance.

Conclusions.—Our data suggest that patients presenting with a UC flare who are infected with *C. difficile* have worse long-term clinical outcomes than those that are *C. difficile*-negative. *C. difficile* testing should be performed for all patients presenting with UC flare. Further studies are warranted to elucidate how infection can alter the natural history of UC.

▶ *Clostridium difficile* infection is a growing concern among patients with inflammatory bowel disease (IBD) presenting with signs and symptoms of disease activity. Rates of infection are higher among IBD patients even in the absence of recent antibiotic use or hospitalization. In-hospital mortality and length of hospitalization are also higher. In this study, among a series of hospitalized patients with active ulcerative colitis (UC) and *C difficile* infection, long-term complications, including colectomy, were higher in the year following hospital admission. Unfortunately, problems in study methodology limit the generalizability of these conclusions. Patients included were those who had a test for *C difficile*, with the assumption made that this would lead to comparisons of similar patients with the key difference being the presence or absence of this infection. Clinician practices regarding which patients and when they were tested during their admission were not given and may have varied. Cyclosporine usage between the 2 groups was similar as were other lab parameters, suggesting that they may have been of similar severity, but this cannot be confirmed. Treatment practices among physicians may have varied. Subsequent hospitalization after initial admission was higher in the *C difficile* group, but the proportion hospitalized for recurrent infection is not known. Recurrence rates for *C difficile* infection are high, and this may explain a large part of the difference in hospitalization rates. Finally, reasons for colectomy were not given and may vary based on the patient and the physician practice. Overall, the findings are interesting and do underscore the need to check for *C difficile* infection among all patients with IBD presenting with diarrhea. More studies are needed to better understand the role of this pathogen in the natural history of IBD.

M. F. Picco, MD, PhD

Colectomy Rate Comparison After Treatment of Ulcerative Colitis With Placebo or Infliximab

Sandborn WJ, Rutgeerts P, Feagan BG, et al (Mayo Clinic, Rochester, MN; Univ Hosp Gasthuisberg, Leuven, Belgium; The Univ of Western Ontario, London, Canada; et al)

Gastroenterology 137:1250-1260, 2009

Background & Aims.—The efficacy of infliximab for treating patients with ulcerative colitis has been established.

Methods.—The Active Ulcerative Colitis Trial (ACT)-1 and ACT-2 randomized, double-blind, placebo-controlled studies evaluated infliximab induction and maintenance therapy in moderately to severely active ulcerative colitis. Overall, 728 patients received placebo or infliximab (5 or 10 mg/kg) intravenously at weeks 0, 2, and 6, then every 8 weeks through week 46 (ACT-1) or 22 (ACT-2). Colectomy, hospitalization, and surgery/procedure data through 54 weeks after the first infusion were obtained from ACT-1, ACT-2, and associated data sources. In the prespecified analysis, all data were combined to ascertain time to colectomy. Kaplan–Meier product-limit method was used to estimate the cumulative incidence of colectomy, and log-rank test was used to compare the combined infliximab group and placebo.

Results.—Eighty-seven percent (630 of 728) of patients had complete colectomy follow-up; 13% (98 of 728) of patients had a median follow-up of 6.2 months. The cumulative incidence of colectomy through 54 weeks was 10% for infliximab and 17% for placebo ($P = .02$), yielding an absolute risk reduction of 7%. Compared with placebo, fewer ulcerative colitis-related hospitalizations and surgeries/procedures per 100 patient-years of treatment occurred with infliximab therapy: 40 vs 20 ($P = .003$) and 34 vs 21 ($P = .03$), respectively. Serious adverse events occurring in infliximab-treated patients included serious infections, tuberculosis, histoplasmosis, listeriosis, and malignancy.

Conclusions.—Patients with moderately to severely active ulcerative colitis treated with infliximab were less likely to undergo colectomy through 54 weeks than those receiving placebo.

▶ This study looked at rates of colectomy for patients enrolled in Active Ulcerative Colitis Trial (ACT)-1 or ACT-2. The investigators should be commended for following up on nearly all patients (87%), including those who discontinued ACT-1 or ACT-2. Rates of colectomy were lower in infliximab groups compared with the placebo groups. However, overall colectomy rates were low. Concomitant corticosteroids and baseline C-reactive protein of at least 2 mg/dL independently increased the risk of colectomy. Hospitalization rates were lower in the infliximab group. Adverse events with infliximab were similar to other published trials. Overall, complete follow-up was more likely in the infliximab group compared with the placebo group, which may have biased the results. It is important to note that these patients were outpatients with moderately active ulcerative colitis (UC). In fact, patients who received intravenous corticosteroids within 2 weeks or "were likely to require colectomy at 12 weeks" were excluded. In practice, infliximab is often given to these more severely active or refractory cases of UC where colectomy rates would be higher and response rates to infliximab likely lower. While the results of this study are important, more information on outcomes is needed in patients with severe disease where infliximab is more likely to be used in clinical practice.

M. F. Picco, MD, PhD

Immunosuppression Impairs Response to Pneumococcal Polysaccharide Vaccination in Patients with Inflammatory Bowel Disease

Melmed GY, Agarwal N, Frenck RW, et al (Univ of California, Los Angeles; Univ of California, Los Angeles, Torrance)

Am J Gastroenterol 105:148-154, 2010

Objectives.—The treatment of inflammatory bowel disease (IBD) often includes immunosuppressive medications, which may increase the risk of vaccine-preventable illnesses. We aimed to assess the impact of immunosuppression on immune responses to pneumococcal vaccination in patients with IBD.

Methods.—The study design consists of a prospective controlled clinical trial. This study was carried out at a tertiary-care IBD clinic. The subjects for the study belonged to one of the following three groups: adult patients with IBD on combination TNF-blockers and immunomodulators (Group A), those without immunosuppressive therapy (Group B), and age-matched healthy controls (Group C). The treatment consisted of immunization with 23-valent pneumococcal polysaccharide vaccines (PSVs). The main outcome was immune response for five serotypes defined as a twofold or greater increase from pre-vaccination titers and $\geq$ 1 μg post-vaccination titer.

Results.—Sixty-four subjects participated in the study: 20 in Group A, 25 in Group B, and 19 in Group C. Pre-vaccination titers were similar among the three groups. Vaccine responses were lower in Group A than in Group B ($P \leq 0.01$ for four out of five antigens) and Group C ($P < 0.01$ for all five antigens). Overall vaccine response was seen in 45, 80, and 85% of Groups A, B, and C ($P = 0.01$), respectively.

Conclusions.—Immune response to PSV-23 is impaired in Crohn's disease (CD) patients on combination immunosuppressive therapy but is normal among non-immunosuppressed patients. Given the unpredictable likelihood for immunosuppressive therapy, newly diagnosed patients with IBD should undergo vaccination before the initiation of immunosuppressive therapy.

▶ Among patients with inflammatory bowel disease (IBD), vaccination is often overlooked. Preventable infections that occur may be more likely to be severe or fatal when patients are taking immunomodulatory or biologic therapy. Vaccination options among patients on immunosuppressive therapies are limited because live vaccines must be avoided.[1] In this study, response to pneumococcal vaccine among patients with IBD on combined immunomodulatory and biologic therapy was significantly lower than patients not taking these medications or healthy controls. It is important to note that nearly half of the immunosuppressed patients responded to the vaccine suggesting that it is still worthwhile among this group. Unfortunately, only those patients on combined immunosuppression could be studied; therefore, neither the effect of monotherapy nor the role of specific therapies could be determined. Also, in the combined immunosuppression group more patients had Crohn's disease (CD). Overall responses in patients with CD were lower, suggesting that vaccine response may also be influenced by the type of IBD and that the study may not be generalizable to patients with ulcerative colitis. Despite these limitations, the message of the study is important. Vaccination of patients with IBD before they require immunomodulatory or biologic therapy results in similar response rates as controls. Patients taking immunomodulatory and/or biologic therapy should be vaccinated with pneumococcal and other dead vaccines and, whereever possible, should have their response measured because of anticipated low response rates.

M. F. Picco, MD, PhD

Reference

1. Sand BE, Cuffari C, Katz J, et al. Guidelines for immunization in patients with inflammatory bowel disease. *Inflamm Bowel Dis.* 2004;10:677-692.

Increased Prevalence of and Associated Mortality With Methicillin-Resistant *Staphylococcus aureus* Among Hospitalized IBD Patients

Nguyen GC, Patel H, Chong RY (Univ of Toronto Faculty of Medicine, Ontario, Canada; Lakeridge Health, Oshawa, Ontario, Canada)

Am J Gastroenterol 105:371-377, 2010

Objectives.—Methicillin-resistant *Staphylococcus aureus* (*MRSA*) infection has become increasingly prevalent in US hospitals, and the impact of *MRSA* on hospitalized inflammatory bowel disease (IBD) patients is unknown.

Methods.—We used the Nationwide Inpatient Sample to identify admissions for IBD ($n = 116{,}842$) between 1998 and 2004. We compared prevalence and in-hospital mortality of *MRSA* among IBD, non-IBD gastrointestinal (GI), and general medical inpatients.

Results.—*MRSA* prevalence increased from 4.5/10,000 to 19.0/10,000 over the 7-year period ($P < 0.0001$). After adjustment for confounders, IBD inpatients were at increased risk of *MRSA* compared with the non-IBD GI (adjusted odds ratio (aOR) 1.61; 95% confidence interval (CI): 1.33–1.96) and general medical (aOR 1.36; 95% CI: 1.11–1.66) groups. Of those with *MRSA*, catheter-related infections were specifically more common among IBD compared with non-IBD GI and general inpatients (28.8% vs. 11.0% and 8.5%, respectively, $P < 0.0002$). Bowel surgery, parenteral nutrition, and health insurance were predictors of *MRSA* infection, but the first two became insignificant after controlling for length of stay (LOS). Compared with LOS ≤ 7days, MRSA was more likely among those hospitalized 8–21 days (aOR 7.40; 95% CI: 4.68–11.7) and 21 days (aOR 58.6; 95% CI: 36.0–95.3). *MRSA* infection was associated with sevenfold increase in mortality (aOR 7.61; 95% CI: 3.33–17.4).

Conclusions.—Hospitalized IBD patients are at increased risk of *MRSA* compared with non-IBD GI and general medical inpatients. Increased mortality in the IBD population associated with *MRSA* reinforces the importance of measures to prevent nosocomial infection and to reduce length of hospitalization.

▶ Methicillin-resistant *Staphylococcus aureus* (MRSA), like *Clostridium difficile* is a common growing problem among hospitalized patients. Risk of *C difficile* infection is increased among patients with inflammatory bowel disease (IBD), leading the authors to investigate whether IBD patients are also at greater risk for MRSA. They used the Nationwide Inpatient Sample (NIS), which is a 20% stratified sample of 90% of acute nonfederal US hospitals, and performed a multivariate analysis adjusting for important factors that may influence MRSA rates. MRSA rates were higher in IBD patients with higher adjusted odds. Higher rates of MRSA translated into increased mortality. While the findings are concerning, they must be interpreted with the limitations of the NIS in mind. Data accuracy could not be verified because there was no patient contact. Coding errors may have also occurred. There was no specific code for MRSA, although the authors' method of identifying cases was reasonable. Length of stay and its relationship to MRSA infection was, as the authors admitted, difficult to sort out. They were not able to determine the length of stay before MRSA infection. It is possible that MRSA may have led to longer length of stay resulting in an erroneous association of length of stay with infection. Length of stay was appropriately relegated to a secondary analysis. However, it likely did influence MRSA rates, and its impact remains an important unanswered question. Overall, the results presented are concerning and, taken with evidence, implicating *C difficile* to suggest a higher rate of hospital-acquired infections among patients with IBD. Clinicians must remain vigilant.

M. F. Picco, MD, PhD

Isotretinoin Is Not Associated With Inflammatory Bowel Disease: A Population-Based Case–Control Study

Bernstein CN, Nugent Z, Longobardi T, et al (Univ of Manitoba IBD Clinical and Res Centre, Winnipeg, Canada)

Am J Gastroenterol 104:2774-2778, 2009

Objectives.—There is anecdotal evidence that isotretinoin use is associated with development of colitis. We aimed at determining whether there is an association between isotretinoin use and development of inflammatory bowel disease (IBD).

Methods.—The population-based University of Manitoba IBD Epidemiology Database and a control group matched by age, sex, and geographical residence were linked to the provincial prescription drug registry, a registry that was initiated in 1995. The number of users and duration of isotretinoin use were identified in both IBD cases and controls.

Results.—We found that 1.2% of IBD cases used isotretinoin before IBD diagnosis, which was statistically similar to controls (1.1% users). This was also similar to the number of IBD patients who used isotretinoin after a diagnosis of IBD (1.1%). There was no difference between isotretinoin use before Crohn's disease compared with its use before ulcerative colitis.

Conclusions.—Patients with IBD were no more likely to have used isotretinoin before diagnosis than were sex-, age-, and geography-matched controls. Although there may be anecdotes of isotretinoin causing acute colitis, our data suggest that isotretinoin is not likely to cause chronic IBD.

► Isotretinoin has long been associated with the development of colitis, yet little evidence exists beyond case reports. In this well-designed nested case-control study, Bernstein et al showed no association of isotretinoin use with the development of inflammatory bowel disease (IBD). The source for the data is population based and well validated. The authors were careful to exclude cases of acute colitis that may be associated with isotretinoin but not IBD. Furthermore, among those patients who took isotretinoin, the median time from last prescription to diagnosis of IBD was nearly 3 years, further casting doubt on any causal association. Unfortunately, the role of this medication in leading to exacerbations of existing IBD is not known. Because it has been associated with the development of acute colitis, it is plausible that it could exacerbate existing IBD. Ultimately, this is probably the more important issue because overall rates of IBD are low regardless of isotretinoin use. Whether isotretinoin use is safe in existing IBD remains an open question.

M. F. Picco, MD, PhD

Linoleic acid, a dietary n-6 polyunsaturated fatty acid, and the aetiology of ulcerative colitis: a nested case–control study within a European prospective cohort study

The IBD in EPIC Study Investigators (Inst of Cancer Epidemiology, Copenhagen, Denmark; Aarhus Univ Hosp, Aalborg, Denmark; et al)

Gut 58:1606-1611, 2009

Objective.—Dietary linoleic acid, an n-6 polyunsaturated fatty acid, is metabolised to arachidonic acid, a component of colonocyte membranes. Metabolites of arachidonic acid have pro-inflammatory properties and are increased in the mucosa of patients with ulcerative colitis. The aim of this investigation was to conduct the first prospective cohort study investigating if a high dietary intake of linoleic acid increases the risk of developing incident ulcerative colitis.

Design and Setting.—Dietary data from food frequency questionnaires were available for 203 193 men and women aged 30–74 years, resident in the UK, Sweden, Denmark, Germany or Italy and participating in a prospective cohort study, the European Prospective Investigation into Cancer and Nutrition (EPIC). These participants were followed up for the diagnosis of ulcerative colitis. Each case was matched with four controls and the risk of disease calculated by quartile of intake of linoleic acid adjusted for gender, age, smoking, total energy intake and centre.

Results.—A total of 126 participants developed ulcerative colitis (47% women) after a median follow-up of 4.0 years (range, 1.7–11.3 years). The highest quartile of intake of linoleic acid was associated with an increased risk of ulcerative colitis (odds ratio (OR) = 2.49, 95% confidence interval (CI) = 1.23 to 5.07, p = 0.01) with a significant trend across quartiles (OR = 1.32 per quartile increase, 95% CI = 1.04 to 1.66, p = 0.02 for trend).

Conclusions.—The data support a role for dietary linoleic acid in the aetiology of ulcerative colitis. An estimated 30% of cases could be attributed to having dietary intakes higher than the lowest quartile of linoleic acid intake.

▶ In this very interesting, carefully conducted, nested, case-control study, increased intake of linoleic acid was associated with developing ulcerative colitis (UC). The European Prospective Investigation into Cancer and Nutrition (EPIC) study is a multicountry cohort study providing longitudinal follow-up data on diet and lifestyle of over 500 000 patients. While questionnaire based, methods for obtaining data on dietary consumption are well validated. Diet information was obtained at least 18 months before the subjects developed UC. This eliminated recall bias and recording changes in diet related to having disease symptoms. These are the major problems in many studies that attempt to determine associations of diet with disease. The finding of lack of association of smoking and development of UC is unusual and attributed to the determination of smoking status at recruitment and not at diagnosis. On average, recruitment occurred 4 years after diagnosis. The assessment of smoking prior to diagnosis was not determined but is essential. It is surprising that these data were not presented. Former smoking is associated with increased risk of UC and might also identify individuals with poorer dietary habits compared with nonsmokers, leading to confounding effects. There may also be a recruitment bias, with smokers less likely to participate in the study. The median age of the UC cases was strikingly high (60 years), which raises the possibility that findings are generalizable. Overall, the findings are intriguing because they are based on a plausible mechanism of increased linoleic acid consumption leading to the production of arachidonic acid metabolites. Further study of this potentially important link of diet to UC is needed.

M. F. Picco, MD, PhD

Maintenance Treatment With Azathioprine in Ulcerative Colitis: Outcome and Predictive Factors After Drug Withdrawal

Cassinotti A, Actis GC, Duca P, et al ("Luigi Sacco" Univ Hosp, Milano, Italy; "Gradenigo" Hosp, Torino, Italy; Univ of Milano, Italy; et al)

Am J Gastroenterol 104:2760-2767, 2009

Objectives.—Whether the duration of maintenance treatment with azathioprine (AZA) affects the outcome of ulcerative colitis (UC) is unclear. We investigated clinical outcomes and any predictive factors after withdrawal of AZA in UC.

Methods.—In this multicenter observational retrospective study, 127 Italian UC patients, who were in steroid-free remission at the time of withdrawal of AZA, were followed-up for a median of 55 months or until relapse. The frequency of clinical relapse or colectomy after AZA withdrawal was analyzed according to demographic, clinical, and endoscopic variables.

Results.—After drug withdrawal, a third of the patients relapsed within 12 months, half within 2 years and two-thirds within 5 years. After multivariable analysis, predictors of relapse after drug withdrawal were lack of sustained remission during AZA maintenance (hazard ratio, HR 2.350, confidence interval, CI 95% 1.434–3.852; $P = 0.001$), extensive colitis (HR 1.793, CI 95% 1.064–3.023, $P = 0.028$ vs. left-sided colitis; HR 2.024, CI 95% 1.103–3.717, $P = 0.023$ vs. distal colitis), and treatment duration, with short treatments (3–6 months) more disadvantaged than >48-month treatments (HR 2.783, CI 95% 1.267–6.114, $P = 0.008$). Concomitant aminosalicylates were the only predictors of sustained remission during AZA therapy ($P = 0.009$). The overall colectomy rate was 10%. Predictors of colectomy were drug-related toxicity as the cause of AZA withdrawal ($P = 0.041$), no post-AZA drug therapy ($P = 0.031$), and treatment duration ($P < 0.0005$).

Conclusions.—Discontinuation of AZA while UC is in remission is associated with a high relapse rate. Disease extent, lack of sustained remission during AZA, and discontinuation due to toxicity could stratify relapse risk. Concomitant aminosalicylates were advantageous. Prospective randomized controlled trials are needed to confirm whether treatment duration is inversely associated with outcome.

▶ Once in remission, patients with inflammatory bowel disease (IBD) maintained on immunomodulatory therapy are often anxious about discontinuing these medications because of the fear of toxicity. This study provides further evidence for maintaining azathioprine therapy among these patients with ulcerative colitis (UC). Patients who attained remission for at least 3 months taking azathioprine and then discontinued the medication had a disturbingly high rate of disease relapse. While shorter duration of therapy increased risk of relapse, high rates of recurrence were also seen among patients who stopped the medication after 48 months. In this retrospective noncontrolled study, the true role of disease duration is difficult to determine because patients who remained in remission on medication longer may have had a better prognosis prior to starting therapy. Other associations found with relapse make sense clinically, but in the absence of controlled data, it is difficult to draw firm conclusions. Regardless, the main finding of this study and others on UC and Crohn's disease should give clinicians pause before stopping azathioprine among patients with IBD in established remission.

M. F. Picco, MD, PhD

Modelling dysplasia detection in ulcerative colitis: clinical implications of surveillance intensity

Awais D, Siegel CA, Higgins PDR (Dartmouth–Hitchcock Med Ctr, Lebanon, NH; West Med Ctr, Ann Arbor, MI)

Gut 58:1498-1503, 2009

Background.—Endoscopic surveillance of chronic colitis uses random biopsies to find dysplastic fields. Enhanced endoscopic methods are more sensitive for dysplasia detection, but their specificity for colorectal cancer risk is unknown.

Aims.—To develop a mathematical model of the sensitivity of random biopsy surveillance, and determine the implications of negative, a single positive, or multiple positive biopsies for dysplasia, and compare the detection threshold to that detectable by enhanced endoscopy.

Methods.—Using mathematical modelling, we calculated the confidence level with which dysplasia can be excluded, the dysplastic field size detection threshold, the predicted area of a dysplastic field, and the number of biopsies needed for a given dysplasia detection threshold and confidence level.

Results.—32 random biopsies provide only 80% confidence that dysplasia involving ≥5% of the colon can be detected. When a single biopsy of 18 is dysplastic, this predicts a dysplastic area (89 cm^2) several orders of magnitude greater than dysplastic fields that are readily detectable by enhanced endoscopy (1 cm diameter), and the predicted field size increases rapidly with multiple positive biopsies.

Conclusions.—Random biopsy surveillance is sufficiently sensitive to detect large dysplastic fields with significant colorectal cancer risk. Enhanced endoscopy can detect much smaller dysplastic fields, but these have unknown (perhaps much lower) colorectal cancer risk. Small dysplastic fields should not be assumed to indicate a high colorectal cancer risk that warrants colectomy. Prospective studies are needed to define the colorectal cancer risk and optimal management of small dysplastic lesions.

▶ Among patients with longstanding ulcerative colitis (UC), colonoscopy with surveillance biopsy has been shown to reduce the risk of colorectal cancer. As endoscopic methods improve, endoscopists are better able to identify dysplastic lesions. Chromoendoscopy in UC has been shown to increase dysplasia detection 4-fold from the conventional white light colonoscopy. The question is whether this enhanced detection rate translates into better patient outcomes. This study suggests that they do not and that standard random biopsy is sufficient. However, this question is far from answered. The authors assume that enhanced endoscopy is only useful in providing higher rates of detection for small dysplastic areas where overall detection of flat lesions is enhanced by this technique. Furthermore, size of the lesion may not indicate the degree of dysplasia. As an example, in a comparison of chromoendoscopy with conventional colonoscopy, Kiesslich[1] reported higher rates of detection of dysplastic lesions with 19 lesions found in 80 patients, 14 only seen on chromoendoscopy compared with 4 lesions in the conventional group (2 polypoid and 2 on random biopsy). While the average size of the lesions seen on chromoendoscopy was small (about 1 cm), 15 were flat, and 7 of 19 were high-grade dysplasia. How many of these could be seen under white light is not clear, but because only 4 abnormalities overall could be seen under white light, at least 3 cases of high-grade dysplasia were detected only under chromoendoscopy. These lesions regardless of the size are important and should be treated by colectomy. Awais et al did not account for targeting visible lesions and based the conclusions on mathematical modeling. From chromoendoscopy publications, the yield of truly random biopsies is about 1 of 1000 for dysplasia. I believe it would be better to take targeted biopsies using advanced imaging techniques. With these enhanced techniques, truly random biopsies may be abandoned in the future and fewer biopsies taken, leading to cost savings. This may lead to more lesions seen on colonoscopy, but these techniques should not be abandoned because we do not know what to do with the findings. The finding of low-grade dysplasia with these techniques and its implications is patient specific, and more natural history studies should be performed. Low-grade dysplasia in this setting may not require colectomy but identify patients for more aggressive surveillance.

M. F. Picco, MD, PhD

Reference

1. Kiesslich R, Goetz M, Lammersdorf K, et al. Chromoscopy-guided endomicroscopy increases the diagnostic yield of intraepithelial neoplasia in ulcerative colitis. *Gastroenterology.* 2007;132:874-882.

Mucosal Healing Predicts Sustained Clinical Remission in Patients With Early-Stage Crohn's Disease

Baert F, for the Belgian Inflammatory Bowel Disease Research Group and the North-Holland Gut Club (H.–Hartziekenhuis Roeselare–Menen vzw, Belgium; et al)

Gastroenterology 138:463-468, 2010

Background & Aims.—Few prospective data are available to support the clinical relevance of mucosal healing in patients with Crohn's disease. This study examined whether complete healing, determined by endoscopy, predicts a better outcome in Crohn's disease.

Methods.—One-hundred thirty-three newly diagnosed and treatment-naïve Crohn's disease patients were given either a combination of immunosuppressive therapy (azathioprine) and 3 infusions of infliximab or treatment with conventional corticosteroids. Patients given azathioprine were given repeated doses of infliximab for relapses, patients given corticosteroids were given azathioprine in cases of corticosteroid dependency and infliximab only if azathioprine failed. A representative subset of 49 patients from the initially randomized cohort underwent ileocolonoscopy after 2 years of therapy. Correlation analysis was performed between different clinical parameters including endoscopic activity (Simple Endoscopic Score) and clinical outcome 2 years after this endoscopic examination. Data were available from 46 patients 3 and 4 years after therapy began.

Results.—Complete mucosal healing, defined as a simple endoscopic score of 0 after 2 years of therapy, was the only factor that predicted sustained, steroid-free remission 3 and 4 years after therapy was initiated; it was observed in 17 of 24 patients (70.8%) vs 6 of 22 patients with lesions detected by endoscopy (27.3%, Simple Endoscopic Score >0) ($P = .036$; odds ratio = 4.352; 95% confidence interval, 1.10–17.220). Fifteen of 17 patients with mucosal healing at year 2 maintained in remission without further infliximab infusions during years 3 and 4 ($P = .032$; odds ratio = 4.883; 95% confidence interval, 1.144–20.844).

Conclusions.—Complete mucosal healing in patients with early-stage Crohn's disease is associated with significantly higher steroid-free remission rates 4 years after therapy began.

▶ This study is a follow-up to the previously published work by the same group on the use of early combined immunosuppression (top down) therapy in newly diagnosed patients with Crohn's disease.[1] This study illustrates the importance of mucosal healing among this newly diagnosed treatment-naïve group. Mucosal healing was the only factor that predicted steroid-free remission. The study was small with mucosal healing only assessed in 49 patients. Endoscopic activity did not correlate with clinical disease activity (CDAI). In fact only half of the patients in clinical remission by CDAI had mucosal healing. Comparisons of efficacy between medications could not be performed primarily because of the small number of patients. The study was conducted from 2001 to 2004 with infliximab used as induction and rescue therapy, unlike how it is currently used as continued maintenance therapy. Continued scheduled infliximab maintenance therapy would have probably led to higher mucosal healing rates. This study adds to the growing body of literature illustrating the importance of mucosal healing after medical and surgical therapy. Assessment of clinical activity is not enough to adequately determine the likelihood of subsequent disease flares or complications. Endoscopy may be necessary among patients with good clinical response but poor predicted long-term outcome. Other noninvasive methods could aid in evaluating mucosal healing. Accurate assessment of both clinical and endoscopic response may become the standard for the future and lead to better long-term outcomes among patients with Crohn's disease. More research is needed.

M. F. Picco, MD, PhD

Reference

1. D'Haens G, Baert F, van Assche G, et al. Early combined immunosuppression or conventional management in patients with newly diagnosed Crohn's disease: an open randomised trial. *Lancet*. 2008;371:660-667.

Once-Daily Dosing of Delayed-Release Oral Mesalamine (400-mg Tablet) Is as Effective as Twice-Daily Dosing for Maintenance of Remission of Ulcerative Colitis

Sandborn WJ, Korzenik J, Lashner B, et al (Mayo Clinic, Rochester, MN; Massachusetts General Hosp, Boston; Cleveland Clinic, OH; et al)
Gastroenterology 138:1286-1296, 2010

Background & Aims.—The practice of dosing mesalamines in divided doses for the treatment of ulcerative colitis (UC) began with sulfasalazine and was driven by sulfapyridine toxicity. This convention and the assumption that dosing multiple times a day is necessary to treat UC had not been challenged until recently. This study was conducted to determine the efficacy and safety of once-daily dosing of delayed-release mesalamine (Asacol 400-mg tablets) compared with twice-daily dosing for maintaining remission in UC patients.

Methods.—A multicenter, randomized, investigator-blinded, 12-month, active-control trial was conducted to assess the noninferiority of delayed-release mesalamine 1.6–2.4 g/day administered once daily compared with twice daily in patients with mild-to-moderate UC currently in clinical remission. The primary end point was maintenance of clinical remission at month 6.

Results.—A total of 1023 patients were randomized and dosed. The primary objective of noninferiority was met. At month 6, 90.5% of patients receiving once-daily dosing had maintained clinical remission, compared with 91.8% of patients receiving twice-daily dosing (95% confidence interval for twice daily - once daily, −2.3 to 4.9). At month 12, 85.4% of patients receiving once-daily dosing had maintained clinical remission, compared with 85.4% of patients receiving twice-daily dosing (95% confidence interval for twice daily - once daily, −4.6 to 4.7). Both regimens had low rates of withdrawals as a result of adverse events and serious adverse events.

Conclusions.—Once-daily dosing of delayed-release mesalamine at doses of 1.6–2.4 g/day was shown to be as effective as twice-daily dosing for maintenance of clinical remission in patients with UC.

▶ Among patients with ulcerative colitis (UC) in remission, mesalamine remains the mainstay of therapy. Compliance is a major issue and is improved by once-daily regimens. Newer preparations such as Lialda and Apriso are marketed with this advantage. Drug delivery systems from these newer medications are thought to be important in allowing once-daily dosing. However, this notion is challenged in this article that compared Asacol (standard preparation) once daily to twice-daily dosing among patients with UC in remission on current maintenance mesalamine. The cumulative daily dose was the same and the efficacy of the regimens was similar. Furthermore, the overall efficacy was similar to the newer preparations. These newer preparations may be more costly than older preparations. This cost may not be justified. The newer preparations do allow for fewer tablets daily, which may be an advantage in compliance, but once-daily dosing regardless of the preparation is probably sufficient in the maintenance of remission among patients with UC. While it is appealing to suggest that once-daily dosing of older preparation such as Asacol may be effective for active disease, more studies are necessary to definitively answer this question.

M. F. Picco, MD, PhD

Photodynamic diagnosis of endoscopically invisible flat dysplasia in patients with ulcerative colitis by visualization using local 5-aminolevulinic acid–induced photosensitization

Watanabe K, Hida N, Ajioka Y, et al (Osaka City Univ Graduate School of Medicine, Japan; Hyogo College of Medicine, Japan; Niigata Univ, Japan)

Gastrointest Endosc 71:1094-1096, 2010

Background.—Patients with ulcerative colitis (UC) are managed clinically with immunomodulators and biologic agents, but must also be monitored for serious problems such as colitis-associated cancer or dysplasia

(CC/D), a fatal condition. Endoscopic methods are used for surveillance colonoscopy in patients with chronic UC, but the official guidelines for these methods include obtaining and analyzing 30 to 40 random (nontargeted) biopsy samples, a daunting task with low diagnostic efficiency. The nontargeted biopsies are needed to detect otherwise invisible CC/D. Fluorescence endoscopy using 5-aminolevulinic acid (5-ALA)-n-induced photosensitization has been reported to be efficacious for CC/D detection and can be used for photodynamic diagnosis (PDD). The efficacy of using 5-ALA with several endoscopic modalities was determined in two cases.

> *Case Reports.*—In the two cases, nontargeted biopsy samples from nearby locations that appeared suspicious for CC/D revealed dysplasia. The endoscopic studies performed included chromoendoscopy with indigo carmine dye spraying, magnifying chromoendoscopic endoscopy with crystal violet solution, narrow-band imaging (NBI) with magnification, and autofluorescence imaging (AFI). The lesion was not visible on any of these studies. PDD was then performed using 1.5 g of 5-ALA dissolved in 125 mL of sodium chloride 0.9% sprayed throughout the colon using the endoscope. Two hours later, fluorescence endoscopy using fiberscopes and a light source delivering white or blue light detected the lesions. A comparison of the details of the biopsy specimens from the PDD-positive and PPD-negative areas delineated the boundaries of the lesions. Postoperative immunohistochemical stains for p53 and Ki-67 revealed the flat lesions were low- or high-grade dysplasia. Even when the area was marked preoperatively with clips using an endoscope during PPD the dysplasia was not detectable using chromoendoscopy, magnifying chromoendoscopy, NBI with magnification, or AFI. Complete resection was accomplished per anum. The lesion was flat against the mucosa and structural atypia was minimal, making it difficult to detect.

Conclusions.—PDD using 5-ALA proved more efficacious than various endoscopic approaches in detecting flat CC/D not apparent on endoscopy. However, PDD using 5-ALA is not appropriate for an initial surveillance colonoscopy because the solution must be sprayed endoscopically throughout the colon 2 hours before observation. Once CC/D has been detected on conventional primary surveillance colonoscopy, PDD with 5-ALA is quite suitable for use during a second, more detailed colonoscopy. The need for surgery will be determined on the basis of this second colonoscopy. More information about the prevalence and characteristics of endoscopically undetectable CC/D should be obtained using the PDD method.

▶ Standard white light surveillance colonoscopy with random biopsy in ulcerative colitis (UC) is commonly practiced but leads to very low dysplasia detection rates. Multiple random biopsies of colonic mucosa without visible dysplastic or polypoid lesions are typically obtained, but the yield for dysplasia in these nontargeted biopsies is very low (0.1%). Overall, dysplasia is found in about 2% of patients with chronic UC through biopsies of visualized lesions. This has led to the development of endoscopic methods to enhance mucosal detail and improve dysplasia detection rates. The most common of these are staining methods through the use of vital dyes (indigo carmine or methylene blue) that are sprayed over the entire colon surface. These methods have resulted in an 8% dysplasia detection rate or 4-fold increase compared with white light alone but can be messy and cumbersome. Other techniques that avoid dye spraying rely on special endoscopes that expose the colon to specific light (narrow band imaging) or make use of natural autofluorescence of the colonic surface. Unfortunately, these techniques are not widely available and are not as effective as staining methods. This case report is interesting because it takes dysplasia detection a step further. They present 2 cases where dysplasia was detected incidentally on nontargeted biopsy samples. The area was re-examined with chromoendoscopy, and the lesion remained invisible. They next applied fluorescence endoscopy by using 5-aminolevulinic acid (5-ALA) sensitization. 5-ALA was sprayed on the area of the abnormality, and in both cases the lesion became visible with a special endoscope. These areas were removed and dysplasia confirmed in both cases. Unfortunately, after spraying it takes 2 hours before the lesion can be seen with this technique, and it can only be used for small areas in the colon. This does make the method impractical for general application as it is presented, but it may be a technique of the future. The clear dramatic improvement in dysplasia detection and ease of use argue that dye-spraying methods should be part of surveillance colonoscopy in UC.

Despite these advantages, controversy exists as to whether this method should be adopted. It is unclear whether detection of these otherwise invisible lesions under white light leads to better overall patient outcomes. Emerging data from the field show how fast technology is advancing.

M. F. Picco, MD, PhD

Trough serum infliximab: a predictive factor of clinical outcome for infliximab treatment in acute ulcerative colitis

Seow CH, Newman A, Irwin SP, et al (Univ of Toronto, Ontario, Canada)
Gut 59:49-54, 2010

Background and Aims.—Antibodies to infliximab reduce serum infliximab with loss of clinical benefit, but undetectable trough serum concentrations of infliximab may occur without antibody formation. The relationship between trough serum infliximab and clinical outcomes was evaluated in acute ulcerative colitis.

Methods.—In a cohort of 115 patients with ulcerative colitis treated with three-dose induction followed by scheduled maintenance infliximab, rates of clinical remission, colectomy, antibodies to infliximab and trough serum infliximab were determined.

Results.—Rates of remission were 32% at week 10 and 37% at week 54. Colectomy occurred in 40% of patients, at a median of 5.3 (IQR 1.9–12.1) months. Detectable trough serum infliximab was present in 39% of patients and, among patients with undetectable infliximab, 41% were antibody positive and 20% were antibody negative. For antibody-positive and antibody-negative patients, rates of remission (18% vs 14%), endoscopic improvement (25% vs 35%) and colectomy (52% vs 59%) were not different. A detectable serum infliximab was associated with higher rates of remission (69% vs 15%; p<0.001) and endoscopic improvement (76% vs 28%, p<0.001). An undetectable serum infliximab predicted an increased risk for colectomy (55% vs 7%, OR 9.3; 95% CI 2.9 to 29.9; p<0.001). Concurrent immunosuppression was not associated with clinical outcomes.

Conclusions.—For patients with ulcerative colitis treated with infliximab, a detectable trough serum infliximab predicts clinical remission, endoscopic improvement and a lower risk for colectomy. An undetectable trough serum infliximab, irrespective of antibody status, is associated with less favourable outcomes.

▶ Lack of response to infliximab among patients with inflammatory bowel disease (IBD) has been attributed to antibody production and resulting absent infliximab levels (trough) prior to the next infusion. In this study, the authors found that serum trough levels were the best predictor of clinical response among patients treated with induction and maintenance therapy for ulcerative colitis (UC). Antibodies to infliximab, while found in most treatment failures, were not universal and not predictive of failure. The authors speculate that this may be due to a delay in antibody formation or some other mechanism leading to early clearance of infliximab and resulting in treatment failure. Regardless of the mechanism, trough levels were a better measure of response than antibody levels. Shortening the interval to every 6 weeks resulted in nearly half obtaining clinical remission with similar trough levels compared with those who received infliximab every 8 weeks. Unfortunately, it is not clear whether those who had to shorten the infusion interval had measurable trough levels at 8 weeks. In those who increased the dose to 10 mg/kg, trough levels were associated with clinical response. Either of these strategies will probably lead to better response rates overall compared with clinical trials with fixed dosing and infusion intervals. While concurrent immunosuppression did not seem to influence trough levels, it is not clear how many patients were immunosuppressant naïve. In Crohn's disease, immunosuppressant naïve patients receiving combined immunomodulator and biologic therapy had a better response than biologic therapy alone. In this study because absent trough levels did predict colectomy, the authors speculated that more aggressive treatment regimens with higher induction dosing and shorter intervals, especially in the UC patients with severe disease, may lead to better clinical outcomes. This clearly warrants further study. It is in this setting that there may be a role for measuring trough levels to guide therapy.

M. F. Picco, MD, PhD

Hemolytic Uremic Syndrome and Death in Persons with *Escherichia coli* O157:H7 Infection, Foodborne Diseases Active Surveillance Network Sites, 2000–2006

Gould LH, the Emerging Infections Program FoodNet Working Group (Ctrs for Disease Control and Prevention, Atlanta, GA; et al)

Clin Infect Dis 49:1480-1485, 2009

Background.—Hemolytic uremic syndrome (HUS) is a life-threatening illness usually caused by infection with Shiga toxin–producing *Escherichia coli* O157 (STEC O157). We evaluated the age-specific rate of HUS and death among persons with STEC O157 infection and the risk factors associated with developing HUS.

Methods.—STEC O157 infections and HUS cases were reported from 8 sites participating in the Foodborne Diseases Active Surveillance Network during 2000–2006. For each case of STEC O157 infection and HUS, demographic and clinical outcomes were reported. The proportion of STEC O157 infections resulting in HUS was determined.

Results.—A total of 3464 STEC O157 infections were ascertained; 218 persons (6.3%) developed HUS. The highest proportion of HUS cases (15.3%) occurred among children aged <5 years. Death occurred in 0.6% of all patients with STEC O157 infection and in 4.6% of those with HUS. With or without HUS, persons aged ≥60 years had the highest rate of death due to STEC O157 infection. Twelve (3.1%) of 390 persons aged ≥60 years died, including 5 (33.3%) of 15 persons with HUS and 7 (1.9%) of 375 without. Among children aged <5 years, death occurred in 4 (3.0%) of those with HUS and 2 (0.3%) of those without.

Conclusions.—Young children and females had an increased risk of HUS after STEC O157 infection. With or without HUS, elderly persons had the highest proportion of deaths associated with STEC O157 infection. These data support recommendations for aggressive supportive care of young children and the elderly early during illness due to STEC O157.

▶ This is an interesting article for all physicians, including gastroenterologists. Shiga toxin-producing *Escherichia coli* O157 (STEC O157) infection is the leading cause of hemolytic uremic syndrome (HUS). HUS is characterized by hemolytic anemia, thrombocytopenia, and renal failure. This article specifically applies to the gastroenterologist when it comes to ordering stool cultures. All stool specimens submitted for the diagnosis of community-acquired diarrhea should be cultured for O157 STEC on selective and differential agar and assayed for O157 STEC. Positive O157 STEC should be reported to public health authorities as well. I think it is important from reading this article that we all make sure our local laboratory has the necessary culture media to perform this test. If not diagnosed, life-threatening cases may be missed.

J. S. Scolapio, MD

Other Inflammatory Bowel Disease

Inflammatory Bowel Disease in the United States from 1998 to 2005: Has Infliximab Affected Surgical Rates?

Cannom RR, Kaiser AM, Ault GT, et al (Univ of Southern California, Los Angeles)

Am Surg 75:976-980, 2009

The treatment costs for patients in the United States with inflammatory bowel disease (IBD) exceed 1.7 billion dollars/year. Infliximab, an antibody to tumor necrosis factor-α, has been extensively used to treat IBD, with 390,000 IBD patients receiving the drug since its FDA approval in 1998. We sought to determine the impact of infliximab on population-based rates of hospitalizations and surgical care for patients with IBD in the United States. We used data from the Nationwide Inpatient Sample to analyze patterns of hospital-based treatment provided to patients with IBD between 1998 and 2005. Data from this analysis were combined with census data to calculate trends in population-based rates of treatment. Overall rates of hospitalization for patients with Crohn's disease and ulcerative colitis increased significantly between 1998 and 2005 (5.1%/year and 3.4%/year respectively, $P < 0.001$ for each). During the same time period there were no changes in the overall rates of surgical care. The expanding use of infliximab has not significantly impacted the use of surgical procedures for patients with either ulcerative colitis or Crohn's disease, and rates of nonsurgical hospitalizations have actually increased. Even in the era of infliximab, surgical care remains a mainstay in the treatment of IBD.

▶ The fundamental question as to whether infliximab has reduced surgical rates in inflammatory bowel disease (IBD) in the United States is difficult to answer. While surgery and hospitalization rates are available through the Nationwide Inpatient Sample, true overall rates of hospitalization and surgery in the US population with IBD are not. In this study, the authors derived overall age-adjusted incidence rates for hospitalizations and surgery based from US census data. While this approach is reasonable, results obtained may not be accurate if the true prevalence of IBD and how it changes with time is not known. The striking conclusion from this study is that despite infliximab use, rates of nonsurgical hospitalizations actually went up and rates of surgery were unchanged. If the prevalence of IBD increased significantly in the study period (as has been reported in Olmsted County) then rates would be overestimated. Alternatively, if we believe that the results are accurate, higher rates of hospitalization may be because disease severity is increasing with time or surgery is being delayed, resulting in more hospitalization as medical management is attempted. Neither interpretation is supported by the current literature. The question remains an important one that unfortunately has yet to be answered.

M. F. Picco, MD, PhD

Lymphoproliferative disorders in patients receiving thiopurines for inflammatory bowel disease: a prospective observational cohort study

Beaugerie L, for the CESAME Study Group (Université Pierre et Marie Curie Paris-VI, France; et al)

Lancet 374:1617-1625, 2009

Background.—Reports of an increased risk of lymphoproliferative disorders in patients receiving thiopurines for inflammatory bowel disease are controversial. We assessed this risk in a prospective observational cohort study.

Methods.—19 486 patients with inflammatory bowel disease, of whom 11 759 (60·3%) had Crohn's disease and 7727 (39·7%) had ulcerative colitis or unclassified inflammatory bowel disease, were enrolled in a nationwide French cohort by 680 gastroenterologists, who reported details of immunosuppressive therapy during the observation period, cases of cancer, and deaths. The risk of lymphoproliferative disorder was assessed according to thiopurine exposure. Median follow-up was 35 months (IQR 29–40).

Findings.—At baseline, 5867 (30·1%) of patients were receiving, 2809 (14·4%) had discontinued, and 10 810 (55·5%) had never received thiopurines. 23 new cases of lymphoproliferative disorder were diagnosed, consisting of one case of Hodgkin's lymphoma and 22 cases of non-Hodgkin lymphoproliferative disorder. The incidence rates of lymphoproliferative disorder were 0·90 per 1000 (95% CI 0·50–1·49) patient-years in those receiving, 0·20/1000 (0·02–0·72) patient-years in those who had discontinued, and 0·26/1000 (0·10–0·57) patient-years in those who had never received thiopurines (p=0·0054). The multivariate-adjusted hazard ratio of lymphoproliferative disorder between patients receiving thiopurines and those who had never received the drugs was 5·28 (2·01–13·9, p=0·0007). Most cases associated with thiopurine exposure matched the pathological range of post-transplant disease.

Interpretation.—Patients receiving thiopurines for inflammatory bowel disease have an increased risk of developing lymphoproliferative disorders.

► Previously disputed, the link of thiopurines to malignancy is now becoming very clear. This is one of several recent studies that have linked malignancy, particularly lymphoproliferative disorders, to thiopurine use among patients with inflammatory bowel disease (IBD). A particular advantage of this study is that it is a prospective study identifying a cohort of patients with IBD followed over time. The patients who had received thiopurines were similar to what one would expect in clinical practice. They tended to have Crohn's disease, were younger, and had a longer disease duration. The association of thiopurines with lymphoproliferative disorders was dramatic even after adjustment for the potential confounding factors of advanced age, male sex, and longer duration of IBD. Unfortunately, information regarding thiopurine therapy prior to study entry and thiopurine dose during the follow-up period was not available. Finally, as with other similar studies, the authors cannot separate whether the thiopurine use led to malignancy or was just a marker of more severe inflammatory disease, which alone may be a risk factor. Overall, the results are important and lead to a growing body of literature pointing out the potential hazards of these drugs. The incidence rate of 1/1000 is higher than other studies and is concerning. However, the rate remains low and needs to be interpreted correctly. The risk-benefit ratio still favors the use of these medications in the appropriate patient, particularly as steroid-sparing agents. Physicians must discuss the risks and benefits of all potential therapies to help their patients make informed decisions.

M. F. Picco, MD, PhD

Venous thromboembolism during active disease and remission in inflammatory bowel disease: a cohort study

Grainge MJ, West J, Card TR (Univ of Nottingham, UK)
Lancet 375:657-663, 2010

Background.—Patients with inflammatory bowel disease who develop deep vein thrombosis or pulmonary embolism often have active disease at the time of thromboembolism. We therefore aimed to quantify the risk of venous thromboembolism prospectively during different activity phases of inflammatory bowel disease.

Methods.—From the General Practice Research Database, we matched patients with prospectively recorded inflammatory bowel disease from November, 1987, until July, 2001 with up to five controls by age, sex, and general practice. A flare was defined as the period 120 days after a new corticosteroid prescription. We used Cox regression analysis with time-varying covariates to accommodate changes in the state of inflammatory bowel disease, and whether patients were at high risk of venous thromboembolism after hospitalisation.

Findings.—13 756 patients with inflammatory bowel disease and 71 672 matched controls were included in the analysis, and of these 139 patients and 165 controls developed venous thromboembolism. Overall, patients with inflammatory bowel disease had a higher risk of venous thromboembolism than did controls (hazard ratio 3·4, 95% CI 2·7–4·3; $p<0 \cdot 0001$; absolute risk 2·6 per 1000 per person-years). At the time of a flare, however, this increase in risk was much more prominent (8·4, 5·5–12·8; $p<0 \cdot 0001$; 9·0 per 1000 person-years). This relative risk at the time of a flare was higher during non-hospitalised periods (15·8, 9·8–25·5; $p<0 \cdot 0001$; 6·4 per 1000 person-years) than during hospitalised periods (3·2, 1·7–6·3; $p=0 \cdot 0006$; 37·5 per 1000 person-years).

Interpretation.—Trials of primary prophylaxis of venous thromboembolism are warranted to find out whether this important complication can be prevented.

▶ The results of this well-done cohort study are sobering. The authors were careful to separate risk of thromboembolism in acute and chronic inflammatory bowel disease (IBD) and also account for hospitalization, which alone is a risk factor for this complication. However, while the relative risk of thromboembolism is high compared with controls, the absolute risk among all nonhospitalized patients was a maximum rate of 6.4/1000 person-years. This highest risk was for outpatients experiencing an acute flare requiring corticosteroids. Unadjusted rates in hospitalized patients, as would be expected, were higher likely because of both increased severity of disease and immobility issues. As the authors admit, it's possible that some of the increased risk is because of bias in detection. Clinicians may be more likely to look for thromboembolism among IBD patients compared with controls, given the known association. This may have led to artificially increased rates. Also, because disease flare was defined as corticosteroid use, results apply to significant flares that may have higher thromboembolism rates overall. Flares treated with biologic therapies may also have been missed. Given the magnitude of the association, it is unlikely that these biases were responsible for the findings. A strength of this study is the consideration of acute and chronic IBD risk, with exclusion of hospitalized patients. While some comfort can be taken in relatively low absolute risks, the overall impact of thromboembolism on this group of patients is significant. While low, individual risk is high compared with risks with other accepted consequences of IBD and IBD therapies.

M. F. Picco, MD, PhD

Colonic Diverticulitis: Does Age Predict Severity of Disease on CT Imaging?

Hall JF, Roberts PL, Ricciardi R, et al (Lahey Clinic, Burlington, MA)

Dis Colon Rectum 53:121-125, 2010

Purpose.—The aim of our study was to determine whether young patients with diverticulitis were more likely to present with abdominal CT evidence of severe disease.

Methods.—We analyzed the abdominal CT scans of 932 patients who presented to our institution with CT scan findings consistent with diverticulitis from January 2002 through June 2007. Radiologists retrospectively reviewed all abdominal scans for the presence of imaging findings consistent with diverticulitis (bowel wall thickness, extraluminal air, free perforation, abscess, or fistula). The cohort was divided into 2 groups; patients ≤50 years of age and patients >51 years of age.

Results.—Two hundred forty-three patients were ≤50 years and 689 patients were >51 years. Young patients were more likely to be male (63% vs 42%, $P < .0001$). Young patients had a higher proportion of scans with extraluminal air than older patients (19.7% vs 12.6%, $P < .008$). Young patients were more likely to present with severe disease found by CT than older patients (19.3% vs 11.5%). When we adjusted for gender, young males had a higher proportion of scans with extraluminal air than older males (22.4% vs 13.1%, $P = .014$). Young males were also more likely to present with severe disease (22% vs 12%).

Conclusion.—Young patients were more likely to have extraluminal air and severe disease found by CT. Young male patients presented more commonly with evidence of severe disease. They did not differ from older patients in rates of free perforation, abscess, or fistula formation.

▶ Colonic diverticulitis occurs predominantly in older individuals; hence, these patients are presumed to have greater severity of disease when compared with their younger counterparts. Abdominal CT remains the gold standard to diagnose diverticular disease. Whether initial abdominal CT scan findings significantly differ between old and young patients is not known. Current diagnostic approaches are attempting to more accurately assess the severity of disease and potential operative risks that are difficult to identify with most clinical criteria.

Hall and associates retrospectively reviewed 932 abdominal CT scans, and the findings were assessed as to the age of the patient (≤50 years vs >51 years). Young patients were more likely to present with severe disease; however, they did not differ from older patients in rates of free perforation, abscess, or fistula formation (Table 3 in the original article).

The strengths of this study include the number of patients (932), their conservative evaluation, the use of well-defined radiographic descriptors, and a new interpretation of radiographic findings without dependence on the initial reports. The results are important as well. Young patients were more likely to present with extraluminal air, increased bowel thickness, and severe disease found by CT.

Limitations of this study include its retrospective design and lack of correlation with concomitant clinical indices. Additionally, it is not known as to whether the initial CT findings led to important changes in treatment decisions and prognosis.

In summary, severe diverticular disease is commonly associated with radiographic findings of extraluminal air and pericolic abscess. These findings are often present in young males. The relevance of these findings as to clinical treatment and prognosis is not known.

J. L. Rombeau, MD

Childhood Trauma Is Associated With Hypothalamic-Pituitary-Adrenal Axis Responsiveness in Irritable Bowel Syndrome

Videlock EJ, Adeyemo M, Licudine A, et al (Univ of California, Los Angeles)
Gastroenterology 137:1954-1962, 2009

Background & Aims.—A history of early adverse life events (EALs) is associated with a poorer outcome and higher levels of distress in adult patients with functional gastrointestinal disorders. An EAL is thought to predispose individuals to develop a range of chronic illnesses by inducing persistent changes in the central stress response systems, including the hypothalamic-pituitary-adrenal (HPA) axis. We sought to determine if

EALs affect the HPA axis response to a visceral stressor in irritable bowel syndrome (IBS) patients and healthy controls, and to determine if this is affected by sex or related to symptoms or quality of life.

Methods.—Forty-four IBS patients (25 women, 19 men) and 39 healthy controls (21 women, 18 men) were assessed for gastrointestinal and psychological symptoms and EALs by validated questionnaires and interview. All subjects underwent a visceral stressor (sigmoidoscopy). Salivary cortisol was collected at baseline and serially for 1 hour poststressor.

Results.—Twenty-one IBS patients and 18 controls had EALs. In subjects with and without IBS, an EAL was associated with higher mean (±SD) cortisol levels (0.32 ± 0.2 vs 0.20 ± 0.1 μg/dL; $P = .003$) and higher area under the curve (28.1 ± 17 vs 18.6 ± 13 μg × min/dL; $P = .005$) after the stressor compared with subjects without EALs. In IBS, a faster resolution of cortisol to basal values corresponded to lower symptom severity ($r = -0.36$, $P < .05$) and better disease-specific quality of life ($r = 0.33$, $P < .05$).

Conclusions.—HPA axis hyperresponsiveness to a visceral stressor is related more to a history of EALs than to the presence of IBS. However, HPA axis reactivity has a moderating effect on IBS symptoms.

▶ It is controversial whether abnormalities of the hypothalamic-pituitary axis play a role in irritable bowel syndrome (IBS), as the literature has been quite conflicting. This issue is important because there is increasing evidence that the presence of an early adverse life event may be able to alter glucocorticoid receptor expression and therefore may act as an epigenetic risk factor for functional gastrointestinal disorders; early adverse life events, such as sexual or physical abuse, occur often in those later afflicted with IBS.[1]

This interesting study from Los Angeles evaluated salivary cortisol responses to a visceral stressor (flexible sigmoidoscopy). The investigators observed that those who had experienced an early adverse life event (whether an IBS patient or control) had a higher cortisol response compared with those who had not been subjected to one of these events. Interestingly, the difference was more pronounced in men compared with women. Furthermore, in IBS there was a slower return of the stimulated cortisol level back to baseline, and this delayed response was associated with an increased IBS symptom intensity and worse quality of life. These data suggest that abnormalities of the hypothalamic-pituitary axis in IBS are not specific to this disorder but rather reflect early adverse life events. However, it does appear that abnormalities of the hypothalamic-pituitary axis may impact on how IBS symptom severity is perceived.

The clinical implication of these data is drugs that centrally and peripherally block the hypothalamic-pituitary axis response (such as the corticotrophin releasing factor-1 antagonists) may not be very effective therapeutically (and some recent empiric evidence supports this contention).[2] Further work to identify the underlying etiopathogenesis of IBS continues, but the biological abnormalities present in these patients are starting to be unraveled, and it appears likely that localized gut abnormalities (such as low-grade inflammations) will be most important.

N. J. Talley, MD, PhD

References

1. Koloski NA, Talley NJ, Boyce PM, et al. A history of abuse in community subjects with irritable bowel syndrome and functional dyspepsia: the role of other psychosocial variables. *Digestion*. 2005;72:86-96.
2. Sweetser S, Camilleri M, Linker Nord SJ, et al. Do corticotropin releasing factor-1 receptors influence colonic transit and bowel function in women with irritable bowel syndrome? *Am J Physiol Gastrointest Liver Physiol*. 2009;296: G1299-G1306.

Continuation of Low-Dose Aspirin Therapy in Peptic Ulcer Bleeding: A Randomized Trial

Sung JJY, Lau JYW, Ching JYL, et al (Chinese Univ of Hong Kong, Sha Tin, New Territories)
Ann Intern Med 152:1-9, 2010

Background.—It is uncertain whether aspirin therapy should be continued after endoscopic hemostatic therapy in patients who develop peptic ulcer bleeding while receiving low-dose aspirin.

Objective.—To test that continuing aspirin therapy with proton-pump inhibitors after endoscopic control of ulcer bleeding was not inferior to stopping aspirin therapy, in terms of recurrent ulcer bleeding in adults with cardiovascular or cerebrovascular diseases.

Design.—A parallel randomized, placebo-controlled noninferiority trial, in which both patients and clinicians were blinded to treatment assignment, was conducted from 2003 to 2006 by using computer-generated numbers in concealed envelopes. (ClinicalTrials.gov registration number: NCT00153725).

Setting.—A tertiary endoscopy center.

Patients.—Low-dose aspirin recipients with peptic ulcer bleeding.

Intervention.—78 patients received aspirin, 80 mg/d, and 78 received placebo for 8 weeks immediately after endoscopic therapy. All patients received a 72-hour infusion of pantoprazole followed by oral pantoprazole. All patients completed follow-up.

Measurements.—The primary end point was recurrent ulcer bleeding within 30 days confirmed by endoscopy. Secondary end points were all-cause and specific-cause mortality in 8 weeks.

Results.—156 patients were included in an intention-to-treat analysis. Three patients withdrew from the trial before finishing follow-up. Recurrent ulcer bleeding within 30 days was 10.3% in the aspirin group and 5.4% in the placebo group (difference, 4.9 percentage points [95% CI, −3.6 to 13.4 percentage points]). Patients who received aspirin had lower all-cause mortality rates than patients who received placebo

(1.3% vs. 12.9%; difference, 11.6 percentage points [CI, 3.7 to 19.5 percentage points]). Patients in the aspirin group had lower mortality rates attributable to cardiovascular, cerebrovascular, or gastrointestinal complications than patients in the placebo group (1.3% vs. 10.3%; difference, 9 percentage points [CI, 1.7 to 16.3 percentage points]).

Limitations.—The sample size is relatively small, and only low-dose aspirin, 80 mg, was used. Two patients with recurrent bleeding in the placebo group did not have further endoscopy.

Conclusion.—Among low-dose aspirin recipients who had peptic ulcer bleeding, continuous aspirin therapy may increase the risk for recurrent bleeding but potentially reduces mortality rates. Larger trials are needed to confirm these findings.

▶ In clinical practice, patients presenting with peptic ulcer bleeding are usually treated endoscopically to stop the bleeding, provided effective antisecretory therapy (with a proton pump inhibitor [PPI]), and advised to discontinue aspirin or other antiplatelet agents until ulcer healing has occurred. However, patients taking aspirin or antiplatelet agents for major cardiovascular and cerebrovascular disease may have a very unfavorable risk-to-benefit ratio if the aspirin is stopped.

This trial aimed to determine how safe the continuation of low-dose aspirin is in those who present with acute peptic ulcer bleeding. The study was a relatively small randomized controlled trial but was elegantly designed. The authors observed that approximately 10% of patients had recurrent ulcer bleeding who were continued on low-dose aspirin (81 mg per day) compared with a rate of 5% in those on placebo. However, more striking was the observation that mortality rates were actually significantly higher in the placebo group overall. Patients who received aspirin had more gastrointestinal complications but lower cardiovascular and cerebrovascular mortality rates, and indeed the mortality rates from the gastrointestinal complications were still lower on aspirin than placebo.

The patients in this population studied here were relatively ill; they had multiple comorbid conditions and were elderly, and therefore, these results may not apply to younger patients or patients who receive aspirin for inappropriate reasons. Notably, all patients in the trial received a PPI, which is the current standard practice. The results cannot be extrapolated to higher doses of aspirin, although presumably most patients should not receive higher doses for cardiovascular or cerebrovascular prophylaxis.

This important study suggests that early resumption of low-dose aspirin should be strongly considered for all patients who need the medication, although due diligence in terms of follow-up is required to ensure recurrent bleeding is not occurring.

N. J. Talley, MD, PhD

Diarrhea-Predominant Irritable Bowel Syndrome Is Associated With Diverticular Disease: A Population-Based Study

Jung H-K, Choung RS, Locke GR III, et al (Mayo Clinic, Rochester, MN)
Am J Gastroenterol 105:652-661, 2010

Objectives.—A subset of patients with colonic diverticular disease have chronic gastrointestinal symptoms, and some have a clinical diagnosis of irritable bowel syndrome (IBS), but whether IBS and diverticular disease are linked is uncertain. We aimed to evaluate this association in the community.

Methods.—A population-based, cross-sectional survey was conducted by mailing a valid symptom questionnaire to the eligible residents of Olmsted County, MN, aged 30–95 years. Colonic diverticular disease (diverticulosis and diverticulitis) was ascertained through a review of the complete medical history of all responders. Subjects with at least one relevant test (colonoscopy, computed tomography (CT) scan, CT colonography, or barium enema) were included. IBS was defined using Rome II criteria.

Results.—Among 2,267 eligible respondents, there were 1,712 subjects who had undergone colon testing (76%): 919 women (54%); mean (±s.d.) age 65 (±11 years). Colonic diverticular disease was identified in 44.4% (95% confidence interval (CI) 42.1–46.8) of the subject. IBS was reported by 8.8% (95% CI 6.9–11.0) of men and 17.0% (95% CI 14.6–19.6) of women. After adjusting for age and gender, the presence of IBS was associated with an increased odds for diverticulosis (odds ratio (OR) = 1.8, 95% CI 1.3–2.4) but not diverticulitis (OR = 1.7, 95% CI 0.9–3.2). In those 65 years of age or older, the presence of IBS was associated with a ninefold higher odds for diverticulosis (OR = 9.4, 95% CI 5.8–15.1). Relative to the non-IBS subgroup, diarrhea-predominant IBS and mixed IBS were significantly associated with an increased odds for diverticular disease (OR = 1.9, 95% CI 1.1–3.2; OR2.6, 95% CI 1.0–6.4, respectively).

Conclusions.—There is a significantly increased odds for colonic diverticulosis in subjects with IBS (relative to those without IBS). These results suggest that IBS and colonic diverticular disease may be connected.

▶ Many patients with diverticulosis have lower abdominal symptoms, although whether the symptoms are caused by the diverticular disease remains controversial. A subset of these patients have symptoms highly consistent with irritable bowel syndrome (IBS), but again the link with diverticulosis remains somewhat obscure. Whether the presence of lower gastrointestinal tract symptoms indicates a higher risk of developing diverticulitis in those with diverticulosis has also been uncertain.

In this population-based study from Olmsted County, MN, subjects who had undergone colon testing and had a diagnosis of diverticulosis or diverticulitis were identified in the community, and the association with IBS symptoms was evaluated as measured by a validated questionnaire data applying standard

Rome II criteria. As diverticulosis has been hypothesized to be linked to a low-fiber diet, one might speculate that any association with IBS would be seen only in those who have constipation-predominant symptoms rather than diarrhea-predominant symptoms. In fact, however, relative to the non-IBS group, those with IBS and diarrhea (or mixed IBS) had a significantly increased risk for diverticular disease. However, IBS symptoms were not linked to an increased risk of developing diverticulitis.

There is some evidence that low-grade inflammatory changes may occur in patients with diverticulosis, and inflammation may precede the development of acute diverticulitis.[1] Low-grade inflammation in the colon has also been linked to the development of IBS, especially diarrhea-predominant IBS.[2] Whether inflammation is the common link between diverticular disease and diarrhea-predominant IBS remains speculative, but it is an area that clearly deserves further work. There are currently ongoing randomized controlled trials testing the hypothesis that the use of 5-aminosalacylic acid drug preparations will reduce the incidence of diverticulitis in patients with diverticulosis, and this work should be watched with great interest.

N. J. Talley, MD, PhD

References

1. Gatta L, Vakil N, Vaira D, et al. Efficacy of 5-ASA in the treatment of colonic diverticular disease. *J Clin Gastroenterol.* 2010;44:113-119.
2. Ohman L, Simrén M. Pathogenesis of IBS: role of inflammation, immunity and neuroimmune interactions. *Nat Rev Gastroenterol Hepatol.* 2010;7:163-173.

Eight year prognosis of postinfectious irritable bowel syndrome following waterborne bacterial dysentery

Marshall JK, Walkerton Health Study Investigators (McMaster Univ, Hamilton, Ontario, Canada; et al)
Gut 59:605-611, 2010

Background.—Although postinfectious irritable bowel syndrome (PI-IBS) is a well-recognised complication of acute gastroenteritis, its prognosis remains poorly defined. The natural history of PI-IBS was assessed among participants in the Walkerton Health Study (WHS), which has followed the long-term effects of a large outbreak of acute gastroenteritis related to municipal water contamination in May 2000.

Methods.—WHS participants were invited to return for annual assessment at a research clinic. Adult residents of Walkerton at the time of the outbreak who enrolled in 2002/2003 and returned for assessment in 2008 were eligible for a PI-IBS study cohort if they had no prior history of IBS or inflammatory bowel disease. A modified Bowel Disease Questionnaire was used to diagnose IBS by Rome I criteria and to identify IBS subtypes.

Results.—Of 4561 WHS participants, 2451 returned for their 8 year assessment and 1166 were eligible for the PI-IBS study cohort (688 females, mean age 46.2 years). The prevalence of IBS among 742 eligible subjects who suffered acute gastroenteritis during the outbreak declined from 28.3% after 2–3 years to 15.4% after 8 years, but remained significantly increased compared with controls who did not have acute gastroenteritis (OR 3.12; 95% CI 1.99 to 5.04). Independent risk factors for PI-IBS at 8 years included female gender, younger age, prior anxiety/ depression, and fever or weight loss during the acute enteric illness. IBS subtypes were not stable over time.

Conclusions.—Acute gastroenteritis can trigger IBS symptoms that persist for at least 8 years. Characteristics of the host and the acute enteric illness can predict the long-term risk of PI-IBS.

▶ This is a very important study of the prognosis of postinfectious irritable bowel syndrome (IBS). It has been increasingly appreciated that many different gastrointestinal infections can lead to irritable bowel symptoms if the small intestine or colon becomes inflamed. After an outbreak of bacterial dysentery in Ontario, the authors followed the population prospectively. They observed that postinfectious IBS will resolve over time in the majority, which is reassuring, but up to 1 in 7 of those affected will have persistent symptoms for at least 8 years after the acute infectious episode (and presumably this won't resolve).

Interestingly, those who were female, younger when the infection hit, and those with premorbid anxiety and depression or with a severe attack (as manifested by fever and weight loss during the acute episode) were more likely to continue to have symptoms 8 years after the initial infection. Another key observation is that among those who developed IBS, the majority had IBS with diarrhea or mixed pattern, but there was a substantial minority who developed constipation-predominant IBS (and some who couldn't be classified based on stool consistency). Perhaps most importantly, persistence of IBS subtype was uncommon, suggesting that the current thinking of some experts that IBS subtypes represent different disease entities may not in fact hold up; IBS appears to be characterized by its erratic nature.

Overall, the information here suggests that clinicians need to be vigilant when prescribing medications for patients with IBS that alter bowel habit, as the disease phenotype can and will change in many cases. For example, the 5HT3 antagonist alosetron, indicated for severe diarrhea-predominant IBS in women, is absolutely contraindicated in the setting of constipation. The new data presented do indicate that physicians can reassure patients with postinfectious IBS that there is a very good chance of improvement over time, although unfortunately a minority will have the disease for the rest of their lives.

N. J. Talley, MD, PhD

Fulminant *Clostridium difficile* Colitis: Patterns of Care and Predictors of Mortality

Sailhamer EA, Carson K, Chang Y, et al (Massachusetts General Hosp, Boston)
Arch Surg 144:433-439, 2009

Hypothesis.—There exist predictors of mortality and the need for colectomy among patients with fulminant *Clostridium difficile* colitis.

Design.—Retrospective study.

Setting.—Academic tertiary referral center.

Patients.—We reviewed the records of 4796 inpatients diagnosed as having *C difficile* colitis from January 1, 1996, to December 31, 2007, and identified 199 (4.1%) with fulminant *C difficile* colitis, as defined by the need for colectomy or admission to the intensive care unit for *C difficile* colitis.

Main Outcome Measures.—Risk of inpatient mortality was determined by multivariate analysis according to clinical predictors, colectomy, and medical team.

Results.—The inhospital mortality rate for fulminant *C difficile* colitis was 34.7%. Independent predictors of mortality included the following: (1) age of 70 years or older, (2) severe leukocytosis or leukopenia (white blood cell count, ≥35 000/μL or <4000/μL) or bandemia (neutrophil bands, ≥10%), and (3) cardiorespiratory failure (intubation or vasopressors). When all 3 factors were present, the mortality rate was 57.1%; when all 3 were absent, the mortality rate was 0%. Patients who underwent colectomy had a trend toward decreased mortality rates (odds ratio, 0.49; 95% confidence interval, 0.21-1.1; $P = .08$). Among patients admitted primarily for fulminant *C difficile* colitis, care in the surgical department compared with the nonsurgical department resulted in a higher rate of operation (85.1% vs 11.2%; $P < .001$) and lower mortality rates (12.8% vs 39.3%; $P = .001$). Patients admitted directly to the surgical department had a shorter mean (SD) interval from admission to operation (0 vs 1.7 [2.8] days; $P = .001$).

Conclusions.—Despite awareness and treatment, fulminant *C difficile* colitis remains a highly lethal disease. Reliable predictors of mortality exist and should be used to prompt aggressive surgical intervention. Survival rates are higher in patients who were cared for by surgical vs nonsurgical departments, possibly because of more frequent and earlier operations.

► This is an excellent article that should be read in its entirety. This retrospective study of 4796 inpatients confirms the increased mortality associated with fulminant *Clostridium difficile*. Predictors of mortality include advanced age greater than 70, WBC above 35 000, and need for cardiopulmonary support. These warning signs should result in aggressive medical and often surgical treatment. This article again provides emphasis on the importance of appropriate use of antibiotics, ie, as a risk factor for developing *C difficile*, and the importance of hospital isolation and universal precautions.

J. S. Scolapio, MD

Miscellaneous

Colonoscopic surveillance improves survival after colorectal cancer diagnosis in inflammatory bowel disease

Lutgens MWMD, On behalf of the Initiative on Crohn and Colitis (ICC) (Univ Med Ctr, Utrecht, The Netherlands; et al)
Br J Cancer 101:1671-1675, 2009

Background.—Colonoscopic surveillance provides the best practical means for preventing colorectal cancer (CRC) in inflammatory bowel disease (IBD) patients. Strong evidence for improved survival from surveillance programmes is sparse.

Method.—The aim of this study was to compare tumour stage and survival of IBD patients with CRC who were a part of a surveillance programme with those who were not. A nationwide pathology database (PALGA (pathologisch anatomisch landelijk geautomatiseerd archief)) was consulted to identify IBD patients with CRC treated in all eight university hospitals in The Netherlands over a period of 15 years. Patients were assigned to the surveillance group when they had undergone one or more surveillance colonoscopies before a diagnosis of CRC. Patients who had not undergone surveillance served as controls. Tumour stage and survival were compared between the two groups.

Results.—A total of 149 patients with IBD-associated CRC were identified. Twenty-three had had colonoscopic surveillance before CRC was discovered. The 5-year CRC-related survival rate of patients in the surveillance group was 100% compared with 74% in the non-surveillance group ($P = 0.042$). In the surveillance group, only one patient died as a consequence of CRC compared with 29 patients in the control group ($P = 0.047$). In addition, more early tumour stages were found in the surveillance group ($P = 0.004$).

Conclusions.—These results provide evidence for improved survival from colonoscopic surveillance in IBD patients by detecting CRC at a more favourable tumour stage.

▶ Surveillance colonoscopy among patients with longstanding chronic ulcerative colitis (UC) and Crohn's colitis is accepted clinical care because of known increased rates of colorectal cancer. However, the evidence for this practice is indirect or based on small studies. This study supports the practice but, while interesting, suffers from the same problems. Survival was improved but the effect was not statistically significant after adjusting for potential confounding factors such as age at cancer diagnosis and the presence of sclerosing cholangitis. Either the small sample size or confounding factors may have been the reason. We are also not given information regarding the extent of UC in the 2 groups. This may have affected colorectal cancer risk. Patients with inflammatory bowel disease (IBD) and cancer, diagnosed concurrently, were initially included in the nonsurveillance group but then appropriately excluded in the multivariate analysis because these patients were not eligible to enter a surveillance program. Patients in the surveillance group did have lower stage tumors, an important finding, but this was not evaluated in a multivariate analysis. In this retrospective study, selection bias may have altered the results. Patients in the surveillance program may have been more likely to report symptoms of colorectal cancer earlier, but the duration of the disease at cancer diagnosis was similar in the 2 groups. Overall, the study findings are important but, as with previous reports, need to be confirmed in larger studies where potential confounding factors can be adequately addressed. This will require the efforts of many centers and is long overdue.

M. F. Picco, MD, PhD

Factors Associated With Septic Complications After Restorative Proctocolectomy

Kiran RP, da Luz Moreira A, Remzi FH, et al (Cleveland Clinic, OH)
Ann Surg 251:436-440, 2010

Objective.—Few studies have evaluated factors that may be associated with the development of septic complications after restorative proctocolectomy. Therefore, the aim of this study is to evaluate preoperative and operative factors that might be associated with septic complications after restorative proctocolectomy.

Methods.—Patients developing abdominal and pelvic septic complications after restorative proctocolectomy were identified from a prospective database. Patients with subclinical leaks and ileostomy closure leak were not included in the septic complication group. A multivariable logistic regression model for sepsis was constructed using a forward stepwise selection with entry criterion of $P < 0.05$.

Results.—From 1983 to 2007, 3233 patients (56% male) were included in the database. Eight-four percent (2597) of patients underwent proximal diversion. Two hundred patients (6.2%) developed septic complications within 3 months of restorative proctocolectomy or within 3 months of ileostomy closure. On multivariate analysis, body mass index > 30 ($P = 0.02$, OR = 1.77), final pathologic diagnosis of ulcerative/indeterminate colitis ($P = 0.02$, OR = 2) or Crohn's disease ($P = 0.02$, OR = 3.6), intraoperative ($P = 0.02$, OR = 1.6), and postoperative transfusions ($P = 0.01$, OR = 1.9) were all independently associated with septic complications. We also demonstrated an independent association among individual surgeons ($P = 0.04$) with decreased septic complications.

Conclusions.—Body mass index greater than 30, final pathologic diagnosis of ulcerative/indeterminate colitis or Crohn's disease, intraoperative and postoperative transfusions, and surgeon were all independent factors associated with septic complications after restorative proctocolectomy.

▶ This interesting study looked at septic complications after restorative proctocolectomy in a very large number of patients from the Cleveland Clinic. Many potential factors that could influence the risk of septic complications were analyzed. Inflammatory bowel disease patients were included among familial adenomatous polyposis patients. Worse outcomes among Crohn's disease patients were found as would be expected. The increased risk among obese patients is important and probably due to the technical challenges of the surgery. The need for blood transfusions was also associated with complications probably related to the underlying disease severity. The individual surgeon's data are important. Even among a very well-trained group of surgeons, performance of less than 150 proctocolectomies was associated with higher rates of septic complications. Also important is what the study did not find. Corticosteroid (>20 mg/d), 6-MP/azathioprine, and infliximab use were not associated with complications. As the authors discuss, this is probably related to the majority of these patients having had a 3-stage pouch procedure. This study is important because it provides information for clinical decision making so that the most appropriate operation can be chosen to limit the risk of complications among patients requiring a restorative proctocolectomy.

M. F. Picco, MD, Phd

Familial Association of Inflammatory Bowel Diseases With Other Autoimmune and Related Diseases

Hemminki K, Li X, Sundquist K, et al (German Cancer Res Ctr (DKFZ), Heidelberg; Lund Univ, Malmö, Sweden; Ctr for Family and Community Medicine, Huddinge, Sweden)

Am J Gastroenterol 105:139-147, 2010

Objectives.—Familial risk estimates are useful for genetic counseling, etiological understanding, and design of gene identification studies. We wanted to estimate the associations of ulcerative colitis (UC) and Crohn's disease (CD) with 32 autoimmune and related diseases among parents and offspring, singleton siblings, twins, and spouses.

Methods.—The Multigeneration Register in Sweden provides reliable access to information on families among 11.5 million individuals throughout the last century. The diseases in individual family members were obtained through linkage to the Hospital Discharge Register. Standardized incidence ratios (SIRs) and 95% confidence intervals were calculated as relative risks for UC/CD in family members of patients diagnosed with any of the 34 diseases compared with those lacking affected family members through years 1964–2004.

Results.—Among a total of 441,642 patients diagnosed with autoimmune and related conditions, 25,846 were diagnosed with UC and 18,885 with CD. Familial cases amounted to 5.4% of all UC patients and 6.5% of CD patients. SIR for UC was 3.9 (95% confidence interval 3.5–4.3) in offspring of affected parents, 4.6 (3.0–7.4) in siblings, 10.4 (6.5–15.8) in families of affected parents and siblings, and 6.3 (1.9–17.7) for monozygotic twins. The respective SIRs for CD were 6.0 (5.4–6.7), 6.3 (4.1–9.8), 34.0 (24.9–45.3), and 23.4 (10.1–51.1). All discordant associations, i.e., those between CD and other diseases, were also found for UC, including ankylosing spondylitis, asthma, polymyalgia rheumatica, psoriasis, and sarcoidosis. For UC, six additional associations were observed. No correlations between specific diseases were found among spouses, but between UC or CD and any disease it was 1.1 (1.0–1.1).

Conclusions.—The concordant familial risks for UC and CD were lower than those commonly cited. Both diseases are associated with several autoimmune and related diseases, suggesting genetic sharing.

▶ This study provides important information on the association of inflammatory bowel diseases with other autoimmune diseases from a very large Swedish disease registry. The method of using standardized incidence ratios to present disease association reports the ratio of observed to expected cases to provide strength of association. It provides no measure of incidence or prevalence of these diseases in inflammatory bowel disease (IBD) and non-IBD patients, which would allow assessment of the overall risk and burden of these diseases in IBD populations. Familial risks were lower than previous studies, possibly due to the study population chosen. The study was based on hospitalized patients, which allowed for better accuracy in establishing disease diagnoses. However, this also selects out a population with potentially more severe disease requiring hospitalization. The authors argue that all hospitalized patients would be subject to the same biases so that the conclusions are valid. However, associations of IBD with other diseases may be overestimated in this cohort. The associations with rheumatoid arthritis and polymyalgia rheumatica rest on the accuracy of these diagnoses, especially because joint manifestations in IBD are common. Similarly, systemic lupus erythematosus may result from antitumor necrosis factor alpha therapy and not IBD itself. This is less likely a problem since the majority of the study time was before the use of infliximab. Overall, the study results are important since they provide estimates of familial risks of IBD in one of the largest (if not the largest) population to date. These results provide more support to expanding studies to establish genetic links between IBD and other diseases. This finding of genetic sharing with other diseases may lead to a better understanding of the genetic basis of IBD.

M. F. Picco, MD, PhD

Trends in Ambulatory and Emergency Room Visits for Inflammatory Bowel Diseases in the United States: 1994-2005

Ananthakrishnan AN, McGinley EL, Saeian K, et al (Med College of Wisconsin, Milwaukee; et al)

Am J Gastroenterol 105:363-370, 2010

Objectives.—Inflammatory bowel diseases (IBDs) require frequent healthcare encounters. Analysis of trends in disease burden is important to study the changing epidemiology of disease. The aim of our study was to examine national trends in IBD-related visits in ambulatory and emergency room (ER) settings.

Methods.—We used data from the National Ambulatory Medical Care Survey (NAMCS) and National Hospital Ambulatory Medical Care Survey (NHAMCS) using the *International Classification of Diseases, 9th Revision, Clinical Modification* codes to identify IBD-related visits. The annualized number of visits was examined in 3-year time periods from 1994 to 2005. We compared the demographic distribution of the inpatient, outpatient, and ER IBD cohorts.

Results.—There were an estimated 1.1 million (95% confidence interval (CI): 0.9–1.4 million) annual IBD-related visits during the period 1994–1996 increasing to 1.8 million (95% CI: 1.4–2.2 million) visits during 2003–2005 (+55%). Correspondingly, there were 28,752 estimated annual ER visits (95% CI: 16,299–41,206) related to IBD during 1994–1996 increasing to 76,374 annual visits (95% CI: 42,498–112,257) during 2003–2005 (+165%). The proportion of outpatient visits by patients older than 50 years increased from 34.1 to 52.0% ($P < 0.0001$). Use of corticosteroids decreased from 26.5% of visits to 14.5% ($P < 0.0001$), with a corresponding rise in immunomodulator/biologic use (2.6–13.8%, $P < 0.0001$). Younger, self-pay patients and those with Crohn's disease were over-represented in the ER IBD cohort compared with inpatients or outpatients.

Conclusions.—There has been an increase in IBD-related ambulatory and ER visits from 1994 to 2005. There is a need for research examining the reasons for the disproportionate representation of certain demographic groups in the ER setting.

▶ In this study, the authors analyze 2 United States national databases maintained by the National Center for Health Care Statistics for the analysis of trends in ambulatory health care utilization. They report striking increases in inflammatory bowel disease (IBD)-related ambulatory and emergency department (ED) visits from 1994-2005. Increases in ambulatory visits over time and disparities between younger and older patients and between self-pay and insured patients are very interesting. Unfortunately, firm conclusions regarding the basis for these trends cannot be made because of limitations of the databases involved. While visit data are provided, rates are calculated by estimates of the US population by census data. Specific individual patient-related information is not available. Increases in outpatient visits could be due to higher IBD prevalence or increase in health care utilization. Whatever the reason, the increase does signal a greater financial burden of IBD on the health care system. Increasing rates of ED visits might reflect increasing severity of IBD or poorer access to outpatient care. Also, nonwhites were overrepresented in the ED cohort compared with outpatients or inpatients. A greater proportion of younger, self-pay, nonwhite patients seeking care in the EDs might suggest health care access problems. Immunomodulator use (including both immunomodulator and biologics) over time increased, while corticosteroid use decreased. This might suggest better management of patients with IBD. A breakdown of medication use among ED versus non-ED patients was not provided but would have been very interesting. One might expect higher corticosteroid use for acute disease and lower immunomodulator use in the ED patients if these patients had poor ambulatory follow-up. Overall, the findings of this study are quite provocative and suggest the need for national IBD databases to understand differences in individual characteristics and access to care that may affect outcomes among patients with IBD.

M. F. Picco, MD, PhD

Increased Short- and Long-Term Risk of Inflammatory Bowel Disease After *Salmonella* or *Campylobacter* Gastroenteritis

Gradel KO, Nielsen HL, Schønheyder HC, et al (Aarhus Univ Hosp, Aalborg, Denmark)

Gastroenterology 137:495-501, 2009

Background & Aims.—Various commensal enteric and potentially pathogenic bacteria may be involved in the pathogenesis of inflammatory bowel diseases (IBD). We compared the risk of IBD between a cohort of patients with documented *Salmonella* or *Campylobacter* gastroenteritis and an age- and gender-matched control group from the same population in Denmark.

Methods.—We identified 13,324 patients with *Salmonella/Campylobacter* gastroenteritis from laboratory registries in North Jutland and Aarhus counties, Denmark, from 1991 through 2003, and 26,648 unexposed controls from the same counties. Of these, 176 exposed patients with IBD before the infection, their 352 unexposed controls, and 80 unexposed individuals with IBD before the *Salmonella/Campylobacter* infection were excluded. The final study cohort of 13,148 exposed and 26,216 unexposed individuals were followed for up to 15 years (mean, 7.5 years).

Results.—A first-time diagnosis of IBD was reported in 107 exposed (1.2%) and 73 unexposed individuals (0.5%). By age, gender, and comorbidity adjusted Cox proportional hazards regression analysis, the hazard ratio (95% confidence interval) for IBD was 2.9 (2.2–3.9) for the whole period and 1.9 (1.4–2.6) if the first year after the *Salmonella/Campylobacter* infection was excluded. The increased risk in exposed subjects was observed throughout the 15-year observation period. The increased risk was similar for *Salmonella* (n = 6463) and *Campylobacter* (n = 6685) and for a first-time diagnosis of Crohn's disease (n = 47) and ulcerative colitis (n = 133).

Conclusions.—In our population-based cohort study with complete follow-up, an increased risk of IBD was demonstrated in individuals notified in laboratory registries with an episode of *Salmonella/Campylobacter* gastroenteritis.

▶ The role of bacteria in the development of inflammatory bowel disease (IBD) has been the subject of intense interest and extensive study. Specific pathogenic bacteria have been implicated, but convincing proof is lacking. In this population-based study from Denmark, the authors conclude that a previous episode of *Salmonella* or *Campylobacter enteritis* is associated with a higher risk of development of IBD. While an intriguing idea, the authors do acknowledge the significant limitations of their data. Patients were retrospectively identified by a national registry, and the association of these infections was demonstrated by comparing the risk of IBD in those with infection (exposed) to those without infection (unexposed). The study design, a population-based cohort study with 15 years of follow-up, strengthens their conclusions. The analysis presenting overall risk and risk after exclusion of the first year of follow-up is important because it addresses the limitations of the article. Exclusion of patients who were diagnosed with IBD within 1 year of infection probably eliminates those with mild existing IBD that was exacerbated by *Salmonella* or *Campylobacter* infection. This is suggested by the finding of a large number of hospitalized exposed patients diagnosed with IBD in the first 2 months after infection. Furthermore, patients with severe symptoms may be more likely to have a stool specimen checked and undergo endoscopy leading to higher rates of diagnosis of IBD. Exclusion of the first year after infection still resulted in an elevated risk strengthening the authors' conclusions. Surveillance bias, as defined by the potential for more stool samples being taken among patients with IBD because of more severe symptoms, was also addressed. This may have led to a higher rate of detection of infection in IBD patients. No such bias was found with most patients being diagnosed with these infections after 1 sample. In summary, the nearly 2-fold increase in risk of IBD among patients with previous *Salmonella* or *Campylobacter* infection is supported by the data with careful methods of data analysis. This provides support for a role of these pathogenic bacteria in the development of IBD.

M. F. Picco, MD, PhD

Time Trends in Therapies and Outcomes for Adult Inflammatory Bowel Disease, Northern California, 1998–2005

Herrinton LJ, Liu L, Fireman B, et al (Kaiser Permanente Northern California, Oakland; et al)

Gastroenterology 137:502-511, 2009

Background & Aims.—The management of inflammatory bowel disease (IBD) has become increasingly complicated, and it is unknown whether poor outcomes (prolonged steroid use, hospitalizations, and surgery) have declined in the general population.

Methods.—This multilevel study used computerized clinical data. The study comprised 2892 adults with Crohn's disease (CD) and 5895 with ulcerative colitis (UC) who received care at 16 medical centers within an integrated care organization in Northern California between 1998 and 2005.

Results.—Time trends included (1) a shift in gastroenterology-related visits from the gastroenterology division to primary care; (2) increased use of IBD-related drugs, except for a 7% decline in use of 5-aminosalicylate in CD and no change in steroid use for CD; (3) for the prevalence of prolonged steroid exposure (120 days of continuous use), a 36% decline for CD with a 27% increase for UC; (4) declines in the hospitalization rates of 33% for CD and 29% for UC; and (5) for the surgery rate, no significant change for CD with a 50% decline for UC.

Conclusions.—Declines in prolonged steroid exposure and the hospitalization rate for CD and in the hospitalization and surgery rate for UC are encouraging; however, the increase in prolonged steroid exposure for UC merits concern and further investigation. The variability in care patterns observed in this study suggests lack of standardization of care and the opportunity to identify targets for quality improvement. These findings should stimulate research to quantify the effect of current trends in IBD management.

▶ This study tracks outcomes among patients with inflammatory bowel disease (IBD) over time in the Kaiser Permanente system. There were no practice guidelines for IBD or mandated referral to a specialist in this system. With exception of prescribing infliximab, which was restricted to gastroenterologists, primary care physicians were free to manage IBD in the manner they deemed appropriate. The patients followed came from a large community-based health system and not a subspecialist or tertiary center practice minimizing referral bias. The finding of a shift of gastroenterology visits from gastroenterologists to primary care physicians is surprising. Equally surprising was that despite an apparent shift, most outcome measures among patients with IBD improved. The reasons could not be defined but are open to speculation. It is not clear whether some patients were managed only by primary care providers and were never seen by a gastroenterologist or alternatively, seen in consultation by a gastroenterologist with ongoing care performed by their primary care provider. The latter is probably the case. Higher rates of primary care visits might reflect improved IBD care or just a shift of routine care in a population with generally mild disease. It is not clear whether gastroenterologists managed more severe cases but the more gastroenterologists at a center, the higher the rate of Crohn's disease (CD) surgery. Where there were more colorectal surgeons there was less immunodulator and steroid supply, which may suggest a greater tendency of patients at these centers to have surgery, although this did not reach statistical significance. Overall, this is an interesting article, but more research is needed to explain the reported trends. Lack of information on disease severity is an important limitation of the study because this probably is the most important issue for subspecialist referral and treatment selection.

M. F. Picco, MD, PhD

Negative capsule endoscopy without subsequent enteroscopy does not predict lower long-term rebleeding rates in patients with obscure GI bleeding

Park JJ, Cheon JH, Kim HM, et al (Yonsei Univ College of Medicine, Seoul, South Korea; Kwandong Univ College of Medicine, Seoul, South Korea)
Gastrointest Endosc 71:990-997, 2010

Background.—Capsule endoscopy (CE) is now widely accepted as a first-line diagnostic modality for obscure GI bleeding (OGIB). However, the clinical implications of negative results of CE studies remain unclear.

Objective.—To investigate long-term (>1 year) outcomes for patients undergoing CE for OGIB and to identify risk factors associated with rebleeding.

Design and Setting.—Retrospective study in a tertiary care hospital.

Methods.—A total of 57 consecutive patients who had undergone CE for OGIB were enrolled and their pre- and post-CE clinical data were collected. Specific treatments were defined as treatments directly aimed at presumed bleeding causes including hemostasis and disease-specific medical therapy, whereas nonspecific treatments were defined as symptomatic treatments for anemia.

Results.—Of the 57 patients, the indication for CE was obscure-overt bleeding in 46 patients and obscure-occult bleeding in 11 patients. Among 51 patients for whom long-term data were available, significant (P2) lesions were found in 23 (45.1%) patients. The overall rebleeding rate was 35.3% during a median follow-up duration of 31.7 months (range 12.8-58.0 months). There was no statistically significant difference in the cumulative rebleeding rate between patients with positive and negative CE results (34.8% vs 35.7%, respectively; $P = .989$). However, specific treatments after CE (hazard ratio, 0.111; 95% CI, 0.013-0.980; $P = .043$) significantly decreased rebleeding.

Limitations.—Small number of patients, retrospective study design.

Conclusions.—The rebleeding rate for patients with OGIB and negative CE results was substantial, indicating that these patients should be closely observed. However, specific treatment after CE significantly reduced the incidence of recurrent bleeding.

► This is a retrospective study of 57 patients from Korea investigating the outcomes for patients undergoing capsule endoscopy (CE) for obscure gastrointestinal (GI) bleeding. This retrospective study makes the point that a negative capsule study does not exclude the possibility that patients may rebleed. I think this study clearly points out that CE can miss significant lesions that may be a source of GI bleeding. I think this study reinforces the point that depending on a patient's clinical history and presentation, further investigation, including a double-balloon enteroscopy (DBE), may be required to locate and treat the bleeding source.

J. S. Scolapio, MD

Efficacy of Ceftriaxone or Meropenem as Initial Therapies in Whipple's Disease

Feurle GE, Junga NS, Marth T (DRK Krankenhaus, Neuwied, Germany; St Josef Krankenhaus, Braunau, Austria; Krankenhaus Maria Hilf, Daun, Germany)

Gastroenterology 138:478-486, 2010

Background & Aims.—Whipple's disease is a chronic infection caused by the actinomycete *Tropheryma whipplei*. We conducted a randomized controlled trial of the efficacy of antimicrobials that are able to cross the blood-brain barrier and to which *T whipplei* is susceptible.

Methods.—Patients from central Europe with previously untreated Whipple's disease (n = 40) were assigned randomly to groups given daily infusions of either ceftriaxone (1 × 2 g, 20 patients) or meropenem (3 × 1 g, 20 patients) for 14 days, followed by oral trimethoprim-sulfamethoxazole for 12 months. The primary outcome measured was maintenance of remission for 3 years, determined by a composite index of clinical and laboratory data as well as histology.

Results.—All patients were observed for the entire follow-up period (median, 89 mo; range, 71–128 mo); all achieved clinical and laboratory remission. Remission was maintained in all patients during the time of observation, except for 2 who died from unrelated causes. A single patient with asymptomatic cerebrospinal infection who was resistant to both treatments responded to chloroquine and minocycline. The odds ratio for the end point (remission for at least 3 years) was 0.95 (95% confidence interval, 0.05–16.29; $P = 1.0$).

Conclusions.—This was a randomized controlled trial to show that treatment with ceftriaxone or meropenem, followed by trimethoprim–sulfamethoxazole, cures patients with Whipple's disease. One asymptomatic individual with infection of the cerebrospinal fluid required additional therapy.

▶ Whipple's disease is rare but very important not to miss, as it is otherwise uniformly fatal. Typical presenting clinical features include migratory arthralgias, weight loss, diarrhea, abdominal pain, hyperpigmentation, and neurological symptoms; small bowel biopsy is diagnostic (if periodic acid-Schiff [PAS]-positive macrophages are present). Tetracycline used to be the primary therapy, but there is a high relapse rate with its use. Thus, treatment of this disease can be difficult and has evolved.

This pivotal randomized controlled trial suggests that either intravenous ceftriaxone or meropenem for 2 weeks followed by trimethoprim-sulfamethoxazole for 1 year is efficacious in terms of curing most patients with Whipple's disease. However, as patients with this rare disease may have an immune defect, regular follow-up of them for life (with annual small bowel biopsy) is recommended once therapy is complete to ensure that there has been no disease relapse. It is important to use antibiotics that will cross the blood-brain barrier in order to potentially cure the disease, and this trial suggests that the microbiological approach used was successful in doing this. Another important point from this study is that a lumbar puncture with examination of the cerebrospinal fluid should be part of the workup for *Tropheryma whipplei*.

Appropriate treatment of this potentially fatal disease is critical, and this research provides additional important information for gastroenterologists faced with these rare patients.

N. J. Talley, MD, PhD

6 Nutrition and Celiac Disease

Bedside postpyloric feeding tube placement: A pilot series to validate this novel technique

Gatt M, MacFie J (Scarborough General Hosp, UK)

Crit Care Med 37:523-527, 2009

Objective.—Postpyloric feeding may facilitate tolerance to enteral nutrition (EN) and offers an alternative route of feed administration when prepyloric EN fails. However, this is constrained by the difficulty of establishing nasojejunal (NJ) tube placement, which may necessitate endoscopy or radiology with the inevitable delay in the instigation of treatment. A bedside technique of NJ tube insertion has, therefore, been developed to permit blind postpyloric intubation. The primary aim of this audit was to validate the success of bedside NJ tube placement using the described technique. Secondary end points included the time taken to establish EN and the value of aspirate pH as an indicator of tube tip placement.

Design.—Observational.

Setting.—District general hospital.

Patients.—Consecutive patients requiring EN.

Measurements and Main Results.—The time taken to insert the tubes, the success rates in achieving the required position, and the time between the decision to feed and commencement of EN were recorded. The pH of any aspirate obtained was related to tube tip placement. Tube position was confirmed radiologically before starting EN. A total of 43 NJ tubes were inserted in 32 patients. Successful postpyloric intubation was achieved in 35 of 43 patients (81%). The median time for tube insertion was 18 (14–30) minutes. Time from the decision to feed to commencement of EN was 6 (5–18) hours. Aspirates were obtained from 26 of 43 (60%) intubations. Gastric aspirate pH readings were obtained for 19 of 43 (44%) of these intubations. Radiology reliably demonstrated the position of the tube tip in all cases.

Conclusions.—By-the-bedside NJ tube placement is possible in more than 80% of patients. This may overcome delays in the commencement of feeds resulting from other methods of postpyloric tube placement.

The use of aspirate pH on its own is not a reliable indicator of tube tip position.

▶ Enteral feeding has been shown to be superior in many studies compared with total parented nutrition (TPN). Enteral access can be the limiting factor in the use of enteral feeding at many hospitals. Enteral nutrition compared with TPN appears to reduce the risk of infection and may maintain the gut mucosal barrier. There is also the risk of aspiration pneumonia when feeding into the stomach in those patients in which you cannot elevate the head of their bed, hence the importance of postpyloric feeding tube placement. In this observation study, the authors report their experience of placing feeding tubes postpyloric with a reported success of near 80%. Their experience as presented in this article is worth reviewing for those clinicians that work in a hospital.

J. S. Scolapio, MD

Malignancies in cases with screening-identified evidence of coeliac disease: a long-term population-based cohort study

Lohi S, Mäki M, Montonen J, et al (Univ of Tampere, Finland; Natl Public Health Inst, Helsinki, Finland; et al)

Gut 58:643-647, 2009

Background and Aims.—The association between diagnosed coeliac disease and malignancy has been established. The present study was conducted to determine whether previously unrecognised and thus untreated adults with screening-identified evidence of coeliac disease carry an increased risk of malignancies.

Methods.—A Finnish population-based adult-representative cohort of 8000 individuals was drawn in 1978–1980. Stored sera of the participants with no history of coeliac disease or any malignancy were tested for immunoglobulin A(IgA), class tissue transglutaminase antibodies (Eu-tTG) in 2001. Positive sera were further analysed by another tissue transglutaminase antibody test (Celikey tTG) and for endomysial antibodies (EMAs). Malignant diseases were extracted from the nationwide database and antibody-positive cases were compared with negative cases during a follow-up of nearly 20 years.

Results.—Altogether 565 of all the 6849 analysed serum samples drawn in 1978–80 were Eu-tTG positive. In further analyses, 202 (2.9%) of the participants were Celikey tTG positive and 73 (1.1%) were EMA positive. The overall risk of malignancy was not increased among antibody-positive cases in the follow-up of two decades; the age- and sex-adjusted relative risk was 0.91 (95% Cl 0.60 to 1.37) for those who were Celikey tTG positive and 0.67 (95% Cl 0.28 to 1.61) for those who were EMA positive.

Conclusions.—The prognosis of adults with unrecognised coeliac disease with positive coeliac disease antibody status is good as regards the overall risk of malignancies. Thus, current diagnostic practice is sufficient and there is no need for earlier diagnosis of coeliac disease by mass screening on the basis of the findings of this study.

▶ Several studies have investigated the association between diagnosed and treated celiac disease and malignancies. It is still not entirely clear if patients with asymptomatic unrecognized celiac disease are at increased risk for cancers. In this Finnish study of 8000 individuals, the prognosis of adults with unrecognized celiac disease was favorable in that there was no additional risk of overall malignancy among untreated adults with celiac disease in a follow-up period of 20 years. I think it is important to not alarm our celiac patients of the malignancy risk, but perhaps to inform them that the scientific data are not conclusive.

J. S. Scolapio, MD

Prophylactic endotracheal intubation in critically ill patients undergoing endoscopy for upper GI hemorrhage

Rehman A, Iscimen R, Yilmaz M, et al (Mayo Clinic, Rochester, MN; Uludag Univ, Bursa, Turkey; Akdeniz Univ, Antalya, Turkey)

Gastrointest Endosc 69:e55-e59, 2009

Background.—Cardiopulmonary complications are common after endoscopy for upper GI (UGI) hemorrhage in the intensive care unit (ICU).

Objective.—To evaluate the practice and outcome of elective prophylactic endotracheal intubation before endoscopy for UGI hemorrhage in the ICU.

Design.—Retrospective, propensity-matched case-control study.

Setting.—A 24-bed medical ICU in a tertiary center.

Patients.—ICU patients who underwent endoscopy for UGI hemorrhage.

Main Outcome Measurements.—Cardiopulmonary complications, ICU and hospital length of stay, and mortality. In a propensity analysis, patients who were intubated for airway protection before UGI endoscopy were matched by probability of intubation to controls who were not intubated before UGI endoscopy.

Results.—Of 307 patients, 53 underwent elective prophylactic intubation before UGI endoscopy. The probability of intubation depended on the Acute Physiology and Chronic Health Evaluation III (APACHE III) score (OR 1.4; 95% CI, 1.2-1.6), age (OR 0.97; 95% CI, 0.95-0.09), the presence of hemetemesis (OR 1.9; 95% CI, 0.8-5.1), previous lung disease (OR 2.1; 95% CI, 0.8-4.9), and the number of transfusions (OR 1.1; 95% CI, 1.0-1.1 per unit). Nonintubated matched controls were identified for all but 4 patients with active massive hemetemesis, who were excluded from matched analysis. Cumulative incidence of cardiopulmonary complications (53% vs 45%, $P = .414$), ICU length of stay (median

2.2 vs 1.8 days, $P = .138$), hospital length of stay (6.9 vs 5.9 days, $P = .785$), and hospital mortality (14% vs 20%, $P = .366$) were similar.

Conclusions.—Cardiopulmonary complications are frequent after endoscopy for acute UGI bleeding in ICU patients and are largely unaffected by the practice of prophylactic intubation.

▶ This is an excellent article that applies to the safety of our gastrointestinal (GI) practice. This retrospective case-control study would suggest that prophylactic intubation for upper GI (UGI) hemorrhage does not improve the risk of cardiopulmonary complications. Prophylactic endotracheal intubation for airway protection during UGI hemorrhage is not standard of practice at most centers despite a reported 20% risk of developing new pulmonary infiltrates on chest X-ray, which would imply increased risk of aspiration. Other studies would suggest fewer cardiac arrests in those that received intubation before an esophagogastroduodenoscopy (EGD) for bleeding. The authors note at the conclusion of their article that prospective studies are needed to clearly answer this question. Until such studies are completed, I believe it is a good idea to work closely with the ICU staff and to intubate the patient that may be unstable and/or is having a large upper GI bleed. Certainly, there is no harm and we may prevent a severe aspiration event, which may be life-threatening.

J. S. Scolapio, MD

Celiac Disease: Predictors of Compliance With a Gluten-free Diet in Adolescents and Young Adults

Errichiello S, Esposito O, Di Mase R, et al (Univ of Magna Graecia, Catanzaro; Univ of Naples "Federico II," Italy)

J Pediatr Gastroenterol Nutr 50:54-60, 2010

Aims.—To identify risk as well as protective factors related to compliance with the gluten-free diet in a cohort of teenagers with celiac disease (CD).

Patients and Methods.—Two hundred four patients with CD (European Society for Pediatric Gastroenterology, Hepatology, and Nutrition criteria) older than or equal to 13 years and residents of Campania (southern Italy) were enrolled in the study. Patients underwent clinical examination and blood sampling, and were interviewed about school performance, social relationships, family integration, smoking habit, and compliance with a gluten-free diet. Anti-tissue transglutaminase antibodies were assayed with an enzyme-linked immunosorbent assay.

Results.—One hundred fifty of 204 (73.5%) reported no dietary transgressions, and 54 of 204 (26.5%) reported occasional or frequent transgressions. During the previous month 29 of 54 (53.7%) poor compliers ate from 0.001 to 1 g of gluten per day, 14 (25.9%) from 1 to 5 g, and 11 (20.4%) more than 5 g. The daily intake of gluten was significantly related to anti-tissue transglutaminase antibodies ($\chi^2 = 38.872$,

$P = 0.000$). Height was below the third percentile in 19 of 204 (9.3%), and weight was above the 97th percentile in 20 of 204 (9.8%). Diet compliance did not seem to influence the weight and height. One hundred eleven of 150 good compliers (74%) and 31of 54 (57.4%) poor compliers were asymptomatic. Most patients reported good family relationships (88.7%), social relationships (91.2%), and school integration (88.2%). Alternatively, 54% of patients reported some limitation in their social life. Compliance was good in patients who reported excellent school integration (83%) and social relationships (81%).

Conclusion.—Optimal school integration significantly contributes to the likelihood of good compliance. A better understanding within the school environment about CD-related issues could improve motivation to adhere to a gluten-free diet.

▶ This is an excellent article that discusses the compliance with a gluten-free diet in young adults from southern Italy. Although it is not possible to determine if these results apply to other cultures, I believe, based on previous US studies, that there is good correlation. This was a cross-sectional study of patients between the ages of 13 and 30. Patients completed a standardized self-administered questionnaire to determine compliance with diet; 26.5% of the patients reported poor compliance with no difference in compliance between the males and females. Interestingly, in this study dietary compliance did not affect weight and height. Also, a large number of the bad compliers tested negative for the tissue transglutaminase (tTG) antibody. This is an interesting observation in that one would expect the tTG to be positive with poor compliance. It is possible that not enough time elapsed for the tTG to revert to positive. Another important observation from this study was that health complaints were more common among the bad compliers, which may have been expected. Those patients with poor school integration tended to be more of the noncompliers. This is perhaps one of the most important observations of this study. If we are trying to help our patients become more compliant with a gluten-free diet, we must not forget to focus on the school environment, especially in the United States where students may be part of hot lunch programs. I think it is important for the physician to communicate to both the students and parents to work closely with their school health official to help promote compliance.

J. S. Scolapio, MD

Endoscopic Clips Prevent Displacement of Intestinal Feeding Tubes: A Long-Term Follow-Up Study

Udorah MO, Fleischman MW, Bala V, et al (Emory Univ, School of Medicine, Atlanta, GA)

Dig Dis Sci 55:371-374, 2010

Background.—Displacement of jejunal feeding tubes is a major problem in enteral feeding. Although endoscopic clips have been used to prevent migration of the tube during placement, the long-term effect of the clips on tube displacement is unknown.

Objectives.—The purpose of this study was to examine the long-term effect of endoscopic clips on preventing displacement of the jejunal feeding tube.

Design.—A retrospective study.

Setting.—A single tertiary medical center.

Main Outcome Measurements.—The success rate of the procedure and the functional duration of the feeding tube.

Results.—About 93% of patients had a percutaneous endoscopic gastrostomy jejunal (PEGJ) tube successfully placed with use of endoscopic clips. About 7% had tube migration and repeat procedures were successful. The mean functional duration of the tube was 55 days.

Limitations.—Retrospective, single-center.

Conclusions.—Use of endoscopic clips can prevent migration during placement of the feeding tube and can also reduce tube displacement in the long term.

▶ Flipping of jejunal feeding tubes back into the stomach is a common clinical problem. This can occur with both nasal jejunal tubes and percutaneous endoscopic gastrostomy jejunal (PEGJ) tubes. Although the tube may appear to be in the jejunum upon withdrawal of the endoscope, the scope can cause displacement of the tube during withdrawal. This is a retrospective study that describes the use of endoclips to prevent migration of a jejunal feeding tube during placement. The authors in this study report a 93% success rate using the endoclips with a mean functional duration of 55 days. I would recommend those who place such tubes to review this well-written article.

J. S. Scolapio, MD

Gastrostomy Tube–Related Complaints in the Pediatric Emergency Department: Identifying Opportunities for Improvement

Saavedra H, Losek JD, Shanley L, et al (Med Univ of South Carolina, Charleston)

Pediatr Emerg Care 25:728-732, 2009

Objective.—To describe the pediatric emergency medicine management of patients who present with gastrostomy tube (G-tube)–related complaints and identify opportunities for improving care and preventing G-tube complications.

Methods.—Retrospective cross-sectional descriptive study of patients (aged <18 years) who received care at an urban children's hospital (110 beds) emergency department (ED) for G-tube–related complaints.

Results.—Over a 23-month period, there were 181 ED patient visits by 77 patients for G-tube–related complaints. The mean number of visits per patient was 2.4. There were 159 (88%) G-tube and 22 (12%) gastrojejunostomy tube (GJ-tube) patient visits. The standard type of G-tube used at the study site ED was an adjustable-length tube. The most common complaint for G-tubes was dislodgement (99, 62%); and for GJ-tubes, malfunction (11, 50%). There were 119 patient visits (75%) needing G-tube replacement. Of these, 115 (97%) were successfully replaced in the ED, 85 (74%) by the pediatric emergency medicine attending physician, and 30 (26%) by the pediatric surgery service. The method of securing or documenting the intragastric depth of the adjustable-length tubes was documented in 15 (10%) of the 157 patients who had G-tubes or foley catheters at the time of ED disposition. The most common major G-tube complication was gastric outlet obstruction (3), and the most common major GJ-tube complication was aspiration pneumonia (3) secondary to gastric malposition (2) or dislodgement (1) of the GJ-tube. Only 9 patient visits (5%) resulted in hospitalization, and there were no deaths.

Conclusions.—Patients with G-tubes had approximately 1.25 mean ED visits per year for G-tube complaints. The most common G-tube complaint was dislodgement. Most dislodged G-tubes were replaced by ED physicians without the assistance of surgeons, but documentation of management and methods of securing the tubes was often incomplete. There were few major complications or hospitalizations. Treatment guidelines are presented that emphasize documentation of confirming G-tube location at the time of disposition from the ED.

▶ This is an excellent article for those gastrointestinal (GI) physicians who care for the pediatric population. To the best of my knowledge, this is the first study to review gastronomy (G)-tube management in the pediatric emergency department (ED). Just as with adults, children may present to the ED with percutaneous endoscopic gastronomy (PEG)-related problems with the most common G-tube complaint being dislodgement and/or clogging of the tube. Most tubes can be replaced via the same tract, provided the site has not closed. This is usually the case if less than 6 to 12 hours has elapsed from the time the tube has fallen out. This study also reports that most ED physicians can manage these problems successfully (97%) without the need of calling a GI physician. It has been our protocol to have patients follow up with their GI physician in the outpatient clinic after being discharged from the ED with PEG-related problems.

J. S. Scolapio, MD

Identifying High-Quality Bariatric Surgery Centers: Hospital Volume or Risk-Adjusted Outcomes?

Dimick JB, Osborne NH, Nicholas L, et al (Univ of Michigan, Ann Arbor)

J Am Coll Surg 209:702-706, 2009

Background.—Payers and professional organizations are expanding accreditation and "centers of excellence" programs in bariatric surgery. Rather than directly measuring outcomes, most programs rely on procedure volume. We sought to determine whether risk-adjusted outcomes or hospital volume were better at predicting future hospital morbidity with bariatric surgery.

Study Design.—We identified all patients who underwent gastric bypass in the New York State Inpatient database (n = 32,381 patients, n = 105 hospitals). Morbidity was ascertained using a previously validated combination of diagnostic and procedure codes. We first calculated the risk-adjusted morbidity and volume at each hospital during a 2-year period (2003 to 2004). We then ascertained the proportion of hospital-level variation explained by each measure using hierarchical modeling techniques. Finally, we compared the ability of each measure to predict future performance, as assessed with risk-adjusted morbidity, in the next 2 years (2005 to 2006).

Results.—Risk-adjusted morbidity explained 83% of future hospital-level variation in morbidity compared with only 21% for hospital volume. When comparing the "best" with the "worst" hospital quartiles, risk-adjusted morbidity predicted a more than fourfold difference in future performance (1.7% versus 7.2%; odds ratio [OR]: 4.5; 95% CI, 3.5 to 5.9). Hospital volume predicted only a twofold difference (2.5% versus 4.5%; OR: 1.9; 95% CI, 1.5 to 2.4) from the best to worst quartile.

Conclusions.—Risk-adjusted morbidity is much better than hospital volume at predicting future performance with bariatric surgery. Rather than focusing on volume, accreditation and centers of excellence programs should focus more on directly measuring outcomes.

▶ Although the use of bariatric procedures continues to increase, concerns of complications have also increased. Private insurers are now steering patients to designated centers of excellence. Most of the accreditation and center of excellence programs rely on procedure volumes as a quality marker. There is now growing evidence that outcome measures, such as morbidity, should replace procedure volumes as a marker of excellence. This article sought to determine whether risk-related outcomes or hospital volumes are a better marker for predicting complications of bariatric surgery. This study supports risk-adjusted morbidity as a better marker of quality care than volume. Since gastroenterologists often have to care for postoperative complications, including strictures, it is imperative that we make sure our patients are referred to quality bariatric programs. This article provides an excellent review and discussion on this topic.

J. S. Scolapio, MD

Indications for Percutaneous Endoscopic Gastrostomy and Procedure-related Outcome

Srinivasan R, Irvine T, Dalzell M (Alder Hey Children's NHS Foundation Trust, Liverpool, UK)

J Pediatr Gastroenterol Nutr 49:584-588, 2009

Objective.—To describe the indications and practice of percutaneous endoscopic gastrostomy (PEG) device insertion for nutritional support and to ascertain procedure-related complications and outcome.

Methods.—Observational study with prospectively collected data on children who underwent PEG-related procedures (PEG insertion, removal, or change to low profile button devices [LPBD]) for a 5-year period (2002–2006) at our centre.

Results.—Six hundred one PEG-related procedures were performed during the study period (384 insertions, 165 conversions to LPBD, 49 permanent PEG removals, and 3 PEG reinsertions). The main indications for PEG insertion were feeding difficulties associated with neurodisability (160/384; 41.6%) and congenital heart disease (CHD 115/384; 30%). Children with CHD required feeding nutritional support at an earlier age than children with neurodisability regardless of underlying cardiac condition. The age of PEG insertion was significantly different between the 2 main groups (neurodisability 3.56 years vs CHD 0.39 years; $P < 0.001$ [t test]). Fifty-nine patients were discharged on the same day as PEG insertion without complications (day case gastrostomy). The median time between PEG insertion to LPBD conversion was 0.83 year (0.12–3.86). Twenty-four of the 49 children having permanent PEG removal had CHD.

Conclusions.—Neurodisabilty and CHD were the main indications for PEG insertion, those with CHD requiring feeding support at an earlier age. Although CHD was an indication for PEG insertion in 30% of instances, a greater percentage of PEG removals (50%) were seen in this group indicating resolution of feeding difficulties.

► This is an excellent article reviewing the indications and outcome of percutaneous endoscopic gastrostomy (PEG)-related procedures in children. Neurodisability, specifically cerebral palsy, was the single most important indication for PEG placement in the 600 children studied. A low incidence of complications was noted in this group, despite being younger at the time of PEG placement. Infection was the most common complication following placement. Overall, this study would support that PEG placement in children is safe with a low procedure-related morbidity. For those gastrointestinal physicians who care for children, this would be an excellent article to review.

J. S. Scolapio, MD

Open-label, sham-controlled trial of an endoscopic duodenojejunal bypass liner for preoperative weight loss in bariatric surgery candidates

Gersin KS, Rothstein RI, Rosenthal RJ, et al (Carolinas Med Ctr, Charlotte; Dartmouth-Hitchcock Med Ctr, Hanover, NH; Cleveland Clinic of Florida, Weston; et al)

Gastrointest Endosc 71:976-982, 2010

Background.—The duodenojejunal bypass liner (DJBL) (EndoBarrier Gastrointestinal Liner) is an endoscopically placed and removable intestinal liner that creates a duodenojejunal bypass resulting in weight loss and improvement in type 2 diabetes mellitus.

Objective.—Weight loss before bariatric surgery to decrease perioperative complications.

Design.—Prospective, randomized, sham-controlled trial.

Setting.—Multicenter, tertiary care, teaching hospitals.

Patients.—Twenty-one obese subjects in the DJBL arm and 26 obese subjects in the sham arm composed the intent-to-treat population.

Interventions.—The subjects in the sham arm underwent an EGD and mock implantation. Both groups received identical nutritional counseling.

Main Outcome Measurements.—The primary endpoint was the difference in the percentage of excess weight loss (EWL) at week 12 between the 2 groups. Secondary endpoints were the percentage of subjects achieving 10% EWL, total weight change, and device safety.

Results.—Thirteen DJBL arm subjects and 24 sham arm subjects completed the 12-week study. EWL was 11.9% ± 1.4% and 2.7% ± 2.0% for the DJBL and sham arms, respectively ($P < .05$). In the DJBL arm, 62% achieved 10% or more EWL compared with 17% of the subjects in the sham arm ($P < .05$). Total weight change in the DJBL arm was −8.2 ± 1.3 kg compared with −2.1 ± 1.1 kg in the sham arm ($P < .05$). Eight DJBL subjects terminated early because of GI bleeding (n = 3), abdominal pain (n = 2), nausea and vomiting (n = 2), and an unrelated preexisting illness (n = 1). None had further clinical symptoms after DJBL explantation.

Limitations.—Study personnel were not blinded. There was a lack of data on caloric intake.

Conclusions.—The DJBL achieved endoscopic duodenal exclusion and promoted significant weight loss beyond a minimal sham effect in candidates for bariatric surgery. (Clinical trial registration number: NPT00469391.).

▶ In this prospective, randomized controlled study of 21 patients, the authors report their outcomes using an endoscopic duodenojejunal bypass liner for weight loss. The authors state in the article that weight loss prior to bariatric surgery may reduce postoperative complications. Although this may be true in super-obese patients (BMI > 50 kg/m^2), it is not the case in those with a BMI in the range of 35 to 40 kg/m^2. In most circumstances, patients are asked to diet and lose weight prior to surgery to ensure postoperative dietary compliance. I would not agree that an endoscopic or other surgical procedure be done prior to the definitive bariatric surgery in the majority of obese patients. Occasionally, in the super-obese patient, a lap-band surgery is done prior to the definitive bypass surgery to reduce postoperative complications. There were significant complications associated with the endoscopic procedure that the authors describe, including a need to remove the device. I would not recommend this endoscopic procedure be performed by a gastroenterologist outside an institutional review board (IRB)-approved research trial.

J. S. Scolapio, MD

Prevalence and Trends in Obesity Among US Adults, 1999-2008

Flegal KM, Carroll MD, Ogden CL, et al (Natl Ctr for Health Statistics, Hyattsville, MD)

JAMA 303:235-241, 2010

Context.—The prevalence of obesity increased in the United States between 1976-1980 and 1988-1994 and again between 1988-1994 and 1999-2000.

Objective.—To examine trends in obesity from 1999 through 2008 and the current prevalence of obesity and overweight for 2007-2008.

Design, Setting, and Participants.—Analysis of height and weight measurements from 5555 adult men and women aged 20 years or older obtained in 2007-2008 as part of the National Health and Nutrition Examination Survey (NHANES), a nationally representative sample of the US population. Data from the NHANES obtained in 2007-2008 were compared with results obtained from 1999 through 2006.

Main Outcome Measure.—Estimates of the prevalence of overweight and obesity in adults. Overweight was defined as a body mass index (BMI) of 25.0 to 29.9. Obesity was defined as a BMI of 30.0 or higher.

Results.—In 2007-2008, the age-adjusted prevalence of obesity was 33.8% (95% confidence interval [CI], 31.6%-36.0%) overall, 32.2% (95% CI, 29.5%-35.0%) among men, and 35.5% (95% CI, 33.2%-37.7%) among women. The corresponding prevalence estimates for overweight and obesity combined (BMI $\geq$25) were 68.0% (95% CI, 66.3%-69.8%), 72.3% (95% CI, 70.4%-74.1%), and 64.1% (95% CI, 61.3%-66.9%). Obesity prevalence varied by age group and by racial and ethnic group for both men and women. Over the 10-year period, obesity showed no significant trend among women (adjusted odds ratio [AOR] for 2007-2008 vs 1999-2000, 1.12 [95% CI, 0.89-1.32]). For men, there was a significant linear trend (AOR for 2007-2008 vs 1999-2000, 1.32 [95% CI, 1.12-1.58]); however, the 3 most recent data points did not differ significantly from each other.

Conclusions.—In 2007-2008, the prevalence of obesity was 32.2% among adult men and 35.5% among adult women. The increases in the prevalence of obesity previously observed do not appear to be continuing at the same rate over the past 10 years, particularly for women and possibly for men.

▶ More and more gastroenterologists are caring for patients with obesity. This has resulted primarly because of the endoscopic procedures required to diagnose and correct postoperative complications. Also obesity may increase the risk of certain gastrointestinal cancers and gastroesophageal reflux disease, according to some studies. This excellent article is a National Health and Nutrition Examination Survey (NHANES) that examines the trends in obesity from 1999 through 2008. Obesity is defined as a body mass index (BMI) of 30.0 or higher. The NHANES data from 1988-1994 showed that the prevalence of obesity in adults had increased by 8% since 1976-1980. The NHANES data from 1999-2000 showed further increase in obesity. This study points out that in 2007-2008 the prevalence of obesity was 32.2% among adult men and 35.5% among adult women. The rate does not appear to be increasing as in previous years. I think it is important for all gastroenterologists to have an understanding of the prevalence of obesity in the United States; therefore, I find this study to be an important reference.

J. S. Scolapio, MD

Radiologic versus Endoscopic Placement of Percutaneous Gastrostomy in Amyotrophic Lateral Sclerosis: Multivariate Analysis of Tolerance, Efficacy, and Survival

Blondet A, Lebigot J, Nicolas G, et al (Centre Hospitalier Universitaire Angers, France)

J Vasc Interv Radiol 21:527-533, 2010

Purpose.—To compare percutaneous radiologic gastrostomy (PRG) and percutaneous endoscopic gastrostomy (PEG) in terms of tolerance, efficacy, and survival in patients with amyotrophic lateral sclerosis (ALS).

Materials and Methods.—Forty patients with ALS (17 men; mean age, 66.1 years; range, 39–83 y) underwent 21 PEG and 22 PRG attempts (including three unsuccessful PEG attempts) from 1999 to 2005. To assess tolerance and efficacy, a successful and well tolerated placement was defined as any successful placement with no major or minor local complications or pain requiring opioid analgesic agents. Univariate analysis was performed for all recorded parameters, followed by multivariate analysis for successful and well tolerated placement, 6-month mortality rate, and survival.

Results.—General success rates were 85.7% for PEG and 100% for PRG. Pain was more frequent in PRGs (81.8% vs 52.4%; $P = .05$). Successful and well tolerated placement was seen in 81.8% of PRGs and 57.1% of PEGs ($P = 0.1$). Advanced age ($P = .02$) and PRG ($P = .07$) were predictive of successful and well tolerated placement. The interval from diagnosis to placement ($P = .001$) and ability to perform spirometry

(P =.002) were predictive of survival. Oximetry measurements (P =.007) and interval from diagnosis to placement (P =.02) were predictive of mortality at 6 months.

Conclusions.—PRG is more efficacious and better tolerated than PEG, essentially because it avoids the respiratory decompensation that may occur in PEG. Therefore, PRG should be preferred in cases of ALS. Survival is linked to ALS evolution and not to the choice of PRG or PEG placement.

▶ Gastrostomy tubes are considered the best choice for long-term care in patients with amyotrophic lateral sclerosis (ALS), as nasogastric tubes present many disadvantages when used for more than 4 weeks. A gastrostomy tube can help prevent aspiration and improve quality of life in almost all patients with ALS. The timing of placement is very important, as a patient's risk of respiratory complications increases with progression of the disease. I find that most neurologists are usually tuned in to when the patient's health and swallow functions begin to decline. In our center, the neurologist or nurse will call the gastrointestinal physician and dietician when they suspect the patient will require a feeding tube. This is usually done when the patient is still able to swallow food and water but beginning to have difficulty. This article would support our practice of having the radiologist place the tube to minimize or avoid respiratory decompensation during the procedure. It has also been our practice to administer 1 L of intravenous fluid the morning of the procedure, as we find many of these patients are dehydrated and may become hypotensive during the procedure. I find this to be an excellent article that reviews a very important clinical management situation.

J. S. Scolapio, MD

Sources of differences in estimates of obesity-associated deaths from first National Health and Nutrition Examination Survey (NHANES I) hazard ratios

Flegal KM, Graubard BI, Williamson DF, et al (Natl Ctr for Health Statistics, Hyattsville, MD; Natl Cancer Inst, Bethesda, MD; Emory Univ, Atlanta, GA)
Am J Clin Nutr 91:519-527, 2010

Background.—Estimates of obesity-associated deaths in the United States for 1991 were published by Allison et al (JAMA 1999;282: 1530–8) and subsequently for 2000 by Mokdad et al (JAMA 2004; 291:1238–45). Flegal et al (JAMA 2005;293:1861–7) then published lower estimates of obesity-associated deaths for 2000. All 3 studies incorporated data from the first National Health and Nutrition Examination Survey (NHANES I).

Objective.—The objective was to clarify the effects of methodologic differences between the 3 studies in estimates of obesity-associated deaths in the US population by using NHANES I hazard ratios.

Design.—The earlier reports used imputed smoking data for much of the NHANES I sample rather than the available reported data and applied a method of calculating attributable fractions that did not adjust for the effects of age, sex, and smoking on mortality in the target US population and did not account for effect modification by age. The effects of these and other methodologic factors were examined.

Results.—The NHANES I hazard ratios in the earlier reports were too low, probably because of the imputed smoking data. The low hazard ratios obscured the magnitude and direction of the bias arising from the incompletely adjusted attributable fraction method. When corrected hazard ratios were used, the incompletely adjusted attributable fraction method overestimated obesity-associated mortality in the target population by >100,000 deaths.

Conclusion.—Methodologic sources of bias in the reports by Allison et al and Mokdad et al include the assessment of smoking status in NHANES I and the method of calculating attributable fractions.

▶ This is a well-written article that gastrointestinal (GI) physicians who care for obese patients should review. There are about 112 000 deaths each year in the United States attributed directly to obesity, defined as a body mass index (BMI) greater than 35 kg/m^2. Some of the data discrepancies regarding the actual death rate from obesity in the United States are the result of bias in the partially adjusted methods for failure to account for the confounding effects of age, gender, and smoking. This study tries to explain the reasons for the effects of methodology on estimating obesity-related deaths in the 3 large studies that have been done to date. For all primary care physicians and GI physicians, this study supports timely referral for obesity surgery in those patients with a BMI greater than 35 kg/m^2.

J. S. Scolapio, MD

The Changing Face of Childhood Celiac Disease in North America: Impact of Serological Testing

McGowan KE, Castiglione DA, Butzner JD (Univ of Calgary, Canada)

Pediatrics 124:1572-1578, 2009

Objective.—The goal was to evaluate the impact of immunoglobulin A endomysial antibody testing on the incidence and clinical presentation of childhood celiac disease.

Methods.—The incidence and clinical presentation of celiac disease in patients <18 years of age in 1990–1996 (pretesting group) versus 2000–2006 (testing group) were compared.

Results.—The median age at diagnosis was 2 years (95% confidence interval: 2–4 years) in the pretesting group ($N = 36$), compared with 9 years (95% confidence interval: 8–10 years) in the testing group ($N = 199$; $P < .001$); the female/male ratios (1.6:1) were similar

($P = .982$). The incidence of celiac disease increased from 2.0 cases per 100 000 children (pretesting group) to 7.3 cases per 100 000 children (testing group; $P = .0256$). The frequency of classic celiac disease presentations decreased from 67% (pretesting group) to 19% (testing group; $P < .001$), but the incidence of classic celiac disease did not differ (0.8 vs 1.6 cases per 100 000; $P = .154$). In the testing group, 13 previously unrecognized clinical presentations were observed in 98 children, including 35 with family history, 18 with abdominal pain, and 14 with type 1 diabetes mellitus. The frequency of Marsh IIIc lesions decreased from 64% (pretesting group) to 44% (testing group; $P = .0403$). In the testing group, classic celiac disease remained predominant (67%) in young children (<3 years), whereas atypical gastrointestinal and silent presentations predominated in older children.

Conclusions.—Antibody testing for celiac disease tripled the incidence of celiac disease and quadrupled the median age at diagnosis.

▶ Pediatric gastrointestinal (GI) physicians may be interested in this well-written article. The take-home message from this article is that serological testing for celiac disease in children with GI tract symptoms, including nonclassic presentations, will increase the diagnostic yield of celiac disease in the pediatric population. Current guidelines for children presenting with chronic abdominal pain in the absence of other symptoms do not recommend testing for celiac disease. This study would suggest that such testing should be done since celiac disease can occur in 0.3% to 1.0 % of children. Since dietary treatment usually results in dramatic improvement in patients' symptoms, this article is very timely and reminds us all to keep celiac disease in the differential diagnosis of children who may have nonclassic GI tract symptoms.

J. S. Scolapio, MD

Time Trends in Age at Onset of Anorexia Nervosa and Bulimia Nervosa

Favaro A, Caregaro L, Tenconi E, et al (Univ of Padova, Italy)

J Clin Psychiatry 70:1715-1721, 2009

Objective.—This study aims to explore the time trends in age at onset of anorexia nervosa and bulimia nervosa.

Method.—The sample was composed of 1,666 anorexia nervosa subjects and 793 bulimia nervosa subjects (according to *DSM-IV* criteria) without previous anorexia nervosa consecutively referred to our outpatient unit in the period between 1985 and 2008. Time trends in illness onset were analyzed according to the year of birth of subjects.

Results.—In both anorexia nervosa and bulimia nervosa, age at onset showed a significant decrease according to year of birth. A regression model showed a significant independent effect of socioeconomic status, age at menarche, and number of siblings in predicting age at onset lower than 16 years.

Conclusion.—Age at onset of anorexia nervosa and bulimia nervosa is decreasing in younger generations. The implications of our findings in terms of long-term outcome remain to be understood. Biologic and sociocultural factors explaining this phenomenon need to be explored in future studies.

▶ This is an excellent article that all gastrointestinal physicians should review. A large part of a gastroenterologist practice is evaluating patients with unexplained weight loss. We may feel uncomfortable suggesting to a patient or family that we suspect the patient may have anorexia nervosa and/or bulimia. These patients can be very difficult to manage and may refuse psychiatric evaluation. This article reviews anorexia nervosa and bulimia and provides information about making a diagnosis. This study is the first to provide evidence in support of a decreasing age at onset in anorexia and bulimia. An earlier age of onset carries a more deleterious impact on specific aspects of general health.

J. S. Scolapio, MD

Update on clinical trials of growth factors and anabolic steroids in cachexia and wasting

Gullett NP, Hebbar G, Ziegler TR (Emory Univ School of Medicine, Atlanta, GA)

Am J Clin Nutr 91:1143S-1147S, 2010

This article and others that focused on the clinical features, mechanisms, and epidemiology of skeletal muscle loss and wasting in chronic diseases, which include chronic kidney disease, cancer, and AIDS, were presented at a symposium entitled "Cachexia and Wasting: Recent Breakthroughs in Understanding and Opportunities for Intervention," held at Experimental Biology 2009. The clinical and anabolic efficacy of specific growth factors and anabolic steroids (eg, growth hormone, testosterone, megestrol acetate) in malnutrition and other catabolic states has been the subject of considerable research during the past several decades. Research on the effects of these agents in cachexia or wasting conditions, characterized by progressive loss of skeletal muscle and adipose tissue, focused on patients with AIDS in the early 1990s, when the devastating effects of the loss of body weight, lean body mass, and adipose tissue were recognized as contributors to these patients' mortality. These same agents have also been studied as methods to attenuate the catabolic responses observed in cancer-induced cachexia and in wasting induced by chronic obstructive pulmonary disease, congestive heart failure, renal failure, and other conditions. This article provides an updated review of recent clinical trials that specifically examined the potential therapeutic roles of growth hormone, testosterone, oxandrolone, and megestrol acetate and emerging data on the orexigenic peptide ghrelin, in human cachexia and wasting.

▶ As gastroenterologists we all see and care for patients with cachexia and wasting for multiple reasons. Feeding tubes and intravenous nourishment (total parenteral nutrition) have been our mainstays of treatment. This article reviews the topic of the use of anabolic steroids and growth hormone in such patients. This type of information is rarely presented in the gastrointestinal (GI) literature. Therefore, I think this is a good article that GI physicians should read. This article discusses the use of growth hormone, ghrelin, megestrol acetate, testosterone, and oxandrolone. It also reviews some of the side effects and contraindications to these medications. My observation from reading this article is that there is a need for additional data in the use of these medications in most patients, and GI physicians should be cautious when prescribing such medications.

J. S. Scolapio, MD

Variability of Histopathological Changes in Childhood Celiac Disease

Weir DC, Glickman JN, Roiff T, et al (Children's Hosp, Boston, MA)

Am J Gastroenterol 105:207-212, 2010

Objectives.—Adult studies of celiac disease (CD) have shown that duodenal mucosal histopathological changes may be patchy, and the diagnostic utility of duodenal bulb biopsies is believed to be limited. Few related pediatric data exist.

Methods.—We assessed the prevalence of variable biopsy findings and duodenal bulb involvement in children with CD, as well as its association with clinical parameters. A total of 198 consecutive cases of CD diagnosed at the Children's Hospital during 2001–2005 were analyzed. All biopsies were scored by a pathologist blinded to the clinical data using the Marsh criteria. Mucosal changes were classified as focal if changes consistent with CD and normal mucosa were found within a single biopsy fragment. Patchiness was defined as variation of at least one Marsh grade between separate fragments in a biopsy set.

Results.—The median age was 9.3 years; 62% were female. An average of 3.6 biopsy samples was obtained per case. In 101 cases, biopsy samples were obtained from the duodenal bulb and the second portion of the duodenum. Focality was present in biopsy samples collected from 36 (18%) cases. Patchiness was found in 105 (53%) cases, and at least 1 normal biopsy fragment was present in 71 (36%) cases. In 10 cases, only the bulb biopsies were diagnostic of CD. There was no association with the clinical features examined.

Conclusions.—Duodenal involvement in pediatric CD is frequently patchy and may show variable severity even within a single biopsy fragment. Variability cannot be predicted by clinical characteristics. Multiple

endoscopic biopsies, including the duodenal bulb, should be obtained in suspected pediatric CD cases to maximize diagnostic yield.

▶ Small bowel biopsy still remains the gold standard for the diagnosis of celiac disease (CD). Although the classical histological picture of intraepithelial lymphocytosis and marked villous atrophy is found in most individuals, some patients may have normal biopsies that may in some cases reflect a sampling error. It has been recognized that mucosal abnormalities in CD can be patchy in adults, with up to 25% variability of at least 1 Marsh grade between duodenal biopsy specimens. In the pediatric CD population, the prevalence, characteristics, and clinicopathological associations of patchy mucosal abnormalities in CD have not been well defined. This study assessed the histopathological changes in childhood celiac disease. This study highlights the fact that duodenal bulb biopsies should be taken with multiple small bowel biopsies (3-6), given the patchy nature of CD in this population of patients.

J. S. Scolapio, MD

7 Gastrointestinal Surgery

A Single Institution's Experience with More than 500 Laparoscopic Heller Myotomies for Achalasia

Rosemurgy AS, Morton CA, Rosas M, et al (Univ of South Florida College of Medicine, Tampa)

J Am Coll Surg 210:637-647, 2010

Background.—Long-term symptom relief and patient satisfaction after Heller myotomy are being reported. Herein, we report the largest experience of laparoscopic Heller myotomy for the treatment of achalasia.

Study Design.—Since 1992, 505 patients have been prospectively followed after laparoscopic Heller myotomy. Until 2004, concomitant fundoplication was undertaken for a patulous hiatus, a large hiatal hernia, or to buttress the repair of an esophagotomy, then concomitant fundoplication became routinely applied. More recently, laparo-endoscopic single site (LESS) Heller myotomy has been performed when possible to improve cosmesis. Before and after myotomy, patients scored their symptoms.

Results.—Before myotomy, 60% of patients underwent endoscopic therapy; of these patients, 27% had Botox (Allergan) therapy alone, 52% underwent dilation therapy alone, and 21% had both. Esophagotomy occurred in 7% of patients. Concomitant diverticulectomy was undertaken in 7%, fundoplication was performed in 59%, and LESS Heller myotomy was done in 12%. Median length of stay was 1 day. With mean follow-up at 31 months, the severity of all symptoms improved significantly. After myotomy, 95% experienced symptoms less than once per week, 86% believed their outcome is satisfying or better, and 92% would undergo myotomy again, if necessary. Symptoms after myotomy are similar with or without fundoplication and regardless of the laparoscopic approach used.

Conclusions.—Laparoscopic Heller myotomy safely and durably relieves symptoms of dysphagia. Confinement is short and satisfaction is very high. Relief of esophageal obstruction is paramount; the approach used or the application of a fundoplication has a lesser impact. Laparoscopic Heller myotomy, preferably with anterior fundoplication using a single site laparoscopic approach, is strongly encouraged for patients

with symptomatic achalasia and is efficacious even after failures of dilation and/or Botox therapy.

▶ This article represents the largest series of patients undergoing surgical treatment of achalasia in the literature today, reporting on over 505 patients undergoing surgery from 1992-2009. That said, the author's surgical treatment has evolved over this time period, leaving the study population of 505 somewhat heterogenous. The treatment evolved from an open technique to a laparoscopic technique, then to a laparoscopic technique through a single incision (laparoendoscopic single-site [LESS] esophagomyotomy), and concomitant anterior fundoplication initially only used in those with a large hiatal hernia or perforation to its use in all patients.

When looking at the methods and results carefully, one is left with essentially a descriptive article outlining the demographics and presenting symptoms of the patients undergoing surgery, the technique used, perioperative outcomes, and then symptom response in a subset of patients in whom follow-up was obtained. Regrettably, it doesn't really add much to the existing knowledge on this topic and raises some significant questions regarding study design, especially the ultimate outcome measure (symptom response) and follow-up (nowhere in the article do the authors report any detail about follow-up other than a "mean follow-up at 31 months"). With this, the article really misses the mark as far as adding substantially to the literature and serves largely as show and tell from a single surgeon promoting a new and unproven technique. Notable is the surgeon's relationship with the company that sells a device for the LESS technique.

Significant findings from this article include:

(1) Sixty percent of patients had undergone endoscopic treatment of their achalasia before coming to surgical intervention—not a new finding

(2) Most patients had symptoms for more than 3 to 4 years before being referred for surgery—not a new finding

(3) Most patients experienced significant improvement in symptom scores (1-10) following myotomy—not a new finding

(4) Average follow-up was short (31 months) considering the 17-year time frame for the study

(5) A new technique being promoted by industry and the senior surgeon appear to be equivalent to traditional technique

I have identified this article as a must-read for several reasons. First, it is the largest series of Heller myotomy patients in the contemporary literature. Next, it confirms in a large series what is already well known: the majority of patients undergoing esophagomyotomy for achalasia will experience significant improvement in their dysphagia and other esophageal and extraesophageal symptoms, and finally, the lack of true outcomes data, which often accompanies articles of this sort. Read carefully and you will find very little data on follow-up, physiologic outcomes, and the outcomes in those who failed this management. These are the areas where we need new information to manage the growing number of patients who have failed this already established option for management.

C. D. Smith, MD

Effect of Transoral Incisionless Fundoplication on Symptoms, PPI Use, and pH-Impedance Refluxes of GERD Patients

Testoni PA, Corsetti M, Di Pietro S, et al (Vita-Salute San Raffaele Univ, Milan, Italy)

World J Surg 34:750-757, 2010

Background.—Three previous studies from the same institution have reported that transoral incisionless fundoplication (TIF) with the EsophyX device is effective for creating a continent gastroesophageal valve and for good functional results as measured only by pH-metry in patients with gastroesophageal reflux disease (GERD). The objective of the present study was to evaluate the effect of TIF on symptoms, use of proton pump inhibitors (PPI), esophageal motility, and pH-impedance in patients with symptomatic GERD.

Methods.—Twenty consecutive patients were enrolled to complete the GERD-HRQL and GERD-QUAL question-naires while on and off PPI. They were also examined by upper gastrointestinal (GI) endoscopy to determine Hill grade and Jobe length of the gastroesophageal valve, and to check for hiatal hernia and esophagitis, esophageal manometry, and pH-impedance before and 6 months after TIF.

Results.—Six months after TIF, the GERD-HRLQ and GERD-QUAL scores off-PPI therapy and the number of total and acid pH-impedance refluxes were significantly reduced ($p < 0.05$). The PPI had been completely stopped in 55% of the patient and was reduced in 22% of the patients.

Conclusions.—At 6-month follow-up, TIF performed using the EsophyX device reduces symptoms and pH-impedance refluxes, allowing interruption or reduction of PPI use in 78% of patients with GERD.

► I selected this article for comment because of the continued interest in endoscopic therapy for gastroesophageal reflux disease (GERD) and the limited data available from which to make decisions about the effectiveness and the role for endoscopic antireflux procedures. Until the recent reintroduction of Stretta, the transoral incisionless fundoplication (TIF—product name Esophyx; Endogastric Solutions, Redmond, Washington) was essentially the only Food and Drug Administration approved and widely available device for endoscopic fundoplication.

The authors of this article review their experience with 20 patients undergoing the TIF, presenting their objective and subjective outcomes at 6 months postprocedure. The authors point out that the 3 articles on which much of the support for this technique is based come from the same institution.[1-3] This represents a series of patients from another European institution attempting to reproduce the results already published. Also, they used impedence-pH to assess physiologic outcomes.

Patients were prospectively enrolled, and all patients had proton pump inhibitor (PPI)-responsive GERD along with objectively confirmed pathologic GERD. Six-month outcomes are as follows:

(1) 55% of patients were off PPIs, and 22% reduced PPI use
(2) GERD health-related quality of life improved
(3) DeMeester Score did not change
(4) By impedence-pH, number of acid reflux episodes decreased
(5) Esophagitis disappeared in 2, was unchanged in 1, and developed in 3

The authors conclude, "In conclusion, the present study found that TIF using the EsophyX device improved patient symptoms and quality of life, and that it significantly reduced the number of cases of gastroesophageal reflux as measured by esophageal pH impedance, enabling about 78% of patients to stop or reduce by less than 50% the PPI use in a 6-month follow-up." This conclusion is generous and borders on overstating the overall result—no change in acid exposure in the distal esophagus at 6 months postprocedure. Anyone wondering if endoscopic GERD via the TIF will replace Nissen—clearly not anytime soon.

C. D. Smith, MD

References

1. Cadière GB, Rajan A, Germay O, Himpens J. Endoluminal fundoplication by a transoral device for the treatment of GERD: a feasibility study. *Surg Endosc.* 2008;22:333-342.
2. Cadière GB, Buset M, Muls V, et al. Antireflux transoral incisionless fundoplication using EsophyX: 12-month results of a prospective multicenter study. *World J Surg.* 2008;32:1676-1688.
3. Cadière GB, Van Sante N, Graves JE, Gawlicka AK, Rajan A. Two-year results of a feasibility study on antireflux transoral incisionless fundoplication using EsophyX. *Surg Endosc.* 2009;23:957-964.

Laparoscopic Nissen fundoplication after failed EsophyX® fundoplication

Furnée EJB, Broeders JAJL, Draaisma WA, et al (Univ Med Centre, Utrecht, The Netherlands; Meander Med Centre, Amersfoort, The Netherlands; et al)
Br J Surg 97:1051-1055, 2010

Background.—Reflux control may be ineffective in a substantial number of patients after endoluminal EsophyX® fundoplication for gastro-oesophageal reflux disease. Subsequent laparoscopic Nissen. fundoplication (LNF) might be required to relieve symptoms. The aim of this study was to evaluate the outcome of LNF after previous EsophyX® fundoplication.

Methods.—EsophyX® failure was defined as recurrence or persistence of typical symptoms, with or without anatomical failure of the wrap or persisting pathological oesophageal acid exposure. Consecutive patients who underwent LNF after failed EsophyX® fundoplication were identified. Symptomatic outcome was obtained by standardized questionnaire, and objective outcome by endoscopy, oesophageal manometry and pH monitoring.

Results.—Eleven patients were included. During LNF, intraoperative gastric perforation occurred in two patients and one developed a subphrenic abscess after operation. Daily heartburn was present in one patient after LNF and three had troublesome daily dysphagia. General quality of life after LNF was not significantly better than that before EsophyX® fundoplication. Oesophageal acid exposure was normalized in all patients after surgery. Oesophagitis was absent after LNF in all except one patient who had persisting grade A oesophagitis.

Conclusion.—Symptomatic and objective reflux control are satisfactory after LNF for a failed EsophyX® procedure. Previous EsophyX® fundoplication, however, is associated with a risk of gastric injury during LNF and a relatively high rate of postfundoplication dysphagia.

▶ In another review in this section,[1] the outcomes of the transoral incisionless fundoplication (TIF) procedure, an endoscopic antireflux procedure, were reviewed. Outcomes at 6 months suggest that this procedure corrects gastroesophageal reflux disease in very few patients, suggesting that patients may ultimately progress to Nissen fundoplication. In this study, the authors reviewed their experience in doing Nissen fundoplication in patients after TIF.

Over a 2-year period (2006-2008), 11 of 88 patients who underwent TIF failed the TIF procedure and underwent Nissen fundoplication. The Nissen fundoplication was performed on average within the first year after TIF. Intraoperatively, adhesions in the area of the TIF resulted in gastric or esophageal perforation in 3 patients (27%) and 1 patient developed a subphrenic abscess requiring exploration. After Nissen fundoplication, quality of life improved but did not reach statistical significance in this small group. Seven of the patients reported subjective improvement but 3 reported new onset of dysphagia after Nissen fundoplication.

Overall, this article presents a 12% rate of failure of the TIF, with patients requiring surgical intervention within 1 year of the TIF, and when a Nissen fundoplication is necessary after a TIF, the risk of perforation and poor outcomes is nearly 5 times what would be realized from Nissen fundoplication alone and double what would be expected after a redo Nissen fundoplication. When considering a patient for TIF, the outcome in the 12% who failed should be considered and communicated to the patient.

C. D. Smith, MD

Reference

1. Testoni PA, Corsetti M, Di Pietro S, et al. Effect of transoral incisionless fundoplication on symptoms, PPI use, and ph-impedance refluxes of GERD patients. *World J Surg*. 2010;34:750-757.

Esophagectomy after anti-reflux surgery

Shen KR, Harrison-Phipps KM, Cassivi SD, et al (Mayo Clinic, Rochester, MN)
J Thorac Cardiovasc Surg 139:969-975, 2010

Objective.—There are few data on whether prior fundoplication has an impact on subsequent esophageal resection and reconstruction. The aim of this study is to review our experience with patients undergoing esophagectomy after previous fundoplication.

Methods.—Medical records were reviewed of all patients undergoing esophageal resection from 1988 to 2008 at the Mayo Clinic. Patients with a fundoplication before esophagectomy were compared with a matched control group who had esophagectomy alone.

Results.—There were 2313 esophageal resections, and 80 patients had undergone at least 1 previous anti-reflux surgery. Indications for esophagectomy were benign stricture/perforation in 41 patients, cancer in 28 patients, and dysplasia in 11 patients. The surgical approach was Ivor Lewis in 38 patients, left thoracoabdominal in 29 patients, transhiatal in 10 patients, and McKeown in 3 patients. The conduit used was stomach in 70 patients, jejunum in 6 patients, and colon in 3 patients; 1 patient had a diversion and cervical esophagostomy only. Operative mortality occurred in 3 patients (3.7%). Postoperative complications occurred in 50 patients (62.5%), including anastomotic leak in 17 (21.5%). Sixteen patients (20%) required reoperation for complications. Complication, anastomotic leak, and reoperation rates were significantly higher in patients with anti-reflux surgery before esophagectomy compared with matched controls.

Conclusion.—Esophagectomy after prior anti-reflux surgery is challenging, but the stomach is usually a suitable conduit for esophageal replacement. Patients with a history of anti-reflux surgery who undergo esophagectomy are at significantly increased risk for postoperative complications, anastomotic leak, and need for reoperation.

▶ This article comes from a center with a long history of esophagectomy. Over 20 years 2313 esophagectomies were performed, and the authors specifically looked at 80 patients who had undergone a fundoplication prior to esophagectomy. They found that even though the prior fundoplication led to a higher complication rate after esophagectomy than in matched patients, the stomach could still be used as the neoesophagus in most patients (70/80), despite the fundus having already been used and distorted.

This article highlights 2 important points. First, even in skilled hands and at accomplished centers with considerable experience with esophageal surgery, esophagectomy has a high rate of complications, especially in reoperative cases. Additionally, the stomach remains the conduit of choice, even when undertaking a case where fundoplication has been performed.

C. D. Smith, MD

Clinicoradiological score for predicting the risk of strangulated small bowel obstruction

Schwenter F, Poletti PA, Platon A, et al (Geneva Univ Hosp and Med School, Switzerland)

Br J Surg 97:1119-1125, 2010

Background.—Intestinal ischaemia as a result of small bowel obstruction (SBO) requires prompt recognition and early intervention. A clinico-radiological score was sought to predict the risk of ischaemia in patients with SBO.

Methods.—A clinico-radiological protocol for the assessment of patients presenting with SBO was used. A logistic regression model was applied to identify determinant variables and construct a clinical score that would predict ischaemia requiring resection.

Results.—Of 233 consecutive patients with SBO, 138 required laparotomy of whom 45 underwent intestinal resection. In multivariable analysis, six variables correlated with small bowel resection and were given one point each towards the clinical score: history of pain lasting 4 days or more, guarding, C-reactive protein level at least 75 mg/1, leucocyte count 10×10^9/l or greater, free intraperitoneal fluid volume at least 500 ml on computed tomography (CT) and reduction, of CT small bowel wall contrast enhancement. The risk of intestinal ischaemia was 6 per cent in patients with a score of 1 or less, whereas 21 of 29 patients with a score of 3 or more underwent small bowel resection. A positive score of 3 or more had a sensitivity of 67·7 per cent and specificity 90·8 per cent; the area under the receiver operating characteristic curve was 0·87 (95 per cent confidence interval 0·79 to 0·95).

Conclusion.—By combining clinical, laboratory and radiological parameters, the clinical score allowed early identification of strangulated SBO.

▶ The management of patients with small bowel obstruction (SBO) remains one of the most vexing and confusing conditions facing the surgeon today. Despite the adage, "the sun should not set on a bowel obstruction," most would agree that not all patients presenting with bowel obstruction should undergo immediate operation, and in many cases an operation is not necessary at all. The decision about if and when to operate relies largely on the judgment of the surgeon. Of course, the goal is to operate only if small bowel necrosis and perforation is imminent and to intervene before the bowel is nonviable or has perforated. On the other hand, many of these patients may have a hostile abdomen making surgical intervention harrowing and complicated by the risks of iatrogenic bowel injury in an already compromised patient.

This study retrospectively looked at patients who presented with bowel obstruction attempting to identify preoperative radiographic and clinical factors that might help predict impending bowel ischemia and perforation, thereby identifying those who should undergo early surgical intervention. The authors specifically looked in detail at those requiring small bowel resection. The study design was robust and included careful patient selection, characterization into subgroups, analysis of multiple clinical and radiographic variables, development of a battery of parameters associated with a high likelihood of need for resection, a scoring system related to these parameters, and a validation strategy to test the specificity and sensitivity of the scoring system.

From this the authors found in a multivariable analysis that 6 variables correlated with small bowel resection and were given 1 point each toward the clinical score: history of pain lasting 4 days or more, guarding, C-reactive protein level at least 75 mg/L, leucocyte count 10×10^9/L or greater, free intraperitoneal fluid volume at least 500 mL on computed tomography (CT), and reduction of CT small bowel wall contrast enhancement. Using this scoring system a score of 1 or less carried a 6% risk of intestinal ischemia, whereas a score of 3 or more carried a greater than 70% likelihood of intestinal ischemia.

This gives us an additional tool when evaluating the patient with SBO to help determine if early surgical intervention is warranted, thereby relieving some of the confusion about if and when surgery is indicated. On the other hand, this study suffers the weakness of any retrospective research, particularly how to manage the bowel obstruction that is evolving over time. While this may provide an initial assessment to help guide first steps in care, it does not address the evolution of a bowel obstruction and the further timing regarding intervention. Alas, surgical judgment will remain an important determinant of the decision and timing regarding surgery for SBO.

C. D. Smith, MD

A meta-analysis comparing conservative treatment versus acute appendectomy for complicated appendicitis (abscess or phlegmon)

Simillis C, Symeonides P, Shorthouse AJ, et al (Imperial College, London, UK; Northern General Hosp, Sheffield, UK)

Surgery 147:818-829, 2010

Background.—No standardized approach is available for the management of complicated appendicitis defined as appendiceal abscess and phlegmon. This study used meta-analytic techniques to compare conservative treatment versus acute appendectomy.

Methods.—Comparative studies were identified by a literature search. The end points evaluated were overall complications, need for reoperation, duration of hospital stay, and duration of intravenous antibiotics.

Heterogeneity was assessed and a sensitivity analysis was performed to account for bias in patient selection.

Results.—Seventeen studies (16 nonrandomized retrospective and 1 nonrandomized prospective) reported on 1,572 patients: 847 patients received conservative treatment and 725 had acute appendectomy. Conservative treatment was associated with significantly less overall complications, wound infections, abdominal/pelvic abscesses, ileus/bowel obstructions, and reoperations. No significant difference was found in the duration of first hospitalization, the overall duration of hospital stay, and the duration of intravenous antibiotics. Overall complications remained significantly less in the conservative treatment group during sensitivity analysis of studies including only pediatric patients, high-quality studies, more recent studies, and studies with a larger group of patients.

Conclusion.—The conservative management of complicated appendicitis is associated with a decrease in complication and reoperation rate compared with acute appendectomy, and it has a similar duration of hospital stay. Because of significant heterogeneity between studies, additional studies should be undertaken to confirm these findings.

▶ The authors perform a meta-analysis in an attempt to bring new knowledge to the management of complicated appendicitis. Options have historically included acute operation for appendectomy versus nonoperative management with antibiotics, percutaneous drainage of any abscess or fluid collection, and interval appendectomy, reserving acute surgery only for those patients who progress despite these measures.

The authors follow a conventional and robust strategy to identify and select studies for inclusion in the analysis. Over a period of nearly 40 years (1969-2007), 17 articles met the study inclusion criteria. A careful analysis of these revealed that nonoperative management of complicated appendicitis resulted in fewer complications and an overall enhanced recovery when compared with patients who underwent immediate operation to manage complicated appendicitis, confirming what many have understood based on anecdotal and personal experience. Specifically, the nonoperative patients had fewer wound infections, abdominal/pelvic abscesses, and ileus/bowel obstructions. Furthermore, the CT group was found to have fewer reoperations compared with the immediate surgery group. No significant differences were found between groups regarding the duration of intravenous antibiotics and the length of first hospitalization. If subsequent admissions (including those for interval appendectomy and complications) were included, still there were no significant differences between the 2 groups. Even though nonoperative management seems more complex and requires multiple procedures and hospitalizations, it is associated with less morbidity and a shorter duration of overall hospital care.

The value in this article is several-fold. First, the compilation and analysis of these data should nearly put to rest the debate about how best to manage complicated appendicitis. All too often, this debate rages at 2:00 AM when the patient with 6 days of periumbilical and right lower quadrant pain finally presents to the hospital with no doubt about the diagnosis, only doubt about the correct next step. The algorithm for management of acute appendicitis being immediate surgery is so ingrained that it is hard to deviate from this algorithm. This study finally gives a name to the real diagnosis and the algorithm that will provide the best care for the majority of these patients.

Equally important, this article highlights how new knowledge can be mined from the existing data, and a well-conceived and well-conducted meta-analysis can bring more clarity with the unrealistic expectation of a prospective randomized controlled trial. This type of study would not be practical, and if we wait for these kind of data, we will not find new knowledge on behalf of improved patient care.

C. D. Smith, MD

Identification of Specific Quality Improvement Opportunities for the Elderly Undergoing Gastrointestinal Surgery

Bentrem DJ, Cohen ME, Hynes DM, et al (Northwestern Univ, Chicago, IL; American College of Surgeons, Chicago, IL; Univ of Illinois at Chicago; et al)
Arch Surg 144:1013-1020, 2009

Hypothesis.—Specific complications occur more frequently in elderly patients undergoing major gastrointestinal (GI) tract operations that may represent opportunities for quality improvement.

Design.—Retrospective cohort study.

Setting.—One hundred twenty-one hospitals participating in American College of Surgeons National Surgical Quality Improvement Program (ACS-NSQIP).

Patients.—Using the ACS-NSQIP participant use file (2005-2006), patients undergoing upper gastrointestinal tract (n = 4115), hepatobiliary or pancreatic (n = 3364), and colorectal (n = 17 268) operations at 121 hospitals were examined.

Main Outcome Measures.—Risk-adjusted 30-day outcomes were assessed using regression modeling adjusting for patient characteristics, comorbidities, and surgical procedures. The elderly were defined as those older than 75 years.

Results.—Between January 1, 2005, and December 31, 2006, a total of 54 747 patients who underwent major GI tract operations were identified from the ACSNSQIP data file. In the elderly, overall perioperative morbidity was 1.2 to 2 times higher and mortality was 2.9 to 6.7 times higher than in younger patients after adjusting for differences in preoperative comorbidities. Irrespective of procedure type, the elderly were significantly more likely to experience cardiac (acute myocardial infarction and cardiac arrest), pulmonary (pneumonia, pulmonary embolism, and respiratory failure), and urologic (urinary tract infection and renal failure) complications. However, surgical site infections, postoperative bleeding events, deep venous thromboses, and rates of return to the operating room did not differ significantly by age.

Conclusions.—Morbidity and mortality are markedly higher in older patients. Quality measures for the elderly currently address only myocardial infarction, surgical site infection, and deep venous thrombosis. If care for the elderly is to be improved, quality improvement initiatives need to be expanded to include postoperative pulmonary and renal complications.

▶ The authors of this article mined the American College of Surgeons National Surgical Quality Improvement Program (ACS-NSQIP) database, specifically analyzing patients older than 75 years who underwent gastrointestinal (GI) procedures (foregut, HPB, and colorectal) to address the hypothesis that complications occur more frequently in elderly patients undergoing major GI tract operations. Further to this, they hoped to identify opportunities to improve care in this subset of patients.

In recognizing this article, it is important to illuminate the NSQIP database and its important current and future role in health care, especially at this time of health care reform and a focus on value (value = outcomes/cost). NSQIP is currently the only risk-adjusted, clinically abstracted, audited, benched-marked, and validated tool for assessing surgical outcomes, including 30-day outcomes. NSQIP is *not* hospital administrative data collected from admission diagnosis and billing documents surrounding hospital stay only. As such, highly credible data are available to analyze outcomes, and importantly, to design quality improvement programs and assess their impact over time.

In this study, the authors have shown conclusively that elderly patients (75 years and older) have a higher mortality and greater number of complications based on their age and independent of other factors. Specifically, cardiac, pulmonary, and urologic complications were more common.

Over the past 20 years, there have been multiple publications detailing outcomes from surgery in the elderly, documenting that complex surgery can be performed in the elderly with outcomes comparable to a younger cohort. Most of these have been single-institution experiences where the institution is notable for its expertise in the area of study. This multi-institutional study confirms what most of us have known anecdotally: the older the patient, the higher the likelihood of complications. This article serves as a framework for future work aimed at better identifying which older patients are most likely to suffer complications from GI surgery, and the areas of focus to limit complications when faced with an elderly patient who must have GI surgery.

C. D. Smith, MD

Outcomes After Fistulotomy: Results of a Prospective, Multicenter Regional Study

Hyman N, O'Brien S, Osler T (Univ of Vermont, Burlington)

Dis Colon Rectum 52:2022-2027, 2009

Purpose.—This study aimed to determine the outcomes and healing rate after fistula surgery across a broad spectrum of colorectal practices.

Methods.—A prospective, multicenter outcomes registry was created by the New England Regional Chapter of The American Society of Colon and Rectal Surgeons. All consecutive patients undergoing surgical treatment of an anal fistula by a participating surgeon from October 1, 2007 to September 30, 2008, were entered. Demographics, fistula characteristics including Parks' classification, smoking history, previous vaginal deliveries, diagnosis of Crohn's disease, Fecal Incontinence Severity Index, and operations performed were noted. A follow-up datasheet recorded postoperative complications, healing at one and three months, and postoperative continence scores. Factors associated with healing and treatment success were compared by use of Fisher's exact test.

Results.—Twenty-five surgeons at 13 hospitals entered 245 patients (162 male, 83 female) in the registry. Seventy-five patients had recurrent fistulas, 51 had multiple tracts, 62 were smokers, and 24 had Crohn's disease. The overall healing rate was 19.5% at one month and 63.2% at three months. Female gender ($P = 0.04$) and recurrent fistula ($P = 0.03$) were associated with nonhealing, and 28.4% of patients required additional surgery. The best healing rate was associated with fistulotomy (87%), whereas a plug had the worst healing rate (32%, $P = 0.001$).

Conclusions.—Surgical treatment of an anal fistula is associated with a substantial risk of nonhealing at three months. Fistulotomy had a high success rate, whereas the bioprosthetic plug had the lowest success rate.

Multicenter studies comparing treatment options for similar fistulas are needed.

▶ This multicenter study assessed management of fistula-in-ano including outcomes across 13 different hospitals in the Northeast. Twenty-five surgeons entered 245 patients in a registry. The group of patients studied was fairly heterogenous, and technique for management was left to the discretion of the surgeon.

Healing rate at 3 months was nearly 65%, and women and those with recurrent fistulas were associated with nonhealing at 3 months. Put differently, a significant number have not healed 3 months after surgical intervention. Nearly 30% needed an additional unplanned procedure. Less than half of the recurrent fistulas were healed at 3 months.

This study highlights the challenges in managing anal fistulae and the reality that many will not be healed 3 months after intervention and less than half of the recurrent fistula will be healed. Interestingly, a newer technique using a bioprosthetic to plug the fistula tract had the worst outcome of all techniques, again indicating the poor healing regardless of technique or surgeon. Patients undergoing management of these fistulae should be warned of the vexing nature of the condition and likely failure.

C. D. Smith, MD

Patterns of recurrence in patients with acute diverticulitis

Eglinton T, Nguyen T, Raniga S, et al (Christchurch Hosp, New Zealand)
Br J Surg 97:952-957, 2010

Background.—The natural history of acute diverticulitis remains unclear, with the role of prophylactic surgery following conservatively managed diverticulitis increasingly controversial. This study investigated recurrence rates, patterns and complications after conservatively managed diverticulitis.

Methods.—This was a retrospective chart review of all patients admitted with diverticulitis between June 1997 and June 2002. Demographic data, management, recurrence rates, complications and subsequent surgery were recorded.

Results.—Some 502 patients were identified, 337 with uncomplicated and 165 with complicated diverticulitis. Median follow-up was 101 (range 60–124) months. Of 320 patients with uncomplicated diverticulitis managed conservatively, 60 (18.8 per cent) had one episode of recurrence, whereas 15 (4.7 per cent) had two or more episodes. After an initial attack of uncomplicated diverticulitis, only 5.0 per cent developed complicated disease. Complicated disease recurred in 24 per cent, compared with a recurrence rate of 23.4 per cent in those with uncomplicated diverticulitis ($P = 0.622$). When recurrence occurred, it usually did so within 12 months of the initial episode.

Conclusion.—Acute diverticulitis has a low recurrence rate and rarely progresses to complications. Any recurrence is usually early, in a pattern more consistent with failure of the index episode to settle. Subsequent elective surgery to prevent recurrence and the development of complications should be used sparingly.

▶ This is a retrospective analysis of over 500 patients treated for diverticulitis over a 5-year period. Patients were categorized as having complicated (33%) or uncomplicated diverticulitis (67%). The eventual outcome and management for each group were followed for at least 5 years in an attempt to further our knowledge of the natural history of diverticulitis, particularly the natural history of medically managed diverticulitis.

This study confirms other work documenting recurrence after medical management of uncomplicated diverticulitis; nearly one fourth of patients will have a recurrence (23.4%). However, most had just a single recurrence, and only 4.7% had more than 2 episodes of diverticulitis. Importantly, the pattern of recurrence in this study suggests that recurrent episodes usually occur early in the first few months after the index episode, falling to a low but persistent rate after 12 months. It seems likely that early recurrence may be a result of failure of the initial episode to settle, as opposed to de novo recurrence. This begs the question of whether aggressive medical therapy might reduce the incidence of these early attacks. Most of these recurrences occurred within 1 year of the index case, suggesting that recurrence was actually incomplete treatment of the initial case.

When considering surgery for uncomplicated diverticulitis, prevention of recurrent acute disease is one of the principal justifications for elective colectomy. This study adds further support to the view that most patients who have diverticulitis will not be affected by recurrence, and so elective surgery to prevent recurrence should be offered sparingly. Also, the number of attacks of diverticulitis has been used as an indication for elective surgery based on the assumption that the risk of recurrence increases with each episode of diverticulitis. Guidelines have recommended elective colectomy after 2 attacks. In this study, the proportion of patients suffering further recurrence did not increase significantly with each recurrent episode, calling into question the recommendation for elective colectomy on the grounds of natural history alone.

This study has the limitations associated with evaluation of a retrospective cohort and the use of readmission data to estimate recurrence. This means that outpatient episodes of recurrent diverticulitis and inpatient treatment elsewhere may not have been captured. However, most significant episodes requiring readmission will have been included in the study, particularly as follow-up was facilitated by the use of national identification numbers. Nonetheless, this article again reminds us that modern management of diverticulitis, and in particular aggressive medical management of initial episodes, results in a natural history that holds surgery for select cases where recurrence would be least tolerated.

C. D. Smith, MD

Sepsis is a Major Predictor of Failure After Ileal Pouch-Anal Anastomosis

Forbes SS, O'Connor BI, Charles Victor J, et al (Univ of Toronto, Ontario, Canada)

Dis Colon Rectum 52:1975-1981, 2009

Purpose.—This study aimed to determine the risk of ileal pouch-anal anastomosis failure and factors predictive of failure overall and in patients with septic complications.

Methods.—Patients were identified through a prospectively maintained patient registry. All patients registered in the Mount Sinai Hospital Inflammatory Bowel Disease database who had an ileal pouch-anal anastomosis for more than 12 months were included in the study. Pouch failure was defined as ileal pouch-anal anastomosis excision or permanent diversion. Cox proportional hazard models with death as a competing risk were created, modeling time to failure as the outcome of interest for all patients and for the subgroup of patients with septic complications.

Results.—The study included 1,554 patients. One hundred six patients experienced an ileal pouch-anal anastomosis failure (6.8%), 49 (46.2%) of these failures were caused by septic complications. Independent predictors of failure included Crohn's disease (hazard ratio 7.5, 95% confidence interval [4.7, 12.0]) and postoperative sepsis (hazard ratio 6.6, 95% confidence interval [4.4, 9.8]). In the subgroup of patients with failure due to postoperative septic complications, independent predictors of failure were Crohn's disease (hazard ratio 2.7, 95% confidence interval [1.3, 5.7]) and presence of a pouch fistula (hazard ratio 2.6, 95% confidence interval [1.3, 5.2]).

Conclusion.—Septic complications are the most common cause of ileal pouch-anal anastomosis failure. Careful patient selection and the prevention of septic complications may decrease the risk of this failure.

▶ This article reports a series of 1554 patients who over a 24-year period (1981-2005) underwent ileal pouch-anal anastomosis (IPAA) for the management of ulcerative colitis. They performed a detailed analysis of outcomes, including univariate and, eventually, multivariate analysis of outcomes determining predictors of pouch failure (need for pouch excision or permanent diverting ileostomy). From this analysis they identified the presence of Crohn's disease (CD) and pelvic sepsis as the 2 factors predictive of failure and recommend careful patient selection preoperatively as well as aggressive management of pelvic sepsis as 2 steps to decrease the chance of pouch failure.

These findings are not particularly new or novel, but this article is a well-done study and contains many other valuable lessons from a 24-year experience with IPAA. For example, they discuss how their management has changed over the years and how this management has decreased the incidence of leaks, fistula, and pelvic sepsis. They outline how changing their technique of creating an S-pouch resulted in a decrease in the leak and pelvic sepsis rate, and how they made this change after an earlier analysis of outcomes and univariate analysis identified the S-pouch as the preferred technique. They also identified the change from hand-sewn anastomosis to the circular stapled anastomosis as having a favorable impact on anastomotic leaks. They also affirm other findings that pouch failure declines as a center gains more experience with the technique of IPAA.

The authors acknowledge that CD remains problematic in that despite a firm policy of *not* performing IPAA on patients with CD, they continue to have patients with unsuspected CD ongoing IPAA. When the CD patient with IPAA develops any postoperative complication related to the pouch or pelvis, the pouch failure rate is over 50%. When centers with this experience continue to have patients with CD slip through screening and have an IPAA, this problem will likely remain unless one takes a very aggressive approach like refusing to perform IPAA in patients with clinical presentations suggestive of CD, despite no pathologic confirmation of this diagnosis.

Overall, this is a well-done study and further confirms and highlights the outcomes after IPAA.

C. D. Smith, MD

Overall Mortality, Incremental Life Expectancy, and Cause of Death at 25 Years in the Program on the Surgical Control of the Hyperlipidemias
Buchwald H, Rudser KD, Williams SE, et al (Univ of Minnesota, Minneapolis)
Ann Surg 251:1034-1040, 2010

Objective.—To present the longest follow-up report of any lipid-atherosclerosis intervention trial.

Summary of Background Data.—The Program on the Surgical Control of the Hyperlipidemias (POSCH), a secondary, clinical/arteriographic, randomized controlled trial, was the first lipid-atherosclerosis trial to demonstrate unequivocally that low density lipoprotein cholesterol reduction reduced the incidence of coronary heart disease death and myocardial infarction.

Methods.—We report POSCH 25 years follow-up for overall mortality, specific cause of death, and certain subgroup analyses, as well as a prediction for increase in life expectancy derived from the POSCH database, supplemented by the 2006 National Death Index, 1989–2006.

Results.—There were 838 patients randomized in POSCH (421 surgery, 417 control). At 25 years follow-up, the difference in the restricted mean survival and the logrank (Mantel-Haenszel) statistic was statistically significant, with survival probabilities of 0.57 (surgery) and 0.51 (controls). Cause of death data indicated a significant increase in cardiovascular deaths in the control group; cancer deaths were also greater in the control group but this was not significant. The most compelling subgroup analysis was a significant increase in survival, starting at 5 years after randomization, in the surgery group for patients with an ejection fraction ≥50%, with relative probabilities of 0.61 (surgery) and 0.51 (control). The estimated incremental increase in life expectancy over more than 25 years of follow-up was 1.0 year overall and 1.7 years in the cohort with an ejection fraction ≥50%.

Conclusions.—A 25-year mortality follow-up in POSCH shows statistically significant gains in overall survival, cardiovascular disease-free survival, and life expectancy in the surgery group compared with the control group.

▶ Henry Buchwald and his colleagues at the University of Minnesota continue their research into the use of the jejunoileal bypass (JIB) (partial ileal bypass) as a therapy for hyperlipidemia refractory to medical management. The JIB was all but dead after thousands of morbidly obese patients underwent this operation to induce weight loss, and many subsequently developed life-threatening metabolic abnormalities and micronutrient deficiencies. Through the 1980s thousands of these operations were reversed. To Dr Buchwald's credit, he recognized a side effect of this operation that provided promise to those with refractory and life-threatening hyperlipidemia, and through a series of modifications, he developed the procedure reported in this article.

Now, after 25 years of careful use and study and enrolling over 800 patients into a prospective randomized clinical trial, these researchers document a reduction in cardiac events and cardiac mortality and an increase in life expectancy, albeit moderate at just less than 2 years, in those patients undergoing the operation versus those randomized to medical management. This prospective randomized study with long-term follow-up is truly a landmark effort considering that surgery is not being used to reestablish normal anatomy or to remove a diseased organ but rather, is being used to alter metabolism and thereby treat a medical condition. This is relatively rare in surgical research.

One could argue that while the difference is statistically significant, the benefit is moderate, is realized only after 20 or more years, and therefore is unlikely to replace medical management of hyperlipidemia. The authors themselves acknowledge that at the individual level these differences may seem inconsequential; looking from a population perspective using this approach, 6 more patients per 100 will be alive 25 years after a myocardial infraction, a potentially significant impact from an overall public health perspective.

Regardless, this is a landmark contribution to the literature, and the authors should be recognized and commended.

C. D. Smith, MD

Outcome of surgery for rectovaginal fistula due to Crohn's disease

Ruffolo C, Penninckx F, Van Assche G, et al (Univ Hosp Gasthuisberg, Leuven, Belgium)

Br J Surg 96:1190-1195, 2009

Background.—This study examined the outcome of surgery for symptomatic Crohn's rectovaginal fistula (RVF) and assessed the effect of therapy with antibody against tumour necrosis factor (TNF) on healing.

Methods.—Fifty-six patients with Crohn's disease underwent surgery for a RVF between January 1993 and December 2006. Outcome analysis was performed in February 2008 in relation to the surgical procedures used and the effect of anti-TNF treatment.

Results.—Four patients with a healed fistula still had a stoma at final follow-up for other reasons and were excluded from the analysis. Fistula closure was achieved in 81 per cent of the remaining 52 patients. Primary and secondary surgical success rates were 56 and 57 per cent respectively. The primary healing rate was similar in patients who received anti-TNF treatment before the first operation (12 of 18 patients) and those who did not (19 of 34). In univariable analysis, duration of Crohn's disease ($P = 0{\cdot}037$) and previous extended colonic resection ($P < 0{\cdot}001$) were significantly related to failure of primary surgery, but only the latter remained significant in multivariable analysis ($P < 0{\cdot}001$). Late recurrence developed in four patients.

Conclusion.—Fistula closure was achieved in most patients, but more than one operation was often required.

► Up to 10% of female patients with Crohn's disease develop rectovaginal fistulas (RVF). These fistulas are usually associated with severe anorectal

Crohn's disease which in turn adversely affects surgical outcomes thus supporting the need for tumor necrosis factor (TNF)-receptor antagonists.

Ruffolo and colleagues reviewed the outcome of 54 patients with Crohn's disease and RVF to determine the effect of anti-TNF on operative repair. They concluded that fistula closure was achieved in most patients (80%), but multiple operations were often needed. Anti-TNF treatments did not appear to significantly impair postoperative outcomes.

The duration and frequency of follow-up are extremely important when evaluating studies such as this. Median follow-up was 109 (range 24-180) months; however, the inclusion of some patients only followed for 2 years may lead to premature conclusions. Regrettably, it is not known as to whether follow-up was uniform among patients. Additionally, one quarter of patients were assessed by telephone interviews. Similar to other studies on this topic, operative repairs (with and without stomas) were heterogeneous emphasizing the need to individualize treatment, however, also confounding the interpretation of results.

Despite these concerns, the high rate of fistula closure is laudable. Moreover, preoperative anti-TNF treatment (based upon often controversial subset analysis) did not appear to significantly impair operative outcome.

J. L. Rombeau, MD

Acute lower gastrointestinal bleeding in 1,112 patients admitted to an urban emergency medical center

Gayer C, Chino A, Lucas C, et al (Wayne State Univ, Detroit, MI)

Surgery 146:600-607, 2009

Background.—This study was performed to elucidate the etiology, effectiveness of diagnostic and therapeutic modalities, and outcomes in patients with acute lower gastrointestinal bleeding.

Methods.—A retrospective review of the medical records of 1,112 consecutive patients admitted to the surgical service of a single urban emergency hospital with lower gastrointestinal bleeding from 1988 to 2006. Two groups were compared: 1988–1997 and 1998–2006.

Results.—All patients underwent colonoscopy, 33.2% within 24 h of admission. Hematochezia was the most frequent presentation (55.5%), followed by maroon stool (16.7%) and melena (11.0%). Most patients, 690 (62.1%) also had upper endoscopy. Sixty-six patients subsequently had barium enemas. Eleven of 27 nuclide scans were positive. Arteriography was performed on 22 patients, with 11 positive results and 2 therapeutic. No statistical difference was found in procedures performed in our 2 time periods. Diverticulosis (33.5%), hemorrhoids (22.5%), and carcinoma (12.7%) were the most common etiologies with the diagnosis of diverticulosis more common in the 1998–2006 time period. The small bowel was the source in 14 total patients. Spontaneous cessation of the bleeding occurred in 863 (77.6%) patients. Endoscopic control increased from 1% in 1997–1998 to 4.4% in 1998–2006 ($P < .05$) with a corresponding decrease in the need for operative control from 22.6% to 16.6% in this same time period ($P < .05$). Furthermore, among elective operations, there was a decrease in right hemicolectomies from 31.6% of total elective cases to 13.9% ($P < .05$). Emergent operations were needed in 3.4% and 4.8% of patients. The readmission rate did not change over time and was 5.2% overall with >50% because of diverticular bleeding.

Conclusion.—In this urban setting, diverticulosis, hemorrhoids, and carcinoma were the most common causes of severe acute lower gastrointestinal bleeding (LGIB) with diverticular bleed causing the highest recurrence. Colonoscopy allows for diagnosis in most patients with severe acute LGIB requiring hospitalization. Furthermore, it is now being used more effectively for hemostasis resulting in less operative intervention to control bleeding.

▶ Patients with acute lower gastrointestinal (LGI) bleeding continue to pose challenges for diagnosis and treatment. Despite advances in colonoscopy, red blood cell scintigraphy, and selective mesenteric angiography, failure to precisely localize the bleeding site is common.

Gayer and colleagues reviewed the outcomes of a large number (1112 patients) with LGI bleeding in an urban emergency medical center. They concluded that colonoscopy confirmed the diagnosis in most patients and even contributed to effective hemostasis.

Accurate localization of LGI bleeding is due to several factors, including the expertise of the diagnosticians, availability of support staff (especially in emergency settings), and the cause of the bleeding. This experienced group of well-trained emergency surgeons undoubtedly was a major factor in obtaining the excellent results. Regrettably, this level of expertise is not consistently available in many hospitals. Additionally, the increased frequency of diverticulosis, hemorrhoids, and cancer presumably contributed to the outstanding results. In other series, angiodysplasias and arteriovenous malformations of the right colon are frequent causes of LGI bleeding and are often difficult to diagnose and treat with colonoscopy. The spontaneous cessation of bleeding in over three fourths of patients underscores the importance of not intervening prematurely.

J. L. Rombeau, MD

Randomized Prospective Study of Endoscopic Rubber Band Ligation Compared With Bipolar Coagulation for Chronically Bleeding Internal Hemorrhoids

Jutabha R, Jensen DM, Chavalitdhamrong D (David Geffen School of Medicine at UCLA)

Am J Gastroenterol 104:2057-2064, 2009

Objectives.—Our purpose was to compare the efficacy, complications, success rate, recurrence rate at 1 year, and crossovers of rubber band ligation (RBL) with those of bipolar electrocoagulation (BPEC) treatment for chronically bleeding internal hemorrhoids.

Methods.—A total of 45 patients of mean age 51.5 years, who had rectal bleeding from grade II or III hemorrhoids and in whom intensive medical therapy failed, were randomized in a prospective study comparing RBL with BPEC. Treatment failure was predefined as continued bleeding, occurrence of a major complication, or failure to reduce the size of all internal hemorrhoidal segments to grade I in ≤ 3 treatments. Patients were followed up for 1 year.

Results.—With similar patients, rectal bleeding and other symptoms were controlled with significantly fewer treatments of RBL than of BPEC (2.3 ± 0.2 vs. 3.8 ± 0.4, $P < 0.05$), and RBL had a significantly higher success rate (92% vs. 62%, $P < 0.05$). RBL had more cases of severe pain during treatment (8% vs. 0%, $P > 0.05$), but significantly fewer failures and crossovers (8% vs. 38%). Symptomatic recurrence at 1 year was 10% RBL and 15% BPEC.

Conclusions.—For patients with chronically bleeding grade II or III internal hemorrhoids that are unresponsive to medical therapy, safety and complication rates of banding and BPEC were similar. The success rate was significantly higher with RBL than with BPEC. Symptom recurrence rates at 1 year were similar.

▶ Gastroenterologists and colorectal surgeons are frequently consulted for treatment of patients with bleeding internal hemorrhoids. When compliant, most of these individuals respond favorably to noninvasive management consisting of stool softeners, fiber supplementation, and alteration of bowel habits.

Invasive treatments are needed for the minority of patients who fail to respond to conservative treatments. Two frequently used treatments include bipolar coagulation (BPEC) and endoscopic rubber band ligation (RBL). The comparative successes of these treatments are unclear.

Jutabha and colleagues from UCLA conducted a prospective, randomized study to compare these treatments in 45 patients with chronically bleeding internal hemorrhoids refractory to standard medical treatment. They noted a significantly higher success rate (absence of recurrent bleeding) with RBL compared with BPEC; however, RBL caused more anorectal pain.

Strengths of this study include its design and detailed follow-up. The higher rate of posttreatment pain in the RBL group was presumably due to too distal placement of the rubber band. It is imperative that the band be placed above the dentate line to avoid the sensory innervation of the anal mucosa. To reduce the frequency of pain, the preplacement site can be tested by applying an angled Alis clamp to the intended areas for RBL. If the patient experiences pain, RBL must be placed more proximal.

Both of these techniques must be repeated to be effective (RBL 2.3 ± 0.2 and BPEC 3.8 ± 0.4 respectively). Patients must be initially informed of the need for several treatments, and the costs of multiple applications should be considered.

J. L. Rombeau, MD

Outcome of surgical treatment for fistula *in ano* in Crohn's disease

van Koperen PJ, Safiruddin F, Bemelman WA, et al (Univ of Amsterdam, The Netherlands)

Br J Surg 96:675-679, 2009

Background.—Recurrence rates and long-term functional outcome after surgical treatment of anal fistula in Crohn's disease were assessed.

Methods.—A consecutive series of patients was treated for Crohn's fistula *in ano*; those without proctitis or active sepsis underwent surgery. Sex, seton usage, infliximab, previous fistula surgery, history of segmental resection and smoking were examined as risk factors for recurrence. Continence was assessed by Vaizey scale and a colorectal Functional outcome questionnaire. Results were compared with institutional data for cryptoglandular fistulas.

Results.—Sixty-one patients were included, with a median follow-up of 79 (range 13–140) months. Twenty-four patients were treated with a seton, 28 by fistulotomy and nine by mucosal advancement. For low fistulas, fistulotomy was used more frequently than the seton, whereas seton drainage was used for most higher fistulas. Recurrence occurred in five of 28 and five of nine patients after fistulotomy and advancement respectively. Soiling was reported by half of the patients treated by seton *versus* two-thirds and three-quarters of those treated by fistulotomy and advancement respectively. Functional outcomes were worse for all patient groups than for cryptoglandular fistulas. No risk factor was significant.

Conclusion.—Surgical outcome for high or complex Crohn's fistula *in ano* remains disappointing, and recurrence is unpredictable.

▶ Anal fistulas in patients with Crohn's disease (CD) are extremely difficult to treat. When compared with the more common cryptoglandular pathogenesis, the postoperative outcome is poor. This is due in part to the severity of rectal disease, impaired wound healing, and side effects of medical therapy such as corticosteroids.

Van Koperen and colleagues reviewed the operative outcome of 61 consecutive patients with CD and anal fistulas without proctocolitis or active sepsis who underwent surgery. Patients were given an array of operative treatments ranging from simple placement of setons to complex transanal mucosal advancement flaps. They concluded that surgical outcome for patients with CD and anal fistulas, particularly if high or complex, is disappointing.

Similar to previous reports on this topic, the study suffers from the heterogeneity of patients and varied surgical treatments. The exclusion of those patients with proctocolitis definitely skews the outcome in favor of surgery. Additionally, it is impossible to determine the effect(s) (either positive or negative) of concomitant pharmacologic treatment. Finally, surgical experience and judgment are major determinants of outcome in most institutions. The number, background, and experience of the operating surgeons are not provided.

An important strength of this study includes the standardized Vaizey scale for continence and the colorectal functional outcomes questionnaire. The median length of follow-up of 79 months is sufficient to evaluate technical failures and early recurrent disease.

This study underscores the difficulty in operative treatment of these patients. Clearly, the operative decision must be tailored to the patient who must be candidly informed of the success rates. More controlled information is needed as to the concomitant effects of the biologic agents and operative treatments.

J. L. Rombeau, MD

Implementing Fast-Track Protocol for Colorectal Surgery: A Prospective Randomized Clinical Trial

Ionescu D, Iancu C, Ion D, et al (Univ of Medicine and Pharmacy, Cluj-Napoca, Romania; Univ of Medicine and Pharmacy, Bucharest, Romania)

World J Surg 33:2433-2438, 2009

Background.—Fast-track protocols are followed by an enhanced recovery, early return to bowel function and to complete nutrition, and a reduced hospital stay. Our study was designed to implement fast-track protocol in our university hospital.

Methods.—The 96 consecutive patients with colorectal neoplasm included in the study were randomized in two equal groups: group 1 (FT) included patients undergoing colorectal surgery in a fast-track protocol, and group 2 (C) included patients undergoing colorectal surgery with a conventional care protocol. As with other fast-track protocols, our protocol included carbohydrate fluids load before operation, early mobilization and oral feeding, regular prokinetics, and multimodal postoperative analgesia. Time to restoration of bowel function, to complete mobilization and feeding, length of hospital stay, and incidence of complications and readmissions were monitored.

Results.—Time to mobilization, restoring of bowel function, and complete oral feeding were significantly shorter with fast-track protocol ($p = 0.001$, $p = 0.042$, and $p = 0.01$, respectively). Hospital stay also was shorter in the fast-track group ($p = 0.001$). The incidence of complications did not significantly differ with the study groups.

Conclusions.—In our study, fast-track protocol resulted in a shorter time to mobilization, complete feeding, and discharge from hospital. Fast-track protocol did not increase the incidence of complications. However, we consider that our data require further confirmation with powered multicenter national studies.

▶ Continued increases in health care costs have led to a need for creative strategies to reduce expenditures in postoperative patients. Based on the seminal investigations of Kehlet and others, the length of postoperative stay (a major component of perioperative cost) can be significantly decreased when the fast-track protocol is implemented. This consists of early removal of nasogastric tubes, early postoperative feeding and ambulation, regular use of prokinetics, and multimodal analgesia. Whether this approach shortens hospital stay in a uniform group of colorectal surgical patients is not known.

Ionescu and colleagues randomized 96 patients who underwent colorectal surgery to a fast-track protocol and a control group given conventional care. Significant shorter hospital stay ($P = .001$) and return to complete oral feeding ($P = .04$) occurred in the fast-track group when compared with the conventional treatment. The fast-track protocol did not increase the complications.

Similar to other reports on this topic, this study has both weaknesses and strengths. It is unclear as to which component of the multimodal fast-track protocol has the greatest effect on the improved results. For example, some prokinetic drugs are expensive and may have a small contribution to the overall results. It is possible that simply applying more appropriate analgesia combined with early feeding and removal of the nasogastric (NG) tube will produce results equivalent to the complete protocol.

Despite the concerns, postoperative fast-track protocol can clearly be applied to colorectal surgical patients with good results. The conventional approach of withholding feeding and leaving NG tube in place until passage of flatus or stool is no longer tenable, particularly in colorectal surgical patients.

J. L. Rombeau, MD

Oncologic Outcomes of Robotic-Assisted Total Mesorectal Excision for the Treatment of Rectal Cancer

Baek J-H, McKenzie S, Garcia-Aguilar J, et al (Gachon Univ of Medicine and Science, Incheon, Korea; City of Hope Natl Med Ctr, Duarte, CA)

Ann Surg 251:882-886, 2010

Objective.—To evaluate local recurrence and survival after robotic-assisted total mesorectal excision (RTME) for primary rectal cancer.

Summary Background Data.—RTME is a novel approach for the treatment of rectal cancer and has been shown to be safe and effective. However, the oncologic results of this approach have not been reported in terms of local recurrence and survival rate.

Methods.—Sixty-four consecutive rectal cancer patients with stage I–III disease treated between November 2004 and June 2008 were analyzed prospectively.

Results.—All patients underwent RTME: 34 had colorectal anastomosis, 18 underwent coloanal anastomosis, and 12 received abdominoperineal resection. Operative mortality rate was 0%. The median operative time was 270 min and median blood loss was 200 mL. The conversion rate was 9.4%. Anastomotic leakage occurred in 4 of 52 (7.7%) patients with anastomosis. Median number of harvested lymph nodes was 14.5. Median distal margin of tumor was 3.4 cm. The circumferential resection margin was negative in all surgical specimens. No port-site recurrence occurred in any patient. Six patients developed recurrence: 2 combined local and distant, and 4 distal alone (mean follow-up of 20.2 months;

range, 1.7–52.5). None of the patients developed isolated local recurrence. The mean time to local recurrence was 23 months. The 3-year overall and disease-free survival rates were 96.2% and 73.7%, respectively.

Conclusions.—RTME can be carried out safely and effectively in terms of recurrence and survival rates. Further prospective randomized trials are necessary to better define the absolute benefits and limitations of robotic rectal surgery.

▶ As the result of laparoscopic surgery's reduced postoperative stay and decreased administration of narcotics coupled with improved cosmesis, surgeons continue to push the envelope for new approaches to minimally invasive surgery. These practices are in turn fueled by the public's demand for innovative operative techniques. Robotic surgery is an example of this advancing technology. It provides 3-dimensional vision, enhanced ergonomics, tremor elimination, superior dexterity, and surgeon's comfort. Whether robotic surgery can be used safely and efficaciously in patients with rectal cancer is not known.

Baek and colleagues reviewed their experience with 64 consecutive patients who underwent robotic-assisted total mesorectal excision for the treatment of rectal cancer. They noted equivalent operative and oncologic outcomes when compared with standard operative resections.

Limitations of this study include the lack of concomitant controls, heterogeneity of operations (abdominal perineal resections, colorectal, and coloanal anastomoses), and variable administration of preoperative neoadjuvant therapy.

One of the most dramatic benefits of robotic colorectal surgery is the quality of exposure in the male pelvis. Experienced surgeons readily recognize the technical difficulty, particularly in the low anterior and lateral rectal planes. Those of us who have witnessed the robotic exposure will attest to its superiority in these settings. Additionally, the study revealed excellent results in obtaining cancer-free lateral margins in all specimens.

This study and other recent publications provide strong rationale in support of prospective, controlled clinical trials. These trials should address the type and adequacy of technical training for surgeons and support personnel, time of setting up the apparatus, and overall costs.

J. L. Rombeau, MD

Prospective randomized controlled trial comparing V–Y advancement flap with primary suture methods in pilonidal disease

Nursal TZ, Ezer A, Çalışkan K, et al (Başkent Univ Dept of General Surgery, Adana, Turkey)

Am J Surg 199:170-177, 2010

Background.—An ideal treatment method for the widely prevalent pilonidal sinus disease is not yet available. The most commonly practiced technique is simple closure following resection of the effected tissue. However, high recurrence rates in some series have led to the search for other methods. One of these methods is the V–Y advancement flap (VYAF), which in theory results in the flattening of the natal cleft without tension in the suture line.

Methods.—In this prospective randomized controlled study, the VYAF method was compared to 2 simple primary closure techniques. In 238 patients, following resection, in the AL (all layers) group, all layers were closed with polypropylene sutures. In the SS (subcutaneous suture) group, polyglactin subcutaneous sutures were used to approximate the wound edges. Skin was closed separately in the SS group. In addition, demographic variables, past history, physical examination findings, defect dimensions, and wound tension were recorded.

Results.—Surgical site infection was observed in 23.9%, 17.4%, and 10.2% of the patients in AL, SS, and VYAF groups, respectively ($P = .129$). Early wound dehiscence without infection was detected in 11.9%, 7.4%, and 10.2% of the patients in groups AL, SS, and VYAF, respectively ($P = .665$). Mean follow-up was 29.7 ± 15.6 months. Survival (time without recurrence) was not significantly different between groups ($P = .648$). In the whole group, independent predictors of recurrence according to logistic regression analysis were younger age, recurrent disease, presence of discharge on physical examination, and development of postoperative surgical site infection.

Conclusions.—VYAF is not superior to simple primary closure techniques in terms of postoperative complications, recurrence, and patient satisfaction. For most cases, simple primary closure would suffice. Patients should be informed of the increased risk of recurrence if any of the independent predictors (being a recurrent case, presence of discharge, development of postoperative infection) are present.

▶ Surgery is the only effective treatment for chronic pilonidal cystic disease. The numbers of proposed operations are many and vary from simple hair removal and drainage to extensive muscle flaps. Controlled reports that objectively compare operative treatments are scarce.

Nursal and colleagues conducted a prospective, randomized controlled study to compare primary suture methods with V-Y advancement flap in 238 patients with pilonidal cystic disease. They concluded that the flap closure was not superior to simple primary closure.

The message in this report is more is not better. In fact, it is worse when one considers the degree of postoperative discomfort and physical limitations in patients undergoing the larger operation (V-Y advancement flaps). The large number of patients (n = 238) and the extensive experience of Turkish surgeons add further validity to the study. Most importantly, it is imperative for surgeons to tailor the operation to the severity of the disease with an emphasis on conservative treatment.

J. L. Rombeau, MD

Randomized clinical trial of symptom control after stapled anopexy or diathermy excision for haemorrhoid prolapse

Nyström P-O, on behalf of the Stapled or Open Pile Procedure (STOPP) trial study group (Karolinska Inst, Stockholm, Sweden; et al)

Br J Surg 97:167-176, 2010

Background.—This multicentre randomized clinical trial studied how symptoms improved after either stapled anopexy or diathermy excision of haemorrhoids.

Methods.—The study involved 18 hospitals in Sweden, Denmark and the UK. Some 207 patients were randomized to either anopexy or Milligan–Morgan haemorrhoidectomy, of whom 90 in each group were operated on. Patients reported symptoms before surgery and after 1 year. Daily postoperative pain scores were recorded in a patient diary. Surgeons evaluated the anal anatomy before surgery and after 1 year.

Results.—Correction of prolapse in the anopexy and haemorrhoidectomy groups was similar at 1 year (88 and 90 per cent respectively; $P = 0{\cdot}80$). Freedom from symptoms was obtained in 44 and 69 per cent respectively ($P = 0{\cdot}002$). Stapled anopexy was associated with less postoperative pain, which resolved more quickly ($P = 0{\cdot}004$). Significant improvements were noted in anal continence and well-being 1 year after both operations ($P < 0{\cdot}001$). Excessive pain was the most common complication after diathermy excision and disturbed bowel function after stapled anopexy.

Conclusion.—Haemorrhoidal prolapse was corrected equally by either operation. Diathermy haemorrhoidectomy gave better symptom relief but was more painful. Neither operation provided complete cure but well-being was greatly improved. Registration number: ISRCTN68315343 (http://www.controlled-trials.com).

▶ Hemorrhoidal disease continues to present many therapeutic challenges for both gastroenterologists and surgeons. A resolution of symptoms occurs in most patients when they reliably adhere to a structured daily regimen of stool softeners and fiber supplements. For the minority of patients unresponsive to conservative treatment, invasive treatments are needed. Excisional hemorrhoidectomy with diathermy is the traditional gold standard. Stapled anopexy has recently been used with increasing frequency. Whether this treatment produces a better outcome than excision with diathermy is not known.

Nyström and colleagues conducted a randomized, multicenter, clinical trial comparing these 2 treatments in 180 patients. Both treatments equally corrected hemorrhoidal prolapse. Diathermy provided better prolonged relief of symptoms but was initially more painful than stapled anopexy.

Limitations of this study include the need for surgeons in 18 different hospitals to accrue sufficient numbers of patients for analyses. Additionally, Ethicon, the parent company for the stapler, provided financial support, although the authors declared no conflict of interest. Nevertheless, the company is to be congratulated for supporting a randomized controlled clinical trial.

This well-controlled, prospective study provides a win for diathermy hemorrhoidectomy. The significant relief of symptoms that continued up to 1 year provides strong support in favor of this treatment. Although cost data are not provided, the stapled anopexy was presumably more expensive.

J. L. Rombeau, MD

Postoperative Complications Following Surgery for Rectal Cancer

Paun BC, Cassie S, MacLean AR, et al (Univ of Calgary, Alberta, Canada)

Ann Surg 251:807-818, 2010

Objective.—This systematic review was designed to determine postoperative complication rates of radical surgery for rectal cancer (abdominal perineal resection and anterior resection).

Summary of Background Data.—Lack of accepted complication rates for rectal cancer surgery may hinder quality improvement efforts and may impede the conception of future studies because of uncertainty regarding the expected event rates.

Methods.—All prospective studies of rectal cancer receiving radical surgery published between 1990 and August 2008 were obtained by searching Ovid MEDLINE, EMBASE, as well as ASCO GI, CAGS, and ASCRS meeting abstracts between 2004 and 2008. There was no language restriction. The outcomes extracted were anastomotic leak, pelvic sepsis, postoperative death, wound infection, and fecal incontinence. Summary complication rates were obtained using a random effects model; the Z-test was used to test for study heterogeneity.

Results.—Fifty-three prospective cohort studies and 45 randomized controlled studies with 36,315 patients (24,845 patients had an anastomosis) were eligible for inclusion. Most of the studies found were based in continental Europe (58%), followed by Asia (25%), United Kingdom (10%), North America (5%), and Australia/New Zealand. The anastomotic leak rate, reported in 84 studies, was 11% (95% CI: 10, 12); the pelvic sepsis rate, in 29 studies, was 12% (9, 16); the postoperative death rate, in 75 studies, was 2% (2, 3); and the wound infection rate, in 50 studies, was 7% (5, 8). Fecal incontinence rates were reported in too few studies and so heterogeneously that numerical summarization was inappropriate. Year of publication, use of preoperative radiation, use of laparoscopy, and use of protecting stoma were not significant variables, but average age, median tumor height, and method of detection (clinical vs. radiologic) showed significance to explain heterogeneity in anastomotic leak rates. Year of publication, study origin, average age, and use of laparoscopy were significant, but median tumor height and preoperative radiation use were not significant in explaining heterogeneity among observed postoperative death rates. With multivariable analysis, only average age for anastomotic leak and year of publication for postoperative death remained significant.

Conclusions.—Benchmark complication rates for radical rectal cancer surgery were obtained for use in sample size calculations in future studies and for quality control purposes. Postoperative death rates showed improvement in recent years.

▶ When compared with foregut surgery, operations for colorectal cancer are associated with frequent complications. This is due to the colon's extensive microflora, attenuated blood supply (when compared with the small intestine), and technical demands, particularly when removing large tumors. One of the problems in interpreting the literature of colorectal surgical complications is the frequent combining of results from rectal and colon surgery. Experienced surgeons readily acknowledge the increased complexity, technical demands, and risks of rectal operations when compared with colonic surgery.

Paun and colleagues performed a systematic review of the literature to determine postoperative complication rates of major operations (abdominal perineal resections and anterior resections) for rectal cancer. These detailed analyses provided benchmark complication rates such as 11% anastomotic leakage, 12% pelvic sepsis, and 2% postoperative mortality.

This report suffers from the standard problems of literature reviews. Prospective cohort and randomized controlled studies were both reviewed. Some studies reported more complete data than others. Additionally, definitions of postoperative complications varied among institutions.

Despite these concerns, this report represents one of the most carefully performed and detailed analyses on this topic. Most importantly, it addresses only rectal cancer. Finally, it provides important information for both surgeons and gastroenterologists to more accurately inform patients preoperatively as to the risk of postoperative complications associated with these major operations.

J. L. Rombeau, MD

Randomized clinical trial of anal fistula plug *versus* endorectal advancement flap for the treatment of high cryptoglandular fistula *in ano*

Ortiz H, Marzo J, Ciga MA, et al (Universidad Pública de Navarra, Pamplona, Spain)

Br J Surg 96:608-612, 2009

Background.—The aim of this randomized study was to compare the results of anal fistula plug and endorectal advancement flap in the treatment of high fistula *in ano* of cryptoglandular origin.

Methods.—Consecutive patients with high trans-sphincteric fistula *in ano* of cryptoglandular aetiology were randomized to treatment with either an anal fistula plug or endorectal advancement flap. Patients agreed to participate in a follow-up programme, which included scheduled visits at 2, 4, 8, 12 and 24 weeks and at 1 year after surgery. The primary endpoint was effectiveness in fistula healing. Recurrence was defined as the presence of an abscess arising in the same area, or obvious evidence of fistulation.

Results.—A large number of recurrences in the fistula plug group led to premature closure of the trial. After 1 year, fistula recurrence was noted in 12 of 15 patients treated with an anal fistula plug compared with two of 16 treated with an endorectal advancement flap (relative risk 6.40 (95 per cent confidence interval 1.70 to 23.97); $P < 0.001$).

Conclusion.—Contrary to other published studies, an anal fistula plug was associated with a low rate of fistula healing, particularly in patients with a history of fistula surgery.

▶ Surgery is the only definitive treatment for high (subsphincteric) cryptoglandular anal fistulas. Traditionally, the endorectal advancement flap has been the most effective operative treatment; however, it is associated with soiling and recurrent postoperative fistulas in up to 40% of patients.

The anal fistula plug is an attractive treatment for this problem due to its ease of placement and purported decreased risk for postoperative recurrence. Ortiz and colleagues conducted a randomized clinical trial to compare the outcomes of these 2 treatments. They observed an inordinate number of fistula recurrences (12 of 15 patients) with the plug thus forcing premature closure of the trial.

There are several lessons to be learned from this report. Most importantly, the value of the randomized clinical trial continues to be confirmed. This innovative treatment was initially embraced, with considerable enthusiasm, by many colorectal surgeons following uncontrolled studies with purported successes. It is unclear why this product was marketed prematurely in the absence of confirmatory controlled data. Regrettably, many patients were subjected to operations that ultimately were unsuccessful.

Despite these disappointing results, the concept of the fistula plug is still intriguing. Perhaps lyophilized porcine material is not the optimal substance for the plug structure. Patient selection is undoubtedly an important outcome variable. It is possible more patients with previous operative repairs were included in this trial when compared with previous studies.

The endorectal advancement flap remains the operative treatment of choice in patients undergoing surgery for high cryptoglandular fistula *in ano*.

J. L. Rombeau, MD

Causes of Mortality in Patients With Peptic Ulcer Bleeding: A Prospective Cohort Study of 10,428 Cases

Sung JJY, Tsoi KKF, Ma TKW, et al (The Chinese Univ of Hong Kong, Shatin)
Am J Gastroenterol 105:84-89, 2010

Objectives.—Despite advances in endoscopic and pharmacological treatment for peptic ulcer bleeding (PUB), mortality remains at 5–10% worldwide. Our aim was to investigate the causes of death in a prospective cohort of PUB in a tertiary referral center.

Methods.—Between 1993 and 2005, all patients with upper gastrointestinal bleeding (UGIB) admitted to the Prince of Wales Hospital were prospectively registered. Demographic data, characteristics of ulcer, and pharmacological, endoscopic, and surgical therapy, were documented. Mortality cases were classified as (A) bleeding-related death (A1: uncontrolled bleeding, A2: within 48 h after endoscopy, A3: during surgery for uncontrolled bleeding, A4: surgical complications or within 1 month after surgery, and A5: endoscopic related mortality) or (B) non-bleeding-related death (B1: cardiac causes, B2: pulmonary causes, B3: cerebrovascular disease, B4: multiorgan failure, and B5: terminal malignancy).

Results.—In all, 18,508 cases of UGIB were enrolled; among them, 10,428 cases from 9,375 patients were confirmed to have PUB, and 577 (6.2%) patients died. There were significantly more patients who died of non-ulcer bleeding causes (79.7%) than bleeding causes (18.4%). The mean (s.d.) age of those who died of bleeding-related causes was higher (75.4 (12.6) years) than that of those who died of non-bleeding causes (71.7 (13.1) years) ($P = 0.010$). Most bleeding-related deaths occurred when immediate control of bleeding failed (29.2%) or when patients died within 48 h after endoscopic therapy (25.5%). Among those who died of non-bleeding-related causes, multiorgan failure (23.9%), pulmonary conditions (23.5%), and terminal malignancy (33.7%) were most common.

Conclusions.—The majority of PUB patients died of non-bleeding-related causes. Optimization of management should aim at reducing the risk of multiorgan failure and cardiopulmonary death instead of focusing merely on successful hemostasis.

▶ This is an excellent article that reviews the causes of mortality in patients with peptic ulcer bleeding. This is a well-written prospective cohort study of over 10 000 patients with bleeding peptic ulcer disease. This article notes that mortality rate from peptic ulcer bleeding is 5% to 10%, and despite the use of acid-suppressing agents, endoscopic hemostasis, and surgery, there is little improvement in patient survival rates. This article points out that 80% of the mortality is not related to bleeding but is the result of multiorgan failure and cardiopulmonary events. The authors emphasize that optimization of management should aim at reducing the risk of multiorgan failure and cardiopulmonary death, instead of a focus mainly on hemostasis. I think this article is a good reminder to all of us who treat gastrointestinal bleeders.

J. S. Scolapio, MD

Early endoscopic balloon dilation in caustic-induced gastric injury

Kochhar R, Poornachandra KS, Dutta U, et al (Postgraduate Inst of Med Education and Res, Chandigarh, India)

Gastrointest Endosc 71:737-744, 2010

Background.—There are no reports on endoscopic balloon dilation (EBD) for caustic-induced gastric outlet obstruction (GOO) in the acute or subacute phase.

Objective.—To study the efficacy of early EBD in patients with caustic-induced gastric injury.

Setting.—Tertiary care center in India.

Design.—Retrospective analysis of data.

Patients.—Out of 41 patients with caustic-induced GOO who reported to us in the subacute phase between January 2001 and December 2008, 31 were treated by EBD. All 31 had ingested an acid 14.39 ± 4.65 days earlier. EBD was achieved by using wire-guided balloons under endoscopic guidance.

Intervention.—The balloon was negotiated across the narrowed segment and inflated for 60 seconds using a pressure gun. Balloons of incremental diameter, up to a maximum of 3 sizes, were used in each sitting. Procedural success was defined as reaching the end point of dilation (15 mm) and absence of symptoms.

Results.—All 31 patients (18 male, mean age 32.06 ± 11.04 years) could be successfully dilated. All but 1 underwent successful dilations to achieve the end point of 15 mm, requiring a median of 9 (range 3-18) dilations over a period of 7 (range 1.5-16) weeks. Complications included self-limiting pain (n = 10), bleeding at the time of the procedure (n = 9), and perforation in 1 patient (3.2%) who required surgery. Thirty patients were followed up for a median of 21 (range 3-72) months with no recurrence.

Conclusion.—Early EBD by an expert endoscopist is a safe and effective treatment modality in the management of caustic-induced GOO.

▶ This is an excellent retrospective study that evaluates the outcome of balloon dilation in caustic-induced gastric injury. Both acids and alkalis can damage both the esophagus and the stomach. There are no reports of early dilation for prevention and treatment of gastric cicatrization. It is thought that early dilation may prevent cicatrization or subsequent scarring of stomach following caustic injury. However, there is concern that early dilation (3 days-3 weeks) may increase the risk of perforation and complications. This study would suggest that it is safe and effective to dilate early using a 15-mm through-the-scope (TTS) balloon. The authors report a 97% success rate at 21-month follow-up. There was only 1 perforation reported of the 41 patients studied. Although more studies may be needed, this study would suggest that early dilation may prevent later scarring and gastric outlet symptoms. This is an interesting article that I think most gastroenterologists would enjoy reading.

J. S. Scolapio, MD

Trends and Outcomes of Hospitalizations for Peptic Ulcer Disease in the United States, 1993 to 2006

Wang YR, Richter JE, Dempsey DT (Temple Univ School of Medicine, Philadelphia, PA)
Ann Surg 251:51-58, 2010

Objectives.—Despite progress in diagnosis and treatment, peptic ulcer disease (PUD) remains a common reason for hospitalization and operation. The purpose of this study was to quantify the time trends of hospitalizations and operations for PUD in the United States (US) since 1993.

Data and Methods.—The Healthcare Cost and Utilization Project Nationwide Inpatient Sample is a 20% stratified sample of all hospitalizations in the United States. It was used to study hospitalizations with PUD as the principal diagnosis during 1993 to 2006, including details on ulcer site, complications, procedures, and mortality. Statistical methods included the χ^2 test and multivariate logistic regression.

Results.—The national estimate of hospitalizations for PUD decreased significantly from 222,601 in 1993 to 156,108 in 2006 (−29.9%), with a larger reduction in duodenal ulcers (95,552 in 1993 vs. 60,029 in 2006, −37.2%) than gastric ulcers (106,987 in 1993 vs. 86,064 in 2006, −19.6%). The inpatient mortality rate of PUD decreased from 3.8% to 2.7% during 1993 to 2006 ($P < 0.001$). Hemorrhage remained the most common complication (71.6% in 1993; 73.3% in 2006) but perforation had the highest mortality (15.1% in 1993; 10.6% in 2006). In comparison to 1993, patients hospitalized for PUD in 2006 more frequently had endoscopic treatment to control bleeding (12.9% vs. 22.2%, $P < 0.001$), similar use of surgical oversewing of ulcer (7.6% vs. 7.4%), less use of gastrectomy (4.4% vs. 2.1%, $P < 0.001$), and less use of vagotomy (5.7% vs. 1.7%, $P < 0.001$). In multivariate logistic regressions, the determinants of mortality were similar in 1993 and 2006.

Conclusions.—Hospitalizations for PUD decreased in the United States from 1993 to 2006, suggesting a decrease in the prevalence and/or severity of ulcer complications over this recent time period. Despite increased patient age and comorbidities, there has been a significant decrease in PUD mortality, a significant increase in the use of therapeutic endoscopy for bleeding ulcer, and a significant decrease in the use of definitive surgery (vagotomy or resection) for ulcer complications.

▶ This is an excellent article that attempts to quantify the time trends of hospitalizations and operations for peptic ulcer disease (PUD) in the United States since 1993. This well-written article concludes that the number of hospital admissions for PUD has significantly decreased since 1993. There has also been a significant decrease in PUD-related mortality. Some limitations of this study include an inability to estimate any change in PUD prevalence. Also, changes in diagnostic criteria and hospital coding practice over time may not allow an adequate estimate of PUD prevalence. Also, a medical history including *Helicobacter pylori* infection treatment and treatment with nonsteroidal anti-inflammatory drugs or proton pump inhibitor therapy is not available in this study. Nevertheless, this is an interesting study that spans a 14-year period that perhaps best supports our current clinical endoscopic practice and medical therapies used to treat PUD.

J. S. Scolapio, MD

8 Liver Disease

Viral Hepatitis

Determination of Immune Memory to Hepatitis B Vaccination Through Early Booster Response in College Students

Jan C-F, Huang K-C, Chien Y-C, et al (Natl Taiwan Univ; Genomic Res Ctr, Taiwan; et al)

Hepatology 51:1547-1554, 2010

The long-term protection of hepatitis B (HB) vaccination has been debated for years. The purpose here was to evaluate the kinetic changes of antibody to HB surface antigen (anti-HBs) and define immune memory of the HB vaccine among college students who had previously received full neonatal immunization against HB. In all, 127 college students aged 18-23 years born after July 1984 who had completed HB vaccination and were seronegative for all three HB viral markers, including HB surface antigen (HBsAg), antibody to HB core protein (anti-HBc), and anti-HBs, were recruited. They received three doses of HB vaccine at enrollment, 1 month and 6 months after enrollment. Their anti-HBs titers were assayed at enrollment, 7-10 days, 1 month, 6 months, and 7 months following the first dose of HB vaccine. The anti-HBs seroprotective rates for subjects 7-10 days, 1 month, 6 months, and 7 months postvaccination were 20.5%, 75.6%, 94.5%, and 99.2%, respectively. Those who were seroprotective at 7 to 10 days after one dose of HB vaccine booster developed significantly higher levels of anti-HBs at 1 and 6 months than those not developing seroprotective anti-HBs response at an earlier timepoint.

Conclusion.—At least one-quarter of HB vaccinees have lost their immune memory to the HB vaccine when entering college. Immune memory to HB vaccine was identified by early seroconversion, which was present in only 20% of vaccinees in the present study. To ensure higher than 90% anti-HBs seroconversion rates, at least 2 doses of HB booster vaccines are recommended for at-risk youths who received complete HB vaccinations in neonatal or infant periods but are seronegative for HBsAg, anti-HBs, and anti-HBc in adolescence.

▶ It has been previously shown that the long-term protection of hepatitis B (HB) vaccine and the need for a booster has not been clearly established. A universal HB immunization program was implemented in Taiwan in 1984.

The coverage rate of HB vaccines in 20 years in Taiwan has been >90%. As a result, there has been a 78% to 87% decrease in seroprevalence of HB surface antigen (HBsAg) carriage in children and a 75% decline in the incidence of hepatocellular carcinoma among children 6 to 9 years of age. The success of this program has been exemplary. There has, however, been a gradual yearly decline in antibody titers among vaccine recipients. This study aimed to evaluate the booster response after HB vaccination in seronegative young adults who had completed neonatal HB immunization in Taiwan before 1992. The seroprotective post-revaccination rates were 20.5% at 7 to 10 days after first dose of vaccine and 99.2% at 7 months. Those who developed early antibody response had the higher levels of HBs antibody at 6 months. To ensure a 90% seroconversion rate, at least 2 doses of HB booster vaccine would be needed for seronegative young adults not responding to neonatal vaccination. The results of this study have important health policy implications. If replicated, it may imply the need for establishing a booster vaccine program. However, this study does not identify if loss of immunity to HB leads to a loss of protection against infection and disease. Future studies are necessary to answer these critical questions.

D. M. Harnois, DO

Efficacy and Safety of Peginterferon Alfa-2a (40KD) Plus Ribavirin in Hepatitis C Patients with Advanced Fibrosis and Cirrhosis

Bruno S, Shiffman ML, Roberts SK, et al (AO Fatebenefratelli e Oftalmico, Milan, Italy; Virginia Commonwealth Univ Med Ctr, Blacksburg; The Alfred Hosp, Melbourne, Australia; et al)
Hepatology 51:388-397, 2010

The objective of this study is to determine the efficacy and safety of peginterferon alfa-2a (40KD)/ribavirin in patients with advanced fibrosis. Data from 341 genotype 1/4 patients (99 with bridging fibrosis/cirrhosis) treated for 48 weeks and 1547 genotype 2/3 patients (380 with bridging fibrosis/cirrhosis) treated for 16 or 24 weeks enrolled in three randomized international studies were analyzed. Sustained virological response (SVR) rates decreased progressively from 60% in genotype 1/4 patients without advanced fibrosis to 51% in those with bridging fibrosis and 33% in those with cirrhosis (trend test $P = 0.0028$); and from 76% to 61% and 57%, respectively, in genotype 2/3 patients treated for 24 weeks (trend test $P < 0.0001$). Irrespective of genotype, patients without advanced fibrosis were more likely to have an earlier response to treatment that was associated with higher SVR rates and lower relapse rates during untreated follow-up. Among patients with or without a diagnosis of advanced fibrosis, rates of SVR and relapse were similar for patients with similar responses in the first 12 weeks.

Conclusion.—Compared with patients with less severe disease, SVR rates are significantly lower in patients with advanced fibrosis. However, irrespective of genotype and degree of fibrosis, the time to become hepatitis C virus (HCV) RNA undetectable was the strongest predictor of SVR.

▶ This study was an important contribution to our understanding of the treatment of hepatitis C in patients because it is one of only a small number of trials that have looked at treatment of patients with hepatitis C virus (HCV) with advanced fibrosis and cirrhosis with peginterferon and ribavirin. The vast majority of all trials in HCV treatment have excluded patients with more advanced disease. Patients in this trial were eligible for enrollment if they had quantifiable HCV RNA in the serum (> 600 IU/mL), had elevated alanine aminotransferase (ALT) levels, and a liver biopsy confirming a diagnosis of chronic hepatitis C. The patients were grouped according to the fibrosis score on the baseline liver biopsy. It is important to note that all cases with cirrhosis were well compensated with a Child-Pugh score of < 7 (Child's A). The primary efficacy outcome in the study was sustained virology response (SVR) defined as undetectable HCV RNA by qualitative polymerase chain reaction (PCR) assay (< 50 IU/mL) at the end of a 24-week untreated follow-up period. Rapid virological response (RVR) was defined as undetectable HCV RNA by qualitative assay after 4 weeks of treatment. Early virological response (EVR) was defined at week 12 on treatment. In this analysis, patients without an RVR at 4 weeks but who achieved an EVR at 12 weeks were divided into 2 groups: those with a complete EVR defined as undetectable HCV RNA by qualitative assay at 12 weeks and those with a slow response at week 12 defined as a detectable level of > 50 IU/mL but a 2-log or more decline in serum HCV RNA level. In addition to the primary efficacy outcome, several secondary efficacy outcomes were evaluated, including assessing the impact of RVR and EVR on achievement of SVR.

D. M. Harnois, DO

Genetic variation in *IL28B* and spontaneous clearance of hepatitis C virus

Thomas DL, Thio CL, Martin MP, et al (Johns Hopkins Univ, Baltimore, MD; SAIC Frederick, Inc, MD; et al)

Nature 461:798-801, 2009

Hepatitis C virus (HCV) infection is the most common blood-borne infection in the United States, with estimates of 4 million HCV-infected individuals in the United States and 170 million worldwide. Most (70–80%) HCV infections persist and about 30% of individuals with persistent infection develop chronic liver disease, including cirrhosis and hepatocellular carcinoma. Epidemiological, viral and host factors have been associated with the differences in HCV clearance or persistence, and studies have demonstrated that a strong host immune response against HCV favours viral clearance. Thus, variation in genes involved in the immune response may contribute to the ability to clear the virus. In a recent genome-wide association study, a single nucleotide polymorphism (rs12979860) 3 kilobases upstream of the *IL28B* gene, which encodes the type III interferon IFN-λ3, was shown to associate strongly with more than a twofold difference in response to HCV drug treatment. To determine the potential effect of rs12979860 variation on outcome to HCV infection in a natural history setting, we genotyped this variant in HCV cohorts comprised of individuals who spontaneously cleared the virus ($n = 388$) or had persistent infection ($n = 620$). We show that the C/C genotype strongly enhances resolution of HCV infection among individuals of both European and African ancestry. To our knowledge, this is the strongest and most significant genetic effect associated with natural clearance of HCV, and these results implicate a primary role for *IL28B* in resolution of HCV infection.

▶ Hepatitis C virus (HCV) infection is the most common blood-borne infection in the United States, with estimates to affect 4 million individuals in the United States. A minority of individuals will spontaneously clear acute HCV infection. Host genetic variations have been assumed to explain the differences in HCV clearance across individuals. A recent genome-wide association study of >1600 individuals chronically infected with hepatitis C identified a strong association with sustained virologic response and the single nucleotide polymorphism (SNP) upstream of the *IL28* gene that encodes the type III interferon IFN-λ3. This study addressed the role of the same rs12979860 SNP in HCV spontaneous clearance in 1008 individuals who cleared virus and individuals with chronic persistent infection. Those patients with the C/C genotype were 3 times more likely to clear HCV relative to patients with C/T and T/T genotypes. These results mirror the protective effect of C/C genotype on sustained virological response after HCV treatment in a previous study by Ge et al in the same volume of *Nature*.[1] Clearly, genetic variability in *IL28B* expression plays an important role in both spontaneous clearance and individual treatment response in HCV infection.

D. M. Harnois, DO

Reference

1. Ge D, Fellay J, Thompson AJ, et al. Genetic variation in IL28B predicts hepatitis C treatment-induced viral clearance. *Nature*. 2009;461:399-401.

Identifying Hepatitis C Virus Genotype 2/3 Patients Who Can Receive a 16-Week Abbreviated Course of Peginterferon Alfa-2a (40KD) Plus Ribavirin

Diago M, Shiffman ML, Bronowicki J-P, et al (Hosp General de Valencia, Spain; Virginia Commonwealth Univ Med Ctr, Richmond; CHU de Nancy, Vandoeuvre-les-Nancy, France; et al)
Hepatology 51:1897-1903, 2010

The objective of this analysis was to compare sustained virological response (SVR) and relapse rates in patients with a rapid virological response (RVR, HCV RNA <50 IU/mL at week 4) randomized to 24 or 16 weeks of treatment with peginterferon alfa-2a (40KD) 180 μg/week plus ribavirin 800 mg/day in the multinational ACCELERATE study. The analysis was restricted to patients who received treatment for 80% or more of the planned duration. Of 1309 eligible patients, 863 individuals (65.9%) achieved an RVR and were included in this analysis (458 assigned to 16 weeks and 405 assigned to 24 weeks). The overall SVR rate was significantly higher in patients randomized to 24 weeks of treatment (91% versus 82%; $P = 0.0006$) and among patients infected with genotype 2 (92% versus 81%; $P = 0.0010$) but not genotype 3 (90% versus 84%; $P = 0.1308$). Relapse rates were significantly lower among all patients randomized to 24 weeks of treatment: overall (6% versus 15%, $P < 0.0001$); in those infected with genotype 2 (5% versus 17%, $P = 0.0001$), and genotype 3 (7% versus 14%, $P = 0.0489$). SVR rates in patients with a vira l load of 400,000 IU/mL or less randomized to 24 and 16 weeks of treatment were similar, 95% and 91% ($P = 0.2012$). Significant pretreatment predictors of SVR included assignment to 24 weeks of treatment ($P = 0.0006$), absence of advanced fibrosis on liver biopsy ($P = 0.0032$), lower HCV RNA level ($P = 0.0017$), and lower body weight ($P < 0.0001$).

Conclusion.—The standard 24-week regimen of peginterferon alfa-2a (40KD) plus ribavirin is significantly more effective than an abbreviated 16-week regimen in genotype 2/3 patients who achieve an RVR. Abbreviated regimens may be considered in patients with a low baseline viral load who achieve an RVR.

▶ This analysis presents the results of the multinational ACCELERATE study, which assessed the sustained virological response (SVR) and relapse rate in patients with rapid virologic response (RVR) for patients undergoing hepatitis C virus (HCV) treatment randomized to 24 weeks or 16 weeks of therapy with peginterferon alfa-2a 180 mg/wk plus ribavirin 800 mg/d. This was a large trial of over 1000 patients, 863 of whom achieved RVR at week 4. The SVR rates exceeded 80% in patients with an RVR regardless of genotype or assigned treatment duration. The SVR rate was significantly lower in patients randomized to 16 weeks versus 24 weeks overall (82% vs 91%). Virological relapse rates were also higher in those with shorter duration therapy. Assignment to 24 weeks of therapy was the most important predictor of SVR. However, there was one group of patients that could be considered for shorter duration therapy. This group consisted of genotype 2/3 individuals with low baseline viral load (HCV RNA level ≤400 000 IU/mL) who achieved an RVR (SVR rates—91% at 16 weeks and 95% at 24 weeks). While dropout rates were higher in the longer duration group, the authors recommend dose reduction in patients not fulfilling the favorable criterion of 16 weeks of therapy to encourage them to complete a full 24 weeks of therapy, if necessary.

D. M. Harnois, DO

Long-Term Efficacy of Tenofovir Monotherapy for Hepatitis B Virus-Monoinfected Patients After Failure of Nucleoside/Nucleotide Analogues

van Bömmel F, de Man RA, Wedemeyer H, et al (Universitätsmedizin Berlin, Germany; Univ Med Ctr Rotterdam, The Netherlands; Hannover Med School, Germany; et al)

Hepatology 51:73-80, 2010

Tenofovir disoproxil fumarate (TDF) has demonstrated high antiviral efficacy in treatment-naive patients with chronic hepatitis B virus (HBV) infection but experience in nucleoside/nucleotide analogue (NA)-experienced patients is limited. In this retrospective multicenter study we therefore assessed the long-term efficacy of TDF monotherapy in patients with prior failure or resistance to different NA treatments. Criteria for inclusion were HBV DNA levels >4.0 $\log_{10}$ copies/mL at the start and a minimum period of TDF therapy for at least 6 months. In all, 131 patients (mean age 42 ± 12 years, 95 male, 65% hepatitis B e antigen [HBeAg]-positive) were eligible. Pretreatment consisted of either monotherapy with lamivudine (LAM; n = 18), adefovir (ADV; n = 8), and sequential LAM-ADV therapy (n = 73), or add-on combination therapy with both drugs (n = 29). Three patients had failed entecavir therapy. Resistance analysis in 113 of the 131 patients revealed genotypic LAM and ADV resistance in 62% and 19% of patients, respectively. The mean HBV DNA level at TDF baseline was 7.6 ± 1.5 $\log_{10}$ copies/mL. The overall cumulative proportion of patients achieving HBV DNA levels <400 copies/mL was 79% after a mean treatment duration of 23 months (range, 6-60). Although LAM resistance did not influence the antiviral efficacy of TDF, the presence of ADV resistance impaired TDF efficacy (100% versus 52% probability of HBV DNA <400 copies/mL, respectively). However, virologic breakthrough was not observed in any of the patients during the entire observation period. Loss of HBeAg occurred in 24% of patients and HBsAg loss occurred in 3%. No significant adverse events were noticed during TDF monotherapy.

Conclusion.—TDF monotherapy induced a potent and long-lasting antiviral response in NA-experienced patients with previous treatment failure. Our data may have implications for current add-on strategies.

▶ Infection with the hepatitis B (HBV) virus affects over 350 million individuals worldwide. A major limitation of nucleoside and nucleotide analog therapy in the treatment of HBV infection is the development of HBV resistance variants. Tenofovir is an antiviral agent with efficacy in the treatment of HIV and HBV infections. This study is a retrospective cohort analysis to assess the efficacy of tenofovir monotherapy in patients with prior failure or resistance to different nucleoside and nucleotide analogs.

Lamivudine resistance did not influence tenofovir efficacy; however, adefovir resistance did impair tenofovir efficacy. Virologic breakthrough was not observed in any of the patients during the observation period. This study demonstrates adequate sustained viral suppression with tenofovir monotherapy in patients with previous lamivudine resistance.

D. M. Harnois, DO

Aging of Hepatitis C Virus (HCV)-Infected Persons in the United States: A Multiple Cohort Model of HCV Prevalence and Disease Progression

Davis GL, Alter MJ, El-Serag H, et al (Baylor Univ Med Ctr, Dallas, TX; Univ of Texas Med Branch, Galveston, TX; Baylor College of Medicine, Houston, TX; et al)

Gastroenterology 138:513-521, 2010

Background & Aims.—The prevalence of chronic hepatitis C (CH-C) remains high and the complications of infection are common. Our goal was to project the future prevalence of CH-C and its complications.

Methods.—We developed a multicohort natural history model to overcome limitations of previous models for predicting disease outcomes and benefits of therapy.

Results.—Prevalence of CH-C peaked in 2001 at 3.6 million. Fibrosis progression was inversely related to age at infection, so cirrhosis and its complications were most common after the age of 60 years, regardless of when infection occurred. The proportion of CH-C with cirrhosis is projected to reach 25% in 2010 and 45% in 2030, although the total number with cirrhosis will peak at 1.0 million (30.5% higher than the current level) in 2020 and then decline. Hepatic decompensation and liver cancer will continue to increase for another 10 to 13 years. Treatment of all infected patients in 2010 could reduce risk of cirrhosis, decompensation, cancer, and liver-related deaths by 16%, 42%, 31%, and 36% by 2020, given current response rates to antiviral therapy.

Conclusions.—Prevalence of hepatitis C cirrhosis and its complications will continue to increase through the next decade and will mostly affect those older than 60 years of age. Current treatment patterns will have little effect on these complications, but wider application of antiviral treatment and better responses with new agents could significantly reduce the impact of this disease in coming years.

► It is currently estimated that up to 4 million persons in the United States have chronic hepatitis C (CHC) infection. We are only now beginning to understand the magnitude of the consequences of chronic infection in these individuals.

Outpatient and hospital visits have doubled in recent years. CHC is the leading indication for liver transplant. The disease contributes to 4600 to 12 000 deaths per year. Hepatocellular carcinoma (HCC), as a consequence of CHC, is one of the fastest-growing cancers in the United States. Several disease-impact models have been developed in the past; however, advances in computer software now permit the development of more complex models. This study uses this technology to predict the future burden to the health care system of CHC infection.

The prevalence of CHC peaked in 2001 at 3.6 million cases. The proportion of CHC patients with cirrhosis will peak at 1 million in 2020. The incidence of hepatitis C virus (HCV)-related HCC is projected to peak in 2019 at approximately 14 000 cases per year. Hepatic deaths due to HCV are predicted to increase through 2022 with 283 378 deaths from 2020-2029. Treatment of all infected persons in 2010 could reduce the risks of cirrhosis-, cancer-, and liver-related death by 16%, 31%, and 36% respectively by 2020 based on currently available antiviral therapy.

This study emphasizes the need to screen, diagnose, and treat individuals with CHC to avoid these devastating consequences.

D. M. Harnois, DO

Entecavir treatment for up to 5 years in patients with hepatitis B e antigen-positive chronic hepatitis B

Chang T-T, Lai C-L, Kew Yoon S, et al (Natl Cheng Kung Univ, Tainan, Taiwan, ROC; Queen Mary Hosp, Hong Kong, China; The Catholic Univ of Korea, Seoul; et al)

Hepatology 51:422-430, 2010

Sustained virologic suppression is a primary goal of therapy for chronic hepatitis B (CHB). In study entecavir (ETV)-022, 48 weeks of entecavir 0.5 mg was superior to lamivudine for virologic suppression for hepatitis B e antigen (HBeAg)-positive CHB. A total of 183 entecavir-treated patients from ETV-022 subsequently enrolled in study ETV-901. We present the results after up to 5 years (240 weeks) of continuous entecavir therapy. The entecavir long-term cohort consists of patients who received ≥1 year of entecavir 0.5 mg in ETV-022 and then entered ETV-901 with a treatment gap ≤35 days. In ETV-901 the entecavir dose was 1.0 mg daily. For patients with samples available at Year 5, proportions with hepatitis B virus (HBV) DNA <300 copies/mL, normal alanine aminotransferase (ALT) levels, HBeAg loss, and HBeAg seroconversion were determined. In all, 146 patients met criteria for inclusion in the entecavir long-term cohort. At Year 5, 94% (88/94) had HBV DNA <300 copies/mL and 80% (78/98) had normal ALT levels. In addition to patients who achieved serologic responses during study ETV-022, 23% (33/141) achieved HBeAg seroconversion and 1.4% (2/145) lost hepatitis B surface antigen (HBsAg) during study ETV-901. Through 5 years, entecavir resistance emerged in one patient. The safety profile of entecavir was consistent with previous reports.

Conclusion.—Extended therapy with entecavir through 5 years maintained or increased rates of HBV DNA suppression and ALT normalization. Additional patients also achieved HBeAg loss and seroconversion.

Entecavir provides sustained viral suppression with minimal resistance during long-term treatment of HBeAg-positive CHB.

► Chronic hepatitis B (CHB) infection affects over 350 million people worldwide. Medications currently approved in the United States include standard interferon, pegylated interferon, lamivudine, adefovir dipivoxil, entecavir, telbivudine, and tenofovir disoproxil fumarate. Interferon therapies have been demonstrated to show a durable serologic response but are limited by the need for parenteral administration and their side effects. Lamivudine demonstrated efficacy initially, but resistance reaches 70% after 4 years of therapy. Current guidelines recommend avoidance of lamivudine as first-line therapy for this reason. Adefovir treatment for 48 weeks resulted in HB virus (HBV) DNA suppression in only 13% of HBe antigen (HBeAg)-positive patients and resistance in 20% of HBeAg patients after 5 years. Patients treated with telbivudine also demonstrated a virologic breakthrough in over 20% of HBeAg-positive patients treated for 2 years. Tenofovir treatment for HBeAg-positive patients with chronic HBV infection has been demonstrated in the past to achieve high levels of virologic suppression, but efficacy and resistance data were only reported through 2 years. Previously, entecavir demonstrated superior histologic and virologic benefit compared with lamivudine in nucleotide-naïve HBeAg-positive HBV-infected patients treated for 48 weeks. This study is an extension of this previous study with results up to 5 years of continuous entecavir therapy. At year 5, 94% of patients had HBV DNA <300 IU/ml, and 80% had normal alanine transaminase (ALT) levels. Through 5 years, entecavir resistance emerged in only 1 patient. This study demonstrates a high level of sustained viral suppression, minimal resistance, and ALT normalization in patients treated with entecavir for CHB.

D. M. Harnois, DO

Genetic variation in *IL28B* and spontaneous clearance of hepatitis C virus

Thomas DL, Thio CL, Martin MP, et al (Johns Hopkins Univ, Baltimore, MD; Harvard Univ, Boston, MA; et al)
Nature 461:798-801, 2009

Hepatitis C virus (HCV) infection is the most common blood-borne infection in the United States, with estimates of 4 million HCV-infected individuals in the United States and 170 million worldwide. Most (70–80%) HCV infections persist and about 30% of individuals with persistent infection develop chronic liver disease, including cirrhosis and hepatocellular carcinoma. Epidemiological, viral and host factors have been associated with the differences in HCV clearance or persistence, and studies have demonstrated that a strong host immune response against HCV favours viral clearance. Thus, variation in genes involved in the immune response may contribute to the ability to clear the virus. In a recent genome-wide association study, a single nucleotide polymorphism (rs12979860) 3 kilobases upstream of the *IL28B* gene, which encodes the type III interferon IFN-λ3, was shown to associate strongly with more than a twofold difference in response to HCV drug treatment. To determine the potential effect of rs12979860 variation on outcome to HCV infection in a natural history setting, we genotyped this variant in HCV cohorts comprised of individuals who spontaneously cleared the virus ($n = 388$) or had persistent infection ($n = 620$). We show that the C/C genotype strongly enhances resolution of HCV infection among individuals of both European and African ancestry. To our knowledge, this is the strongest and most significant genetic effect associated with natural clearance of HCV, and these results implicate a primary role for *IL28B* in resolution of HCV infection.

▶ Chronic infection with the hepatitis C virus (HCV) affects 170 million people worldwide. Current therapy for HCV includes peginterferon and ribavirin. It has been understood for some time that length of treatment and likelihood of response is related to genotype of the HCV. There are, however, significant variations in response to therapy within genotype 1 in particular that have not to date been clearly explained. In this report, the genetic polymorphism near the interleukin 28 (*IL28*) gene encoding interferon λ3 (INF-λ3) is associated with treatment response in patients of European ancestry and African Americans. Polymorphism on chromosome 19, rs12979860, was associated with variability in the sustained virological response (SVR) of patients with genotype 1 HCV. The polymorphism was found to reside upstream of the *IL28* gene encoding INF-λ3. The genotypes identified were CC, CT, and TT. In patients of European or African American ancestry the CC genotype was associated with a 2-fold or greater rate of SVR than the TT genotype. It is estimated that approximately half of the differences in SVR between populations can be accounted for by the frequency of the C allele. This test is not yet commercially available but may become an important tool in distinguishing the likelihood of response to INF treatment, much like the HCV genotype (eg, genotype one fourth vs genotype two thirds) that is currently being used.

D. M. Harnois, DO

Peginterferon Alfa-2a/Ribavirin for 48 or 72 Weeks in Hepatitis C Genotypes 1 and 4 Patients With Slow Virologic Response

Ferenci P, for the Austrian Hepatitis Study Group (Med Univ, Vienna, Austria; et al)

Gastroenterology 138:503-512, 2010

Background & Aims.—This randomized multicenter trial evaluated individualization of treatment duration with peginterferon alfa-2a 180 μg/wk plus ribavirin 1000/1200 mg/day in patients with chronic hepatitis C genotype 1/4 based on the rapidity of virologic response (VR).

Methods.—Patients with a rapid VR (RVR; undetectable hepatitis C virus [HCV]-RNA level (<50 IU/mL at week 4) were treated for

24 weeks, those with an early VR (EVR; no RVR but undetectable HCV-RNA level or ≥2-$\log_{10}$ decrease at week 12) were randomized to 48 (group A) or 72 weeks of treatment (group B; peginterferon alfa-2a was reduced to 135 μg/wk after week 48). Patients without an EVR continued treatment until week 72 if they had undetectable HCV-RNA levels at week 24. The primary end point was relapse; sustained VR (SVR; undetectable HCV-RNA level after 24 weeks of follow-up evaluation) was a secondary end point.

Results.—Of 551 genotype 1/4 patients starting treatment, 289 were randomized to group A (N = 139) or group B (N = 150). The relapse rate was 33.6% in group A (95% confidence interval [CI], 24.8%–43.4%) and 18.5% in group B (95% CI, 11.9%–27.6%; P = .0115 vs group A) and the SVR rate was 51.1% (95% CI, 42.5%–59.6%) and 58.6% (95% CI, 50.3%–66.6%; $P > .1$), respectively. The overall SVR rate was 50.4% (278 of 551; 95% CI, 46.2%–54.7%), including 115 of 150 patients with an RVR treated for 24 weeks and 4 of 78 patients without an EVR.

Conclusions.—Extending therapy with peginterferon alfa-2a/ribavirin to 72 weeks decreases the probability of relapse in patients with an EVR. If they can be maintained on extended-duration therapy, SVR rates also may improve.

▶ The current treatment regimen for hepatitis C virus (HCV) is a combination of pegylated interferon (PEG-IFN) plus ribavirin. The probability of eradication and recommended length of treatment varies by genotype. Guidelines for treatment for genotype 2 and 3 are 24 weeks of therapy and 48 weeks for genotype 1 and 4. Response to treatment can be used to evaluate duration of treatment and likelihood of a sustained virological response (SVR). Once treatment is initiated, those with a rapid virological response (RVR) are most likely to attain an SVR and may be considered for shorter duration therapy. Similarly, there is evidence that extending the duration of therapy increases the chance of achieving an SVR.

This randomized multicenter trial evaluated an individualized length of treatment duration based on virological response. All patients were genotype 1 or 4. Those achieving RVR at 4 weeks received 24 weeks of therapy. Those with no RVR at 4 weeks (detectable HCV RNA) but undetectable HCV-RNA or ≥2-$\log_{10}$ decrease at 12 weeks of therapy (early virological response [EVR]) were randomized to 48 weeks versus 72 weeks of therapy. The primary end points were rate of relapse and SVR. Of the 551 genotype 1 or 4 patients, 289 were randomized to 48 weeks or 72 weeks of therapy. The relapse rate was 33.6% for those patients treated for 48 weeks of therapy and 18.5% for those treated for 72 weeks (P = .0115). The SVR rate was 51.1% and 58.6%, respectively ($P > .1$).

In conclusion, extending therapy with PEG-INF/ribavirin to 72 weeks decreases the probability of relapse in genotype 1 and 4 patients achieving an EVR at 12 weeks of therapy.

D. M. Harnois, DO

Cholestatic Liver Disease

Failure to Perform Cholecystectomy for Acute Cholecystitis in Elderly Patients Is Associated with Increased Morbidity, Mortality, and Cost

Riall TS, Zhang D, Townsend CM Jr, et al (The Univ of Texas Med Branch, Galveston)

J Am Coll Surg 210:668-679, 2010

Background.—Cholecystectomy during initial hospitalization is the current recommended therapy for acute cholecystitis. The rate of cholecystectomy and subsequent health care trajectory in elderly patients with acute cholecystitis has not been evaluated.

Study Design.—We used 5% national Medicare sample claims data from 1996 to 2005 to identify a cohort of patients aged 66 years and older, requiring urgent or emergent admission for acute cholecystitis. We evaluated cholecystectomy rates on initial hospitalization, factors independently predicting receipt of cholecystectomy, factors predicting further gallstone-related complications, and 2-year survival in the cholecystectomy and no cholecystectomy groups in univariate and multivariate models.

Results.—There were 29,818 Medicare beneficiaries who were urgently or emergently admitted for acute cholecystitis from 1996 to 2005. Mean age was 77.7 ± 7.3 years, 89% of patients were white, and 58% were female. Twenty-five percent of patients did not undergo cholecystectomy during the index admission. Lack of definitive therapy was associated with a 27% subsequent cholecystectomy rate and a 38% gallstone-related readmission rate in the 2 years after discharge; the readmission rate was only 4% in patients undergoing cholecystectomy ($p < 0.0001$). No cholecystectomy on initial hospitalization was associated with worse 2-year survival (hazard ratio 1.56, 95% CI 1.47 to 1.65) even after controlling for patient demographics and comorbidities. Readmissions led to an additional $7,000 in Medicare payments per readmission.

Conclusions.—Our study demonstrated that 25% of cholecystectomies on Medicare beneficiaries were not performed on initial hospitalization, leading to readmissions in 38% of surviving patients. For patients requiring readmission, the percentage of open procedures was increased, and the additional Medicare payment was $7,000 per re-admission. Cholecystectomy for acute cholecystitis in elderly patients should be performed during initial hospitalization to prevent recurrent episodes of cholecystitis, multiple readmissions, higher readmission rates, and increased costs.

▶ Approximately 20 million people in the United States have gallstones leading to 700 000 operative procedures annually. The prevalence of gallstones increases with age. The management of gallstones in the elderly presents increased challenges. Claims data from Medicare from 1996-2005 were used to identify the cohort of patients for this analysis. In this study, a higher percentage of patients who did not undergo cholecystectomy during their initial hospitalization required readmission to the hospital. In addition, patients who did not have their gallbladder removed were 56% more likely to die within 2 years of this initial event than those who had their gallbladder removed. Authors conclude that cholecystectomy for acute cholecystitis should be performed during initial hospitalization in elderly patients who are candidates for surgery.

D. M. Harnois, DO

Long-Term Outcomes of Positive Fluorescence *In Situ* Hybridization Tests in Primary Sclerosing Cholangitis

Bangarulingam SY, Bjornsson E, Enders F, et al (Mayo Clinic, Rochester, MN)
Hepatology 51:174-180, 2010

Patients with primary sclerosing cholangitis (PSC) are at increased risk for developing cholangiocarcinoma (CCA). Fluorescence *in situ* hybridization (FISH) is a cytological test designed to enhance early CCA diagnosis. The long-term outcome of PSC patients with a positive FISH test (polysomy, trisomy/tetrasomy) are unclear. All PSC patients with at least one FISH test were identified and defined to have CCA if they had a positive tissue biopsy, positive cytology, or evidence of cancer in the explant after liver transplantation. A total of 235 PSC patients had at least one FISH test performed, and 56 patients had CCA on histopathology (n = 35) or cytology (n = 21). Overall, 120 of 235 (51%) of PSC patients tested for FISH were positive, but only one third of these positive patients had CCA. Sensitivity and specificity for FISH polysomy were 46% and 88%, and for trisomy/tetrasomy they were 25% and 67%, respectively. Survival analysis showed that patients with FISH polysomy had an outcome similar to patients with CCA; whereas FISH trisomy/tetrasomy patients had an outcome similar to patients with negative FISH tests. The FISH polysomy patients without cancer compared with those with CCA had lower serum bilirubin, lower carbohydrate antigen 19-9 (CA 19-9), lower Mayo risk score, and lower occurrence of dominant strictures.

Conclusion.—In PSC patients, the presence of a dominant stricture plus FISH polysomy has a specificity of 88% for CCA. Patients with FISH showing trisomy or tetrasomy have a similar outcome to patients with negative FISH. FISH testing should be used selectively in patients with other signs indicating CCA and not as a screening tool in all PSC patients undergoing endoscopic retrograde cholangiopancreatography (ERCP).

▶ Bangarulingam et al report their experience in a large cohort of patients with primary sclerosing cholangitis (PSC) undergoing endoscopic retrograde cholangiopancreatography (ERCP). A number of these ERCP procedures were performed in patients as part of diagnosis or management of PSC but not all were in the setting of a dominant stricture or mass lesions on cross-sectional imaging to support a diagnosis of cholangiocarcinoma. A total of 235 patients with PSC underwent 1 or more fluorescence in situ hybridization (FISH) analyses over an almost 5-year time period. A total of 56 of 235 (24%) patients had biopsy or cytologic evidence of cholangiocarcinoma during the period of study. Although 120/235 (51%) patients had a positive FISH test at some point during the period of study, only one third (40/120, 33%) of these were ultimately diagnosed with cholangiocarcinoma by tissue analysis. The authors note the very low sensitivity and specificity of tetrasomy or trisomy FISH results; only 14 of 73 patients (19%) were FISH positive. The sensitivity and specificity were improved with polysomy results; 26 of 47 patients (55%) with positive polysomy FISH had cholangiocarcinoma.

Establishing the diagnosis of cholangiocarcinoma in the setting of PSC can be extremely difficult. The FISH analysis can assist in the diagnosis if polysomy is present. However, the results reported in this study caution against the sole use of a positive FISH in the absence of other supporting evidence in diagnosing cholangiocarcinoma. The authors provide a useful algorithm for interpreting the results of FISH in the setting of PSC.

D. M. Harnois, DO

High Dose Ursodeoxycholic Acid for the Treatment of Primary Sclerosing Cholangitis

Lindor KD, Kowdley KV, Luketic VAC, et al (Mayo Clinic Rochester, MN; Virginia Mason Med Ctr, Seattle, WA; Virginia Commonwealth Univ School of Medicine, Richmond; et al)

Hepatology 50:808-814, 2009

Background.—Previous controlled trials are inconclusive regarding the efficacy of ursodeoxycholic acid (UDCA) for treating primary sclerosing cholangitis (PSC).

Methods.—One hundred fifty adult patients with PSC were enrolled in a long-term, randomized, double-blind controlled trial of high-dose UDCA (28–30 mg/kg/day) versus placebo. Liver biopsy and cholangiography were performed before randomization and after 5 years. The primary outcome measure was development of cirrhosis, varices, cholangiocarcinoma, liver transplantation or death.

Results.—The study was terminated after six years because of futility. At enrollment, the UDCA (n=76) and placebo (n=74) groups were similar with respect to gender, age, duration of disease, serum aspartate aminotransferase (AST) and alkaline phosphatase (AP) levels, liver histology and Mayo risk score. During therapy, AST and AP levels decreased more in the UDCA than the placebo group ($p<0.01$) but improvements in liver tests were not associated with decreased endpoints. By the end of the study, 30 patients in the UDCA group (39%) versus 19 patients in the placebo group (26%) had reached one of the pre-established clinical endpoints. After adjustment for baseline stratification characteristics, the risk of a primary endpoint was 2.3 times greater for patients on UDCA than for those on placebo ($p<0.01$) and 2.1 times greater for death, transplantation, or minimal listing criteria ($p=0.038$). Serious adverse events were more common in the UDCA than placebo group (63% vs 37%: $p<0.01$).

Conclusions.—Long-term high-dose UDCA therapy is associated with improvement in serum liver tests in PSC but does not improve survival and was associated with higher rates of serious adverse events.

► Primary sclerosing cholangitis (PSC) is a chronic cholestatic liver disease of unknown etiology characterized by fibrosing inflammation and destruction of the extrahepatic and/or intrahepatic bile ducts. No effective medical therapy exists for people with PSC. An earlier published pilot study had demonstrated the potential benefit of higher dose ursodeoxycholic acid (UDCA) in the treatment of these patients and provided the basis of this randomized, double-blind, placebo-controlled trial of high-dose UDCA (28-30 mg/kg/d) in PSC. The results of this trial surprised many within the field of hepatology. Serious adverse events including death, transplantation, or meeting minimal listing criteria were more common in the UDCA group versus placebo. Though patients on therapy had improvement in serum liver levels, survival was not improved and a greater number of adverse events were seen in the higher dose UDCA group. At this time, high-dose (28-30 mg/kg/d) UDCA therapy is not recommended for patients with PSC.

D. M. Harnois, DO

Diagnosis and Management of Primary Sclerosing Cholangitis

Chapman R, Fevery J, Kalloo A, et al (John Radcliffe Hosp, Headington, Oxford, UK; Univ Hosp Gasthuisberg, Leuven, Belgium; The Johns Hopkins Hosp, Baltimore, MD; et al)
Hepatology 51:660-678, 2010

Background.—Primary sclerosing cholangitis (PSC) is a chronic cholestatic liver disease. Characteristics include inflammation, fibrosis of both intrahepatic and extrahepatic bile ducts, and the formation of multifocal bile duct strictures. This progressive disorder is probably immune mediated and can develop into cirrhosis, portal hypertension, and hepatic decompensation. Forms of PSC include large duct and small duct disease, overlap syndromes, and secondary sclerosing cholangitis (SSC). Guidelines approved by the American Association for the Study of Liver Diseases for PSC are intended to be flexible approaches to diagnostic, therapeutic, and preventative care.

Recommendations.—To diagnose PSC in patients with a cholestatic biochemical profile, cholangiography is used. Magnetic resonance cholangiography (MRC) is an indirect, noninvasive technique; endoscopic retrograde cholangiography (ERC) is a direct, invasive technique. Routine liver biopsy is not recommended for patients with typical cholangiographic findings, rarely adding useful diagnostic data. If the ERC or MRC is normal, liver biopsy may help to diagnose small duct PSC. Liver biopsy may also help to diagnose or exclude overlap syndrome (conditions with diagnostic features of both PSC and other immune-mediated liver diseases) in patients with disproportionately elevated aminotransferase levels. All patients with possible PSC should have serum IgG4 levels measured to rule out IgG4-associated sclerosing cholangitis. No prognostic model for predicting clinical outcomes has proved best for a specific patient.

A prompt ERC can exclude the presence of a dominant stricture in patients with increased serum bilirubin levels and/or worsening pruritus accompanying progressive bile duct dilatation on imaging studies and/or cholangitis. If the patient has dominant strictures with PSC, endoscopic dilatation with or without stenting is done initially. If this is unsuccessful, biliary tract dilatation by percutaneous cholangiography with or without stenting is considered. Brush cytology and/or endoscopic biopsy is recommended before endoscopic therapy for dominant strictures to rule out a superimposed malignancy. Surgery is needed for some patients without cirrhosis whose dominant strictures are refractory to endoscopic and/or percutaneous management. Antimicrobial therapy and correction of bile duct obstruction in dominant strictures should resolve the cholangitis. With recurrent bacterial cholangitis, recommendations include prophylactic long-term antibiotics and an evaluation for liver transplantation.

Bone density examinations to exclude osteopenia or osteoporosis are done at PSC diagnosis and every 2 to 3 years thereafter. Patients with hepatic osteopenia are given daily therapy with calcium 1.0 to 1.5 g and vitamin D 1000 IU. For hepatic osteoporosis, bisphosphonate therapy is added. Parenteral rather than oral forms of bisphosphonate therapy are given to patients with osteoporosis and esophageal varices.

Full colonoscopy and biopsies are recommended for newly diagnosed PSC patients with no history or symptoms of inflammatory bowel disease (IBD). Patients with PSC and IBD require surveillance colonoscopy with biopsies every 1 to 2 years to exclude colorectal neoplasia. Ursodeoxycholic acid (UDCA) is not recommended for medical therapy or to prevent colorectal cancer in patients with ulcerative colitis and PSC. The guidelines for IBD are appropriate for patients with coexisting PSC. Corticosteroids and other immunosuppressants are given to adult patients with PSC and overlap syndrome.

Annual ultrasound examinations can detect mass lesions in the gallbladder. When mass lesions are found and the patient's underlying liver disease permits, cholecystectomy is recommended.

Patients whose constitutional performance status or liver biochemical-related parameters decline should be evaluated for cholangiocarcinoma (CCA). Surgical resection is appropriate for patients with CCA and no cirrhosis. Liver transplantation is considered for patients with early stage CCA not amenable to surgical resection whose neoadjuvant therapy was performed by experienced transplant centers. Liver transplantation is also useful for patients with advanced liver disease. Biliary strictures caused by other conditions are excluded in posttransplant patients before recurrent PSC is diagnosed.

Special Patient Groups.—Women of childbearing age with no portal hypertension can safely carry a pregnancy under close medical supervision. For children, a liver biopsy is used to diagnose overlap syndrome with PSC and autoimmune hepatitis. The treatment for overlap syndrome is immunosuppressive agents. Screening and surveillance to detect biliary tract cancer in children with PSC are not needed. A PSC diagnosis should not influence the choice of colorectal cancer screening performed in children with IBD. Liver transplantation is effective for children with end-stage liver disease caused by PSC.

Conclusions.—The guidelines for diagnosing and managing primary sclerosing cholangitis are based on relevant published information, the American College of Physicians Manual for Assessing Health Practices and Designing Practice Guidelines, guideline policies, and the experience of the authors in the various topics. Rather than standards of care, which are inflexible policies to be followed in every case, the guidelines are designed to be used judiciously as indicated for the specific patient.

▶ Perhaps no other article has as much impact on clinical practice as the guidelines developed through consensus by experts in the field and approved by the society. In February 2010, guidelines for diagnosis and management of primary sclerosing cholangitis (PSC) were published in *Hepatology*. The guidelines are a comprehensive review of PSC and its potential complications in both adults and children and are required reading for anyone treating these patients.

D. M. Harnois, DO

Liver Transplantation

Sirolimus-Based Immunosuppression Is Associated with Increased Survival After Liver Transplantation for Hepatocellular Carcinoma

Toso C, Merani S, Bigam DL, et al (Univ of Alberta, Edmonton, Canada)
Hepatology 51:1237-1243, 2010

Liver transplantation is an important treatment option for selected patients with nonresectable hepatocellular carcinoma (HCC). Several reports have suggested a lower risk of posttransplant tumor recurrence with the use of sirolimus and a higher one with calcineurin inhibitors, but the selection of an ideal immunosuppression protocol is still a matter of debate. The aim of this study was to define the immunosuppression associated with the best survival after liver transplantation for HCC. It was based on the Scientific Registry of Transplant Recipients and included 2,491 adult recipients of isolated liver transplantation for HCC and 12,167 for non-HCC diagnoses between March 2002 and March 2009. All patients remained on stable maintenance immunosuppression protocols for at least 6 months posttransplant. In a multivariate analysis, only anti-CD25 antibody induction and sirolimus-based maintenance therapy were associated with improved survivals after transplantation for HCC (hazard ratio [HR] 0.64, 95% confidence interval [CI]: 0.45-0.9, $P \leq 0.01$; HR 0.53, 95% CI: 0.31-0.92, $P \leq 0.05$, respectively). The other studied drugs, including calcineurin inhibitors, did not demonstrate a significant impact. In an effort to understand whether the observed effects were due to a direct impact of the drug on tumor or more on liver transplant in general, we conducted a similar analysis on non-HCC patients. Although anti-CD25 induction was again associated with a trend toward improved survival, sirolimus showed a trend toward lower rates of survival in non-HCC recipients, confirming the specificity of its beneficial impact to cancer patients.

Conclusion.—According to these data, sirolimus-based immunosuppression has unique posttransplant effects on HCC patients that lead to improved survival.

▶ In May 2010, the journal *BMC Cancer* published the hypothesis and methods of a randomized open-label trial comparing sirolimus-containing immunosuppression versus mTOR inhibitor-free immunosuppression in patients undergoing liver transplantation for hepatocellular cancer (HCC). This study will be conducted throughout Europe, Canada, and Australia. It will answer an important question on the benefit of mTOR inhibition-based immunosuppression in patients transplanted with HCC.

The theoretical benefits of mTOR inhibition, with its antiproliferative properties in HCC, have been clearly published. In the last year, 2 important trials were published demonstrating the benefit of sirolimus-based immunosuppression in patients transplanted with HCC. These trials add further, although not yet definitive, evidence supporting the use of mTOR inhibition-based immunosuppression in patients transplanted with HCC.

D. M. Harnois, DO

Liver Transplantation Following Donation After Cardiac Death: An Analysis Using Matched Pairs

Pine JK, Aldouri A, Young AL, et al (St James's Univ Hosp, UK)
Liver Transpl 15:1072-1082, 2009

Grafts from donation after cardiac death (DCD) donors are used to increase the number of organs available for liver transplantation. There is concern that warm ischemia may impair graft function. We compared our DCD recipients with a case-matched group of donation after brain death (DBD) recipients. Between January 2002 and April 2008, 39 DCD grafts were transplanted. These were matched with 39 DBD recipients on the basis of identified variables that had a significant impact on mortality. These were used to individually match DCD and DBD patients with similar predictive mortality. We compared patient/graft survival, primary non-function (PNF), and rates of complications. Of all liver transplants, 6.1% were DCD grafts. PNF occurred twice in the DCD group. The incidence of nonanastomotic biliary strictures (NABS; 20.5% versus 0%, $P = 0.005$) and hepatic artery stenosis (HAS; 12.8% versus 0%, $P = 0.027$) in the DCD group was higher. One-year (79.5% versus 97.4%, $P = 0.029$) and 3-year (63.6% versus 97.4%, $P = 0.001$) graft survival was lower in the DCD group. Three-year patient survival was also lower (68.2% versus 100%, $P < 0.0001$). Our study is the first to use case-matched patients and compare groups with similar predictive mortality. There was a higher incidence of NABS and HAS in the DCD group. NABS were likely a result of warm ischemia. HAS may have been due to ischemia or arterial injury during retrieval. The DCD group had significantly poorer outcomes, but DCD grafts remain a valuable resource. With careful donor/recipient selection, minimization of ischemia, and good postoperative care, acceptable results can be achieved.

▶ The list of patients requiring liver transplant continues to increase yearly. Attempts to increase the donor pool have included expansion of donor selection, use of split liver grafts, and initiation of living donor liver transplant. Perhaps the most significant potential expansion of the donor pool would include use of grafts from donation after cardiac death (DCD). The current standard for organ graft donation is donation after brain death (DBD). DCD grafts are procured from donors for whom death is declared on the basis of cardiopulmonary criteria rather than cessation of whole brain function. These organs are perceived as being at higher risk for graft failure. In this article by Pine et al from the United Kingdom, case-matched analysis of DCD and DBD donor organs was performed. There was a higher incidence of nonanastomotic biliary strictures and hepatic artery thrombosis in the DCD group, with evidence of a poorer outcome in these patients. This article and the article by Grewal et al[1] review the experience of centers using grafts from DCD donors. Both articles emphasize that DCD graft remain a valuable resource for liver transplantation, and with careful donor and recipient selection, acceptable results can be achieved.

D. M. Harnois, DO

Reference

1. Grewal HP, Willingham DL, Nguyen J, et al. Liver transplantation using controlled donation after cardiac death donors: an analysis of a large single-center experience. *Liver Transpl.* 2009;15:1028-1035.

Impact of Sirolimus on the Recurrence of Hepatocellular Carcinoma After Liver Transplantation

Chinnakotla S, Davis GL, Vasani S, et al (Baylor Univ Med Ctr, Dallas, TX)
Liver Transpl 15:1834-1842, 2009

Tumor recurrence after liver transplantation for hepatocellular carcinoma is associated with a poor prognosis. Because immunosuppression is a well-known risk factor for tumor growth, it is surprising that its possible role in the outcome of liver transplantation has been poorly evaluated. We performed a case-control review of prospectively collected data and compared 2 groups of patients according to the type of immunosuppression after liver transplantation for hepatocellular carcinoma at a single center. One hundred six patients received tacrolimus and mycophenolate mofetil, and 121 received sirolimus. Patients in the sirolimus group had significantly higher recurrence-free survival rates than patients in the tacrolimus group ($P = 0.0003$). The sirolimus group also had significantly higher patient survival rates than the tacrolimus group at 1 year (94% versus 79%), 3 years (85% versus 66%), and 5 years (80% versus 59%; $P = 0.001$). Sirolimus was well tolerated, and the patients in this study did not have the increase in surgical complications noted by other investigators. Leukopenia was the most common side effect, but it typically resolved with dose reduction. Dyslipidemia and mouth ulcers were common but were easily controlled. In summary, the data suggest a beneficial effect of sirolimus immunosuppression on recurrence-free survival, which translates into patient survival benefits.

▶ In May 2010, the journal *BMC Cancer* published the hypothesis and methods of a randomized open-label trial comparing sirolimus-containing immunosuppression versus mTOR inhibitor-free immunosuppression in patients undergoing liver transplantation for hepatocellular cancer (HCC). This study will be conducted throughout Europe, Canada, and Australia. It will answer an important question on the benefit of mTOR inhibition-based immunosuppression in patients transplanted with HCC.

The theoretical benefits of mTOR inhibition with its antiproliferative properties in HCC have been clearly published. In the last year, 2 important trials were published demonstrating the benefit of sirolimus-based immunosuppression in patients transplanted with HCC. These trials add further, although not yet definitive, evidence supporting the use of mTOR inhibition-based immunosuppression in patients transplanted with HCC.

D. M. Harnois, DO

Liver Transplantation Using Controlled Donation After Cardiac Death Donors: An Analysis of a Large Single-Center Experience

Grewal HP, Willingham DL, Nguyen J, et al (Mayo clinic, Jacksonville, FL; et al)

Liver Transpl 15:1028-1035, 2009

The use of donation after cardiac death (DCD) donors may provide a valuable source of organs for liver transplantation. Concerns regarding primary nonfunction (PNF) and intrahepatic biliary stricture (IHBSs) have limited the enthusiasm for their use. A retrospective analysis of 1436 consecutive deceased donor liver transplants performed between December 1998 and October 2006 was conducted. These included 108 DCD liver transplants, which were compared to 1328 transplants performed with organs from donors meeting the criteria for donation after brain death (DBD). The median follow-up was 48 months. The 1-, 3-, and 5-year patient survival and graft survival for DCD donors were 91.5%, 88.1%, and 88.1% and 79.3%, 74.5%, and 71.0%, respectively. The 1-, 3-, and 5-year patient survival and graft survival for DBD donors were 87.3%, 81.1%, and 77.2% and 81.6%, 74.7%, and 69.1%, respectively. Patient survival and graft survival were not significantly different between DCD donors less than 60 years old, DCD donors greater than 60 years old, and DBD donors. Causes of graft loss included IHBSs (n = 9), PNF (n = 4), recurrent hepatitis C virus (n = 4), hepatic artery thrombosis (n = 1), rejection (n = 2), and patient death (n = 13). Contrary to previously published data, excellent long-term patient survival and graft survival can be obtained with DCD allografts, and in our experience, they are equivalent to those obtained from DBD allografts.

▶ The list of patients requiring liver transplant continues to increase yearly. Attempts to increase the donor pool have included expansion of donor selection, use of split liver grafts, and initiation of living donor liver transplant. Perhaps the most significant potential expansion of the donor pool would include use of grafts from donation after cardiac death (DCD). The current standard for organ graft donation is donation after brain death (DBD). DCD grafts are procured from donors for whom death is declared on the basis of cardiopulmonary criteria rather than cessation of whole brain function. These organs are perceived as being at higher risk for graft failure. In this article by Grewal et al from the Mayo Clinic in Florida, patient and graft survival was not significantly different between DCD donors and DBD donors. However, they note that approximately 10% of recipients developed nonanastomotic biliary strictures. The use of DCD grafts represents a potentially valuable resource for liver transplantation, and with careful donor and recipient selection, results can be favorable.

D. M. Harnois, DO

Non-Alcoholic Fatty Liver Disease

Nonobese Population in a Developing Country Has a High Prevalence of Nonalcoholic Fatty Liver and Significant Liver Disease

Das K, Das K, Mukherjee PS, et al (Inst of Postgraduate Med Education and Res, Kolkata, India; Liver Foundation, West Bengal, India; et al)
Hepatology 51:1593-1602, 2010

There is a paucity of community-based epidemiological data on nonalcoholic fatty liver (NAFL) among nonaffluent populations in developing countries. Available studies are radiological and/or biochemical and lack histological assessment, limiting their strength. We conducted a prospective epidemiological study comprising a 1:3 subsample of all adult (>18 years) inhabitants of a rural administrative unit of West Bengal, India. Subjects positive for hepatitis B virus and/or hepatitis C virus infection and consuming any amount of alcohol were excluded. Diagnosis of NAFL was by dual radiological screening protocol consisting of ultrasonographic and computed tomographic examination of the liver. Transient elastographic examination and liver biopsy were performed in a subset to identify significant liver disease. The risk factors of having NAFL were analyzed. A total of 1,911 individuals were analyzed, 7% of whom were overweight and 11% of whom had abdominal obesity. The prevalence of NAFL, NAFL with elevated alanine aminotransferase, and cryptogenic cirrhosis was 8.7%, 2.3%, and 0.2%, respectively. Seventy-five percent of NAFL subjects had a body mass index (BMI) <25 kg/m^2, and 54% were neither overweight nor had abdominal obesity. The subjects with the highest risk of having NAFL were those with a BMI >25 kg/m2 (odds ratio 4.3, 95% confidence interval 1.6-11.5). Abdominal obesity, dysglycemia (fasting plasma glucose >100 mg/dL or elevated homeostatic model assessment of insulin resistance), and higher income were the other risk factors. Even having a normal BMI (18.5-24.9 kg/m^2) was associated with a 2-fold increased risk of NAFL versus those with a BMI <18.5 kg/m^2.

Conclusion.—There is a significant prevalence of NAFL and potentially significant liver disease, including cryptogenic cirrhosis, in this predominantly nonobese, nonaffluent population in a developing country. NAFL will be a major determinant of future liver disease burden in countries of the developing world.

▶ Nonalcoholic fatty liver (NAFL) has been associated with visceral fat and insulin resistance. It encompasses a spectrum of pathology from steatosis to nonalcoholic steatohepatitis (NASH) to cirrhosis. Most of the studies of NAFL have concentrated in developed countries of the West. Very little is known about the disease in developing countries. In this study in West Bengal, India, NAFL is found to be prevalent among individuals without the typically understood risk factors of obesity and sedentary life style. Studies have demonstrated a high prevalence of type 2 diabetes and insulin resistance in Asian Indians. This may play a role in the higher prevalence rate of NAFL in these individuals. In this analysis, patients with normal weight and active life style still had a risk of NAFL. This study suggests a need to individualize the assessment of risk of NAFL in different ethnic populations and concludes that the prevalence of NAFL may be greater than previously estimated.

D. M. Harnois, DO

Pioglitazone, Vitamin E, or Placebo for Nonalcoholic Steatohepatitis

Sanyal AJ, for the NASH CRN (Virginia Commonwealth Univ, Richmond; et al)

N Engl J Med 362:1675-1685, 2010

Background.—Nonalcoholic steatohepatitis is a common liver disease that can progress to cirrhosis. Currently, there is no established treatment for this disease.

Methods.—We randomly assigned 247 adults with nonalcoholic steatohepatitis and without diabetes to receive pioglitazone at a dose of 30 mg daily (80 subjects), vitamin E at a dose of 800 IU daily (84 subjects), or placebo (83 subjects), for 96 weeks. The primary outcome was an improvement in histologic features of nonalcoholic steatohepatitis, as assessed with the use of a composite of standardized scores for steatosis, lobular inflammation, hepatocellular ballooning, and fibrosis. Given the two planned primary comparisons, P values of less than 0.025 were considered to indicate statistical significance.

Results.—Vitamin E therapy, as compared with placebo, was associated with a significantly higher rate of improvement in nonalcoholic steatohepatitis (43% vs. 19%, $P = 0.001$), but the difference in the rate of improvement with pioglitazone as compared with placebo was not significant (34% and 19%, respectively; $P = 0.04$). Serum alanine and aspartate aminotransferase levels were reduced with vitamin E and with pioglitazone, as compared with placebo ($P<0.001$ for both comparisons), and both agents were associated with reductions in hepatic steatosis ($P = 0.005$ for vitamin E and $P<0.001$ for pioglitazone) and lobular inflammation ($P = 0.02$ for vitamin E and $P = 0.004$ for pioglitazone) but not with improvement in fibrosis scores ($P = 0.24$ for vitamin E and $P = 0.12$ for pioglitazone). Subjects who received pioglitazone gained more weight than did those who received vitamin E or placebo; the rates of other side effects were similar among the three groups.

Conclusions.—Vitamin E was superior to placebo for the treatment of nonalcoholic steatohepatitis in adults without diabetes. There was no benefit of pioglitazone over placebo for the primary outcome; however, significant benefits of pioglitazone were observed for some of the secondary outcomes. (ClinicalTrials.gov number, NCT00063622.)

▶ Nonalcoholic steatohepatitis (NASH) is characterized histologically by hepatic steatosis and lobular inflammation with hepatocellular ballooning. The progression to cirrhosis in these individuals is 15%. There are no current effective therapies. The disease is associated with insulin resistance providing the basis for looking at pioglitazone and vitamin E in the treatment of NASH.

This was a multicenter, randomized, placebo-controlled, double-blind clinical trial conducted by the NASH Clinical Research Network (CRN) established by the National Institute of Diabetes and Digestive and Kidney Diseases (NIDDK) in the treatment of patients with NASH without diabetes mellitus. A total of 83 patients received placebo, 84 received vitamin E (800 IU daily), and 80 received pioglitazone (30 mg daily). While there was improvement noted in serum liver tests and inflammation in the pioglitazone-treated patients, the study demonstrated no benefit of pioglitazone over placebo in the primary outcome of improvement in histologic findings and the established targets for reduction in activity score. In addition, the patients treated with pioglitazone had a significant gain in weight. Vitamin E at a dose of 800 IU daily did appear to demonstrate improvement over placebo.

The Pioglitazone versus Vitamin E versus Placebo for the Treatment of Nondiabetic Patients with Nonalcoholic Steatohepatitis (PIVENS) trial demonstrated some improvement in certain outcomes in the treatment of NASH, but unfortunately, it still leaves us short of a proven truly effective therapy for these patients.

D. M. Harnois, DO

The Incidence and Risk Factors of Hepatocellular Carcinoma in Patients with Nonalcoholic Steatohepatitis

Ascha MS, Hanouneh IA, Lopez R, et al (The Cleveland Clinic, OH)

Hepatology 51:1972-1978, 2010

Nonalcoholic steatohepatitis (NASH) is a well-recognized cause of cirrhosis and has been increasingly associated with the development of hepatocellular carcinoma (HCC). The aims of this study were to (1) estimate the incidence of HCC in patients with NASH-related cirrhosis, (2) compare incidence in NASH-related cirrhosis with hepatitis C virus (HCV)-related cirrhosis, and (3) identify risk factors of HCC in patients with NASH-related cirrhosis compared with HCV-related cirrhosis. Adult patients with cirrhosis secondary to chronic HCV (n = 315) or NASH (n = 195) were evaluated at our hepatobiliary clinic between 2003 and 2007. To assess for HCC development, all patients were monitored using serial abdominal computed tomography and serum alpha-fetoprotein every 6 months. Kaplan-Meier analysis was performed to estimate the cumulative incidence of HCC. Descriptive statistics were computed for all factors. Univariate and multivariate Cox regression analysis were used to assess associations between HCC and factors of interest. The median follow-up was 3.2 years (25th percentile [P25], 75th percentile [P75]: 1.7, 5.7) during which 25/195 (12.8%) of NASH-cirrhotic and 64/315 (20.3 %) of HCV-cirrhotic patients developed HCC ($P = 0.03$). Yearly cumulative incidence of HCC was found to be 2.6% in patients with NASH-cirrhosis, compared with 4.0% in patients with HCV cirrhosis ($P = 0.09$). Multivariate regression analysis revealed that older age ($P = 0.006$) and alcohol consumption ($P = 0.002$) were independent variables associated with development of HCC in patients with NASH-cirrhosis. Compared with nondrinkers, patients who reported any regular alcohol consumption were at greater risk for HCC development (hazard ratio: 3.6; P25, P75: 1.5, 8.3).

Conclusion.—Patients with NASH cirrhosis have a greatly increased risk of liver cancer. Alcohol consumption, a modifiable risk factor, appears to be the most significant factor associated with risk of HCC development in our study population.

▶ The incidence of hepatocellular cancer (HCC) has doubled in the United States in the last 2 decades. The majority of cancers are detected in patients with chronic liver disease and cirrhosis. The prevalence of nonalcoholic fatty liver disease (NAFLD) is rising in the United States and will progress to cirrhosis in 5% to 15% of patients. While previous studies have demonstrated NAFLD as a risk factor for HCC, none were a large population study in patients with nonalcoholic steatohepatitis (NASH). This study compares the incidence of HCC in cirrhotic patients with NASH ($N = 195$) and chronic HCV ($N = 315$). The estimated annual cumulative risk for HCC in patients with NASH was 2.6% per year versus 4.0% per year in patients with HCV cirrhosis. In this study, obesity was not an independent predictor of HCC. Older age at diagnosis was a risk factor for HCC, emphasizing the importance of screening in these individuals. In addition, the most significant and potentially modifiable risk factor for HCC in patients with NASH-related cirrhosis was alcohol consumption. In both the NASH and HCV groups, social alcohol intake increased the risk of HCC compared with nondrinkers (HCV, $P = .002$; NASH, $P = .001$). This article highlights the need for HCC screening in patients with NASH-related cirrhosis and identifies a potential modifiable factor (alcohol consumption) to reduce the risk of developing HCC.

D. M. Harnois, DO

Apolipoprotein C3 Gene Variants in Nonalcoholic Fatty Liver Disease

Petersen KF, Dufour S, Hariri A, et al (Yale Univ School of Medicine, New Haven, CT)

N Engl J Med 362:1082-1089, 2010

Background.—Nonalcoholic fatty liver disease is associated with hepatic insulin resistance and type 2 diabetes mellitus. Whether this association has a genetic basis is unknown.

Methods.—In 95 healthy Asian Indian men, a group known to have a high prevalence of nonalcoholic fatty liver disease, we genotyped two single-nucleotide polymorphisms (SNPs) in the gene encoding apolipoprotein C3 (*APOC3*) that are known to be associated with hypertriglyceridemia (rs2854116 [T-455C] and rs2854117 [C-482T]). Plasma apolipoprotein C3 concentrations, insulin sensitivity, and hepatic triglyceride content were measured. We also measured plasma triglyceride concentrations and retinyl fatty acid ester absorption as well as plasma triglyceride clearance after oral and intravenous fat-tolerance tests. Liver triglyceride content and *APOC3* genotypes were also assessed in a group of 163 healthy non–Asian Indian men.

Results.—Carriers of the *APOC3* variant alleles (C-482T, T-455C, or both) had a 30% increase in the fasting plasma apolipoprotein C3 concentration, as compared with the wildtype homozygotes. They also had a 60% increase in the fasting plasma triglyceride concentration, an increase by a factor of approximately two in the plasma triglyceride and retinyl fatty acid ester concentrations after an oral fat-tolerance test, and a 46% reduction in plasma triglyceride clearance. The prevalence of nonalcoholic fatty liver disease was 38% among variant-allele carriers and 0% among wild-type homozygotes ($P<0.001$). The subjects with nonalcoholic fatty liver disease had marked insulin resistance. A validation study involving non-Asian Indian men confirmed the association between *APOC3* variant alleles and nonalcoholic fatty liver disease.

Conclusions.—The polymorphisms C-482T and T-455C in *APOC3* are associated with nonalcoholic fatty liver disease and insulin resistance.

▶ Several studies have previously demonstrated the strong relationship between nonalcoholic fatty liver disease (NAFLD) and insulin resistance. What has been less clear is the nature of this relationship. There has been no established genetic basis for the relationship between insulin resistance and NAFLD and no biomarkers of the disease.

Previous studies have identified 2 single-nucleotide polymorphisms (SNPs) in the gene encoding apolipoprotein C3 (APOC3) associated with hypertriglyceridemia. Asian Indian men are a group of individuals shown to have a high risk of NAFLD and insulin resistance. In this study, investigators screened a group of healthy Asian Indian men for the 2 APOC3 SNPs. They measured the effects of the SNPs on insulin resistance, triglyceride levels, and functional testing of fat absorption and clearance. They then validated the results in healthy non-Asian Indian men.

What they found was a correlation in APOC3 variant alleles (C-484T and T-455C) and NAFLD and insulin resistance in both Asian Indian and non-Asian Indian men. In addition, this study demonstrated that a reduction in weight (approximately 6 kg) in Asian Indian men eliminated hepatic steatosis and resulted in an improvement in insulin sensitivity. This is one of the first studies to identify a gene for NAFLD and insulin resistance.

D. M. Harnois, DO

Cirrhosis and Complications

Randomized Controlled Trial of Carvedilol Versus Variceal Band Ligation for the Prevention of the First Variceal Bleed

Tripathi D, Ferguson JW, Kochar N, et al (Royal Infirmary, Edinburgh, UK; et al)
Hepatology 50:825-833, 2009

Current therapy for preventing the first variceal bleed includes beta-blocker and variceal band ligation (VBL). VBL has lower bleeding rates, with no differences in survival, whereas beta-blocker therapy can be limited by side effects. Carvedilol, a non-cardioselective vasodilating beta-blocker, is more effective in reducing portal pressure than propranolol; however, there have been no clinical studies assessing the efficacy of carvedilol in primary prophylaxis. The goal of this study was to compare carvedilol and VBL for the prevention of the first variceal bleed in a randomized controlled multicenter trial. One hundred fifty-two cirrhotic patients from five different centers with grade II or larger esophageal varices were randomized to either carvedilol 12.5 mg once daily or VBL performed every 2 weeks until eradication using a multibander device. Seventy-seven patients were randomized to carvedilol and 75 to VBL. Baseline characteristics did not differ between the groups (alcoholic liver disease, 73%; median Child-Pugh score, 8; median age, 54 years; median follow-up, 20 months). On intention-to-treat analysis, carvedilol had lower rates of the first variceal bleed (10% versus 23%; relative hazard 0.41; 95% confidence interval 0.19-0.96 [$P = 0.04$]), with no significant differences in overall mortality (35% versus 37%, $P = 0.71$), and bleeding-related mortality (3% versus 1%, $P = 0.26$). Six patients in the VBL group bled as a result of banding ulcers. Per-protocol analysis revealed no significant differences in the outcomes.

Conclusion.—Carvedilol is effective in preventing the first variceal bleed. Carvedilol is an option for primary prophylaxis in patients with high-risk esophageal varices.

▶ In previous studies, nonselective beta blockers (NSBB), namely propranolol and nadolol, have been demonstrated in carefully conducted randomized control trials to be highly effective in decreasing the risk of bleeding from portal hypertensive gastropathy. Many studies have also shown NSBB therapy to be beneficial in the prevention of variceal bleeding. However, drug side effects often result in dose reduction or discontinuation. In this study, carvedilol, a drug combination of propranolol and prazosin, was effective in preventing the first variceal bleeding when compared with variceal band ligation (VBL) every 2 weeks, with no significant differences in overall mortality or bleeding-related mortality. This is the first study to demonstrate effectiveness of this therapy against a trial of band ligation for the prevention of variceal bleeding.

D. M. Harnois, DO

Rifaximin Treatment in Hepatic Encephalopathy

Bass NM, Mullen KD, Sanyal A, et al (Univ of California, San Francisco; Case Western Reserve Univ, Cleveland, OH; Virginia Commonwealth Univ, Richmond; et al)

N Engl J Med 362:1071-1081, 2010

Background.—Hepatic encephalopathy is a chronically debilitating complication of hepatic cirrhosis. The efficacy of rifaximin, a minimally absorbed antibiotic, is well documented in the treatment of acute hepatic encephalopathy, but its efficacy for prevention of the disease has not been established.

Methods.—In this randomized, double-blind, placebo-controlled trial, we randomly assigned 299 patients who were in remission from recurrent hepatic encephalopathy resulting from chronic liver disease to receive either rifaximin, at a dose of 550 mg twice daily (140 patients), or placebo (159 patients) for 6 months. The primary efficacy end point was the time to the first breakthrough episode of hepatic encephalopathy. The key secondary end point was the time to the first hospitalization involving hepatic encephalopathy.

Results.—Rifaximin significantly reduced the risk of an episode of hepatic encephalopathy, as compared with placebo, over a 6-month period (hazard ratio with rifaximin, 0.42; 95% confidence interval [CI], 0.28 to 0.64; $P<0.001$). A breakthrough episode of hepatic encephalopathy occurred in 22.1% of patients in the rifaximin group, as compared with 45.9% of patients in the placebo group. A total of 13.6% of the patients in the rifaximin group had a hospitalization involving hepatic encephalopathy, as compared with 22.6% of patients in the placebo group, for a hazard ratio of 0.50 (95% CI, 0.29 to 0.87; $P=0.01$). More than 90% of patients received concomitant lactulose therapy. The incidence of adverse events reported during the study was similar in the two groups, as was the incidence of serious adverse events.

Conclusions.—Over a 6-month period, treatment with rifaximin maintained remission from hepatic encephalopathy more effectively than did placebo. Rifaximin treatment also significantly reduced the risk of hospitalization involving hepatic encephalopathy. (ClinicalTrials.gov number, NCT00298038.)

▶ The number of persons within the United States with cirrhosis is currently estimated at 5.5 million. This number is expected to significantly increase over the next 2 decades. Hepatic encephalopathy is a complication of cirrhosis with significant life-altering effects. In 2004, 50 000 patients were hospitalized with hepatic encephalopathy.

The current standard of care for patients with hepatic encephalopathy is treatment with a nonabsorbable disaccharide lactulose. All antibiotics, such as neomycin, vancomycin, paromomycin, and metronidazole are not recommended for long-term use because of significant toxicity.

Rifaximin is a minimally absorbed oral antimicrobial agent that is concentrated in the gastrointestinal tract. In this phase 3 randomized, double-blind, placebo-controlled trial, patients received either rifaximin at a dose of 550 mg twice daily or placebo. Rifaximin significantly reduced the risk of an episode of hepatic encephalopathy as compared with placebo and resulted in less breakthrough episodes. The drug was well tolerated with a low side effect profile. It must be noted that more than 90% of patients received concomitant lactulose therapy. This study confirms the efficacy of rifaximin in reducing the complications of hepatic encephalopathy associated with liver failure secondary to cirrhosis.

D. M. Harnois, DO

Simvastatin Lowers Portal Pressure in Patients With Cirrhosis and Portal Hypertension: A Randomized Controlled Trial

Abraldes JG, Albillos A, Bañares R, et al (Univ of Barcelona, Spain; Centro de Investigación Biomédica en Red de Enfermedades Hepáticas y Digestivas, Spain)

Gastroenterology 136:1651-1658, 2009

Background & Aims.—Simvastatin improves liver generation of nitric oxide and hepatic endothelial dysfunction in patients with cirrhosis, so it could be an effective therapy for portal hypertension. This randomized controlled trial evaluated the effects of continuous simvastatin administration on the hepatic venous pressure gradient (HVPG) and its safety in patients with cirrhosis and portal hypertension.

Methods.—Fifty-nine patients with cirrhosis and portal hypertension (HVPG >12 mm Hg) were randomized to groups that were given simvastatin 20 mg/day for 1 month (increased to 40 mg/day at day 15) or placebo in a double-blind clinical trial. Randomization was stratified according to whether the patient was being treated with β-adrenergic blockers. We studied splanchnic and systemic hemodynamics and variables of liver function and safety before and after 1 month of treatment.

Results.—Simvastatin significantly decreased HVPG (−8.3%) without deleterious effects in systemic hemodynamics. HVPG decreases were observed in patients who were receiving β-adrenergic blockers (−11.0%; $P = .033$) and in those who were not (−5.9%; $P = .013$). Simvastatin improved hepatic, fractional, and intrinsic clearance of indocyanine green, showing an improvement in effective liver perfusion and function. No significant changes in HVPG and liver function were observed in patients receiving placebo. The number of patients with adverse events did not differ significantly between groups. No patient was withdrawn from the study based on adverse events.

Conclusions.—Simvastatin decreased HVPG and improved liver perfusion in patients with cirrhosis. These effects were additive with those of

β-adrenergic blockers. The beneficial effects of simvastatin should be confirmed in long-term clinical trials for portal hypertension.

▶ This is a randomized, placebo-controlled, double-blind clinical trial showing the beneficial effects of simvastatin in lowering portal pressures in individuals with portal hypertension. Simvastatin has been shown to improve liver generation of nitric oxide (NO) and hepatic endothelial dysfunction in patients with cirrhosis. Experimental data in humans and animal models have suggested that statin therapy can decrease intrahepatic vascular resistance and improve flow-mediated vasodilation of liver vasculature in the cirrhotic liver through up-regulation of NO production. This study demonstrates that 1 month of simvastatin administration significantly decreased hepatic venous portal gradient (HVPG) in some patients with cirrhosis and severe portal hypertension. Thirty-two percent of patients achieved an HVPG reduction of 20% or greater (>12 mm Hg). This level of reduction has been shown in previous studies to reduce portal hypertension complications and mortality and is the standard goal for any therapy in the treatment of portal hypertension. This trial was conducted without the use of β-blocker therapy, and it suggests that the combination of simvastatin and nonselective β-blocker therapy may be of even greater benefit. Simvastatin may also provide benefits for those patients intolerant of β-blocker therapy.

D. M. Harnois, DO

Liver Lesions

The diagnostic and economic impact of contrast imaging techniques in the diagnosis of small hepatocellular carcinoma in cirrhosis

Sangiovanni A, Manini MA, Iavarone M, et al (Univ of Milan, Italy)

Gut 59:638-644, 2010

Background.—Contrast-enhanced ultrasound (CE-US), contrast CT scan and gadolinium dynamic MRI are recommended for the characterisation of liver nodules detected during surveillance of patients with cirrhosis with US.

Aim.—To assess the sensitivity, specificity, diagnostic accuracy and economic impact of all possible sequential combinations of contrast imaging techniques in patients with cirrhosis with 1–2 cm liver nodules undergoing US surveillance.

Patients/Methods.—64 patients with 67 de novo liver nodules (55 with a size of 1–2 cm) were consecutively examined by CE-US, CT, MRI, and a fine-needle biopsy (FNB) as diagnostic standard. Undiagnosed nodules were re-biopsied; non-malignant nodules underwent enhanced imaging follow-up. The typical radiological feature of hepatocellular carcinoma (HCC) was arterial phase hypervascularisation followed by portal/venous phase washout.

Results.—HCC was diagnosed in 44 (66%) nodules (2, <1 cm; 34, 1–2 cm; 8, >2 cm). The sensitivity of CEUS, CT and MRI for 1–2 cm

HCC was 26, 44 and 44%, with 100% specificity, the typical vascular pattern of HCC being identified in 22 (65%) by a single technique versus 12 (35%) by at least two techniques carried out at the same time point (p=0.028). Compared with the cheapest dual examination (CE-US+CT), the cheapest single technique of stepwise imaging diagnosis of HCC was equally expensive (€26 440 vs €28 667), but led to a 23% reduction of FNB procedures (p=0.031).

Conclusions.—In patients with cirrhosis with a 1–2 cm nodule detected during surveillance, a single imaging technique showing a typical contrast pattern confidently permits the diagnosis of HCC, thereby reducing the need for FNB examinations.

▶ In the last few years, 2 of the liver disease societies, European Association for the Study of the Liver (EASL) and American Association for the Study of Liver Diseases (AASLD), have published guidelines for the diagnosis and management of hepatocellular cancer (HCC). Lesions greater than 2 cm can generally be accurately diagnosed on imaging alone; lesions between 1 and 2 cm pose the greatest diagnostic dilemma. The guidelines state that lesions 1 to 2 cm require either confirmation on 2 contrast imaging examinations or a biopsy to confirm diagnosis.

This study provided a prospective head-to-head comparison of CT, MRI, and contrast-enhanced ultrasound (commonly available throughout centers in Europe) in the diagnosis of small HCC lesions 1 to 2 cm in size. The specificity was 100% for these techniques when the pattern of vascular enhancement was typical for HCC. There was no added benefit in sensitivity by the use of 2 contrast imaging studies versus a single study. The authors state that sequential use of contrast imaging studies to obtain a diagnosis of HCC in a suspected but not confirmed lesion 1 to 2 cm in size was economically better than a fine needle biopsy procedure. In addition, a typical pattern of vascular enhancement on a single-contrast imaging study was sufficient to accurately diagnose lesions 1 to 2 cm in size. If validated, these findings may significantly alter the recommended guidelines for management in small HCC lesions 1 to 2 cm in size.

D. M. Harnois, DO

Autoimmune Liver Disease

Diagnosis and Management of Autoimmune Hepatitis

Manns MP, Czaja AJ, Gorham JD, et al (Med School of Hannover, Germany; Mayo Clinic College of Medicine, Rochester, MN; Dartmouth Med School, Lebanon, NH; et al)

Hepatology 51:2193-2213, 2010

Clinical practice guidelines are defined as "systematically developed statements to assist practitioner and patient decisions about appropriate heath care for specific clinical circumstances." (All references are available in the Supporting Information.) These guidelines on autoimmune hepatitis provide a data-supported approach to the diagnosis and management of this disease. They are based on the following: (1) formal review and analysis of the recently-published world literature on the topic [Medline search]; (2) American College of Physicians Manual for Assessing Health Practices and Designing Practice Guidelines; (3) guideline policies, including the AASLD Policy on the Development and Use of Practice Guidelines and the American Gastroenterological Association Policy Statement on Guidelines; and (4) the experience of the authors in the specified topic.

These recommendations, intended for use by physicians, suggest preferred approaches to the diagnostic, therapeutic and preventive aspects of care. They are intended to be flexible, in contrast to standards of care, which are inflexible policies to be followed in every case. Specific recommendations are based on relevant published information. To more fully characterize the quality of evidence supporting the recommendations, the Practice Guidelines Committee of the AASLD requires a class (reflecting benefit versus risk) and level (assessing strength or certainty) of evidence to be assigned and reported with each recommendation. The grading system applied to the recommendations has been adapted from the American College of Cardiology and the American Heart Association Practice Guidelines, and it is given below (Table 1 in the original article).

▶ Perhaps no other article has as much impact on clinical practice as the guidelines developed through consensus by experts within the field and approved by the society. In June 2010, the long-awaited guidelines for diagnosis and management of autoimmune hepatitis were published in *Hepatology*. The guidelines are a comprehensive review of autoimmune hepatitis in both adults and children and are required reading for anyone treating these patients.

D. M. Harnois, DO

Miscellaneous

Early Laparoscopic Cholecystectomy Improves Outcomes After Endoscopic Sphincterotomy for Choledochocystolithiasis

Reinders JSK, Goud A, Timmer R, et al (St Antonius Hosp, Nieuwegein, The Netherlands; et al)

Gastroenterology 138:2315-2320, 2010

Background & Aims.—Patients with choledochocystolithiasis generally undergo endoscopic sphincterotomy (ES) followed by laparoscopic cholecystectomy (LC). However, many patients receive this surgery 6–8 weeks after ES. There is a high conversion rate of elective LC after ES, and patients can develop recurrent biliary events during the waiting period. We investigated whether the timing of surgery influences outcome.

Methods.—We performed a randomized trial of patients with choledochocystolithiasis who underwent successful ES. Patients were randomly assigned to groups that received early LC (within 72 hours after ES, n = 49) or delayed LC (after 6–8 weeks, n = 47), based on an expected difference in conversion rate of 25% vs 5%, respectively. Conversion rate, biliary events during follow-up, duration and difficulty of surgeries, postoperative morbidity, and hospital stay were scored. Intention-to-treat analyses were performed.

Results.—Groups were comparable in age, sex, and comorbidity. There was no difference between groups in conversion rate (4.3% in early vs 8.7% in delayed group) nor were there differences in operating times and/or difficulties or hospital stays. During the waiting period for LC, 17 patients in the delayed group (36.2%) developed recurrent biliary events compared with 1 patient in the early group ($P < .001$).

Conclusions.—In a randomized trial to evaluate timing of LC after ES, recurrent biliary events occurred in 36.2% of patients whose LC was delayed for 6–8 weeks. Early LC (within 72 hours) appears to be safe and might prevent the majority of biliary events in this period following sphincterotomy.

▶ Randomized controlled trials have demonstrated superior outcome in laparoscopic cholecystectomy (LC) after endoscopic sphincterotomy (ES) for choledochocystolithiasis rather than a wait-and-see approach. Patients in these trials who were allocated to surgery underwent LC 4 to 6 weeks after ES. There has been a retrospective study, which showed a lower conversion rate to open procedures in patients who underwent LC within 2 weeks after ES versus those who had LC 4 to 6 weeks after ES. This is the first randomized trial to look at the outcome of LC within 72 hours after ES or delayed LC after 6 to 8 weeks. In the delay to surgery, 36.2% of the patients developed a recurrent biliary event compared with 1 patient in the early group. There were no differences in conversion rate, complications, or length of stay. This study concluded that early LC is safe and may prevent recurrent biliary events.

D. M. Harnois, DO

Genetic Modifiers of Liver Disease in Cystic Fibrosis

Bartlett JR, for the Gene Modifier Study Group (Univ of North Carolina at Chapel Hill; et al)

JAMA 302:1076-1083, 2009

Context.—A subset (≈3%-5%) of patients with cystic fibrosis (CF) develops severe liver disease with portal hypertension.

Objective.—To assess whether any of 9 polymorphisms in 5 candidate genes (α_1- antitrypsin or α_1-antiprotease [*SERPINA1*], angiotensin-converting enzyme [*ACE*], glutathione S-transferase [*GSTP1*], mannose-binding lectin 2 [*MBL2*], and transforming growth factor β1 [*TGFB1*]) are associated with severe liver disease in patients with CF.

Design, Setting, and Participants.—Two-stage case-control study enrolling patients with CF and severe liver disease with portal hypertension (CFLD) from 63 CF centers in the United States as well as 32 in

Canada and 18 outside of North America, with the University of North Carolina at Chapel Hill as the coordinating site. In the initial study, 124 patients with CFLD (enrolled January 1999-December 2004) and 843 control patients without CFLD were studied by genotyping 9 polymorphisms in 5 genes previously studied as modifiers of liver disease in CF. In the second stage, the *SERPINA1* Z allele and *TGFB1* codon 10 genotype were tested in an additional 136 patients with CFLD (enrolled January 2005-February 2007) and 1088 with no CFLD.

Main Outcome Measures.—Differences in distribution of genotypes in patients with CFLD vs patients without CFLD.

Results.—The initial study showed CFLD to be associated with the *SERPINA1* Z allele (odds ratio [OR], 4.72; 95% confidence interval [CI], 2.31-9.61; $P = 3.3 \times 10^{-6}$) and with *TGFB1* codon 10 CC genotype (OR, 1.53; 95% CI, 1.16-2.03; $P = 2.8 \times 10^{-3}$). In the replication study, CFLD was associated with the *SERPINA1* Z allele (OR, 3.42; 95% CI, 1.54-7.59; $P = 1.4 \times 10^{-3}$) but not with TGFB1 codon 10. A combined analysis of the initial and replication studies by logistic regression showed CFLD to be associated with *SERPINA1* Z allele (OR, 5.04; 95% CI, 2.88-8.83; $P = 1.5 \times 10^{-8}$).

Conclusions.—The *SERPINA1* Z allele is a risk factor for liver disease in CF. Patients who carry the Z allele are at greater risk (OR, ≈ 5) of developing severe liver disease with portal hypertension.

▶ The authors studied a subset of patients with cystic fibrosis (CF) and portal hypertension secondary to liver disease. Their analysis of candidate genes demonstrated that the *SERPINA1* Z allele was a risk factor for liver disease in CF patients. Patients who carried the Z allele were at greatest risk of developing severe liver disease complicated by portal hypertension (odds ratio = 5). The significance of this discovery is a hope of identifying markers early in life for the development of severe liver disease in patients with CF.

In addition, by studying a large number of patients with CF, severe liver disease, and portal hypertension, the authors were also able to increase our understanding of the clinical features of these patients. In most patients with CF and liver disease, hepatic synthetic function is preserved for a long time. Liver biochemistry tests were poor predictors of severe liver disease and portal hypertension. In pediatric patients with CF, severe liver disease may occur as early as 10 to 12 years of age. In addition, the prevalence of severe liver disease in patients with CF does not increase in adults with CF, despite an increase in longevity. The vast majority of patients in this study were diagnosed with liver disease by age 20 with a mean and median age of diagnosis from 10 to 11 years.

D. M. Harnois, DO

Etiology, Management, and Outcome of the Budd-Chiari Syndrome

Darwish Murad S, for EN-Vie (European Network for Vascular Disorders of the Liver) (Erasmus MC Univ Hosp Rotterdam, the Netherlands; et al)

Ann Intern Med 151:167-175, 2009

Background.—The Budd–Chiari syndrome (BCS) is hepatic venous outflow obstruction. What is known about the syndrome is based on small studies of prevalent cases.

Objective.—To characterize the causes and treatment of incident BCS.

Design.—Consecutive case series of patients with incident BCS, enrolled from October 2003 to October 2005 and followed until May 2006.

Setting.—Academic and nonacademic hospitals in France, Spain, Italy, Great Britain, Germany, Belgium, the Netherlands, Portugal, and Switzerland.

Patients.—Persons older than 16 years with definite hepatic outflow obstruction diagnosed by imaging. Persons with hepatic outflow obstruction due to heart failure, sinusoidal obstruction syndrome, cancer, or liver transplantation were excluded.

Measurements.—Signs and symptoms; laboratory and imaging findings; diagnosis; treatment; and overall, transplantation-free, and intervention-free survival.

Results.—163 incident cases of BCS were identified. Median follow-up was 17 months (range, 0.1 to 31 months). Most patients (84%) had at least 1 thrombotic risk factor, and many (46%) had more than 1; the most common was myeloproliferative disorders (49% of 103 tested patients). Patients were mainly treated with anticoagulation (140 patients [86%]), transjugular intrahepatic portosystemic shunting (56 patients [34%]), or liver transplantation (20 patients [12%]), and 80 patients (49%) were managed noninvasively. Only 3 patients underwent surgical shunting. The survival rate was 87% (95% CI, 82% to 93%) at 1 year and 82% (CI, 75% to 88%) at 2 years.

Limitation.—Treatment was not standardized across all centers, and data on important clinical variables were missing for some patients.

Conclusion.—Most patients with BCS have at least 1 thrombotic risk factor, and many have more than 1; myeloproliferative disorders are most common. One- and 2-year survival rates are good with contemporary management, which includes noninvasive therapies (anticoagulation and diuretics) and invasive techniques. Transjugular intrahepatic portosystemic shunting seems to have replaced surgical shunting as the most common invasive therapeutic procedure.

▶ This study looked at the etiology, management, and short-term outcomes of Budd-Chiari syndrome in 163 patients accrued through 39 hospitals throughout 9 western European countries. In the majority of cases, 1 or more thrombotic risk factors were diagnosed. Almost half of the patients had more than 1 underlying clotting disorder, emphasizing the need to complete a thorough evaluation for hypercoaguable state and that the workup should not stop because of an identification of a single etiology. The majority of patients were safely managed with noninvasive treatments, including anticoagulation, or with minimally invasive treatments, such as transjugular intrahepatic portosystemic shunting, which is now replacing surgical shunting as the treatment of choice.

D. M. Harnois, DO

Article Index

Chapter 1: Esophagus

Chapter 2: Gastrointestinal Motility Disorders/ Neurogastroenterology

Chapter 3: Pancreaticobiliary Disease

Chapter 4: Gastrointestinal Cancers and Benign Polyps

Chapter 5: Inflammatory Bowel Disease

Chapter 6: Nutrition and Celiac Disease

Chapter 7: Gastrointestinal Surgery

Chapter 8: Liver Disease

Author Index

U

V

W

Y

Z

FSC
www.fsc.org
MIX
Papier | Fördert gute Waldnutzung
FSC® C083411

Kolibri 360 GmbH
Ferdinand-Jühlke-Straße 7
99095 Erfurt, Deutschland
produktsicherheit@kolibri360.de